Ultrasound Teaching Module
TRANSVAGINAL SCAN IN GYNECOLOGY

Ultrasound Teaching Module
TRANSVAGINAL SCAN IN GYNECOLOGY

Kuldeep Singh
MBBS FAUI FICMCH FICMU
Consultant Ultrasonologist
Dr Kuldeep's Ultrasound and Color Doppler Clinic
D-80, East of Kailash, New Delhi, India

Special interest in obstetric sonology
in detailed anomaly scanning and
color Doppler for management and
gynecological scanning

For Appointments:
Routine call: 098111966613
Level II call: 09811977372
Fectal Echo call: 09911196613
Ultrasound Training: 09811977372
E-mail: singhdrkuldeep@rediffmail.com

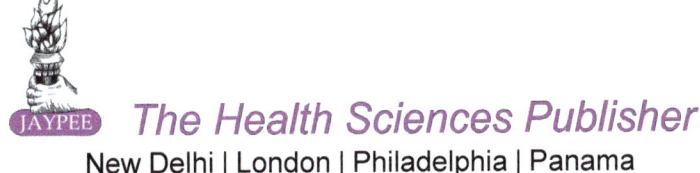

The Health Sciences Publisher
New Delhi | London | Philadelphia | Panama

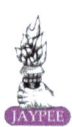 **Jaypee Brothers Medical Publishers (P) Ltd.**

Headquarters
Jaypee Brothers Medical Publishers (P) Ltd.
4838/24, Ansari Road, Daryaganj
New Delhi 110 002, India
Phone: +91-11-43574357
Fax: +91-11-43574314
E-mail: jaypee@jaypeebrothers.com

Overseas Offices

J.P. Medical Ltd.
83, Victoria Street, London
SW1H 0HW (UK)
Phone: +44-20 3170 8910
Fax: +44 (0) 20 3008 6180
E-mail: info@jpmedpub.com

Jaypee Medical Inc.
325, Chestnut Street
Suite 412, Philadelphia, PA 19106, USA
Phone: +1 267-519-9789
E-mail: support@jpmedus.com

Jaypee Brothers Medical Publishers (P) Ltd.
Bhotahity, Kathmandu, Nepal
Phone: +977-9741283608
E-mail: kathmandu@jaypeebrothers.com

Jaypee-Highlights Medical Publishers Inc.
City of Knowledge, Bld. 237, Clayton
Panama City, Panama
Phone: +1 507-301-0496
Fax: +1 507-301-0499
E-mail: cservice@jphmedical.com

Jaypee Brothers Medical Publishers (P) Ltd.
17/1-B Babar Road, Block-B, Shaymali
Mohammadpur, Dhaka-1207
Bangladesh
Mobile: +08801912003485
E-mail: jaypeedhaka@gmail.com

Website: www.jaypeebrothers.com
Website: www.jaypeedigital.com

© 2016, Jaypee Brothers Medical Publishers

The views and opinions expressed in this book are solely those of the original contributor(s)/author(s) and do not necessarily represent those of editor(s) of the book.

All rights reserved. No part of this publication may be reproduced, stored or transmitted in any form or by any means, electronic, mechanical, photocopying, recording or otherwise, without the prior permission in writing of the publishers.

All brand names and product names used in this book are trade names, service marks, trademarks or registered trademarks of their respective owners. The publisher is not associated with any product or vendor mentioned in this book.

Medical knowledge and practice change constantly. This book is designed to provide accurate, authoritative information about the subject matter in question. However, readers are advised to check the most current information available on procedures included and check information from the manufacturer of each product to be administered, to verify the recommended dose, formula, method and duration of administration, adverse effects and contraindications. It is the responsibility of the practitioner to take all appropriate safety precautions. Neither the publisher nor the author(s)/editor(s) assume any liability for any injury and/or damage to persons or property arising from or related to use of material in this book.

This book is sold on the understanding that the publisher is not engaged in providing professional medical services. If such advice or services are required, the services of a competent medical professional should be sought.

Every effort has been made where necessary to contact holders of copyright to obtain permission to reproduce copyright material. If any have been inadvertently overlooked, the publisher will be pleased to make the necessary arrangements at the first opportunity.

Inquiries for bulk sales may be solicited at: jaypee@jaypeebrothers.com

Ultrasound Teaching Module: Transvaginal Scan in Gynecology

First Edition: **2016**

ISBN 978-93-85999-26-0

Dedicated to

My parents
Mrs Yoginder Kaur
Mr KJ Singh
Who are with God

In fond remembrance of my pet Suzi

Preface

Technical advances in diagnostic ultrasound lead to a better understanding of gynecological pathologies. This happened with transvaginal scanning, better resolution, color Doppler and three-dimensional/four-dimensional ultrasound that helped us in accurate diagnosis. It is now onto us to learn and practice these advances in diagnostic ultrasound. The book endeavors the same, so that we do not lag behind. Careful glance of the images will help in better understanding and clinching the diagnosis. This is due to inclusion of a corresponding ultrasound image for most of the pathologies. In addition, other topics are also covered in Ultrasound Teaching Module: *Transvaginal Scan in Gynecology*.

Kuldeep Singh

Acknowledgments

I am thankful to my family, Nishu (wife), Jaanvi (daughter) and Ramanjeet (son). My sincere thanks to Shri Jitendar P Vij (Group Chairman), for his confidence, Mr Ankit Vij (Group President) and Mr Tarun Duneja (Director–Publishing), for their persistent support and the team, Mr KK Raman (Production Manager), Ms Samina Khan (Executive PA to Director-Publishing), Mr Lalit Kumar (DTP Operator), Mr Ashwani Kumar and Gyanendra Kumar (Proofreaders) of M/s Jaypee Brothers Medical Publishers (P) Ltd, New Delhi, India.

Thanks to my seniors, well-wishers and colleagues.

Contents

1. **Role of Ultrasound**   1
2. **Indications**   2
3. **Approach and Preparation**   3
4. **Common Pathologies Seen on Ultrasound**   5
5. **Normal Pelvis**   7
   - 5.1. *Normal Endometrium* 8
   - 5.2. *Normal Myometrium* 24
   - 5.3. *Normal Cavity* 27
   - 5.4. *Normal Contour* 31
   - 5.5. *Normal Intrauterine Contraceptive Device* 34
   - 5.6. *Normal Vaginal Vault* 41
   - 5.7. *Normal Adnexa* 44
6. **Uterocervical Abnormalities**   50
   - 6.1. *Congenital Uterine Defects* 51
   - 6.2. *Fibroids* 67
   - 6.3. *Fibroid Polyp* 94
   - 6.4. *Adenomyosis* 107
   - 6.5. *Asherman's Syndrome* 120
   - 6.6. *Endometrial Polyp* 125
   - 6.7. *Endometrium: Abnormal Thickness and Echo Pattern* 141
   - 6.8. *Cervical Polyp* 160
   - 6.9. *Cervical Mass* 164
7. **Adnexal Abnormalities**   167
   - 7.1. Small Ovaries 168
   - 7.2. *Dysfunctional Cysts* 172
   - 7.3. *Hemorrhagic Cyst* 179
   - 7.4. *Cyst with Fluid-fluid Level* 190
   - 7.5. *Cyst with Clot* 193
   - 7.6. *Ovarian Tumor* 200
   - 7.7. *Dermoid* 211
   - 7.8. *Polycystic Ovaries* 218
   - 7.9. *Endometriosis* 226
   - 7.10. *Adnexal Mass* 242
   - 7.11. *Hydrosalpinx* 250
   - 7.12. *Pouch of Douglas* 256
   - 7.13. *Ectopic* 258
   - 714. *Free Fluid* 266

CHAPTER 1

ROLE OF ULTRASOUND

- To examine the uterus, ovaries, cervix, vagina and adnexae.
- Classification of a mass identified on other modalities, e.g. solid, cystic, and mixed.
- Assistance with *in vitro* fertilization (IVF).
- To identify the relationship of normal anatomy and pathology to each other.

CHAPTER 2

INDICATIONS

- Menstrual irregularities
  - Menorrhagia
  - Metrorrhagia (irregular uterine bleeding)
  - Polymenorrhea
  - Menometrorrhagia (excessive irregular bleeding)
  - Amenorrhea
  - Oligomenorrhea
  - Precocious puberty
  - Delayed menses
  - Postmenopausal bleeding
- Pelvic pain
- Dysmenorrhea (painful menses)
- F/H uterine or ovarian cancer
- Palpable lump
- Infertility—primary or secondary (evaluation, monitoring and/or treatment)
- Anomalies/evaluation
- Signs/symptoms of pelvic infection
- IUCD localization (intrauterine contraceptive device)
- Urinary incontinence or pelvic organ prolapse.

CHAPTER 3

APPROACH AND PREPARATION

- Transabdominal approach—a full bladder is required.
- Transvaginal approach—the patient empties her bladder before the transvaginal scan is started.
- Transperineal approach

TRANSABDOMINAL APPROACH

This is a generalized overview to identify the cervix, uterus and ovaries:
- Check for the orientation of the uterus (anteverted vs retroverted)
- Assess the uterine size and contour
- Assess the myometrium
- Assess the endometrial status and measure the thickness
- Assess the cervix and vagina
- Look for abnormalities in the pouch of Douglas
- Check the ovaries and adnexae
- Assess bladder and lower ureters.

Start the scan sagittally in the midline immediately above the pubis. The bladder should be adequately full and you should be able to see the fundus of the uterus. In this plane you should be able to assess the uterus, cervix and vagina. Depending on resolution of your equipment, change the depth and zoom to get the best image possible. Rotate perpendicularly into transverse and scan the complete uterus. Angle laterally and look for the ovaries.

TRANSVAGINAL APPROACH

Inserting the Transvaginal Probe

- Before letting the patient empty their bladder, inform the procedure and show them the transvaginal (TV) probe. Definitely explain the importance of a transvaginal scan because it is the gold standard in gynecological ultrasound because of its superior accuracy and improved diagnostic resolution.
- Cover the probe with a latex-free TV sheath/condom and lubricate with sterile gel on the outside.

- If required elevate the patients bottom with a pillow to assist the scan. The examination table can also be used.
- Be extremely gentle even if there is some resistance as the probe is being inserted.
- Check with the patients if they are okay.
- When maneuvering the probe to visualize the adnexae, withdraw slightly then angle the probe towards the fornix. This avoids unnecessary patient discomfort.

CHAPTER 4

COMMON PATHOLOGIES SEEN ON ULTRASOUND

VAGINAL
- Gartners duct cyst.

CERVICAL
- Nabothian (retention) cysts
- Polyps
- Cervical fibroids
- Cervical carcinoma
- Cervical stenosis.

UTERINE
- Fibroids (leiomyoma)
  - Submucosal
  - Intramural
  - Subserosal
  - Pedunculated
- Adenomyosis.

ENDOMETRIAL
- Endometrial polyps
- Endometrial carcinoma
- Endometrial hyperplasia
- Endometritis
- Cystic hyperplasia secondary to Tamoxifen
- Adhesions—Asherman's syndrome
- Submucosal fibroids
- Arteriovenous malformation (AVM)
- Hydro/hematometra
- Blood/fluid/infection or retained products of conception (RPOC)

OVARIAN

- Ovarian cysts
  - Simple vs complex (hemorrhagic, corpus luteal, ruptured, septated)
  - Any mural nodules
- Dermoid
- Ovarian tumors:
  - Cystadenoma (serous/mucinous)—benign
  - Cystadenocarcinoma (serous/mucinous)—malignant
- Polycystic ovarian disease
- Endometrioma
- Torsion
- Hyperstimulation syndrome
- Ectopic pregnancy.

POUCH OF DOUGLAS AND ADNEXAE

- Fluid
- Pelvic inflammatory disease (PID)
- Ectopic pregnancy
- Endometriosis
- Pelvic venous congestion
- Bowel pathology may be seen (but cannot be excluded).

FALLOPIAN TUBES

- Pelvic inflammatory disease (PID)
- Pyosalpinx
- Hydrosalpinx
- Ectopic pregnancy
- Cyst
- Endometriosis.

CHAPTER 5

NORMAL PELVIS

5.1. Normal Endometrium
5.2. Normal Myometrium
5.3. Normal Cavity
5.4. Normal Contour
5.5. Normal Intrauterine Contraceptive Device
5.6. Normal Vaginal Vault
5.7. Normal Adnexa

5.1. NORMAL ENDOMETRIUM

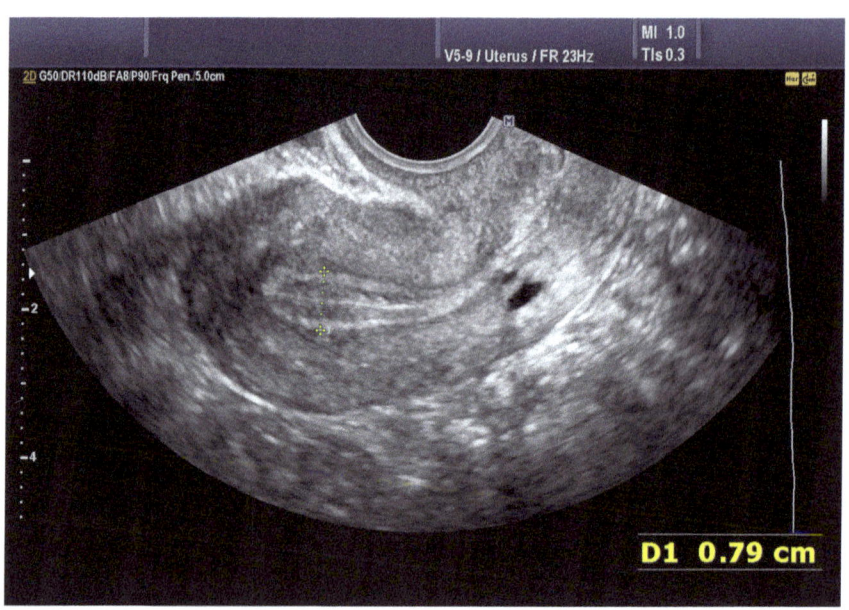

5.1. Normal Endometrium

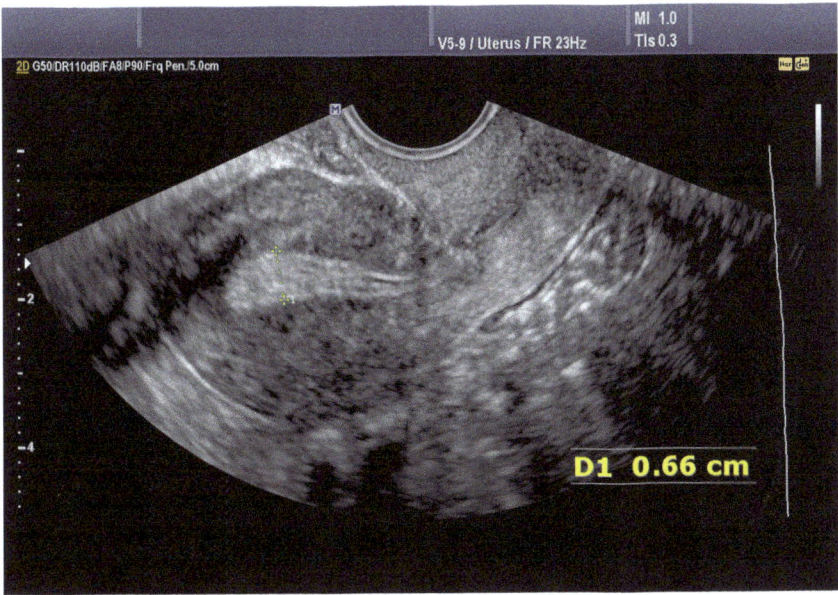

Fig. 5.1.1: Evaluate the endometrium for any collection or focal thickening

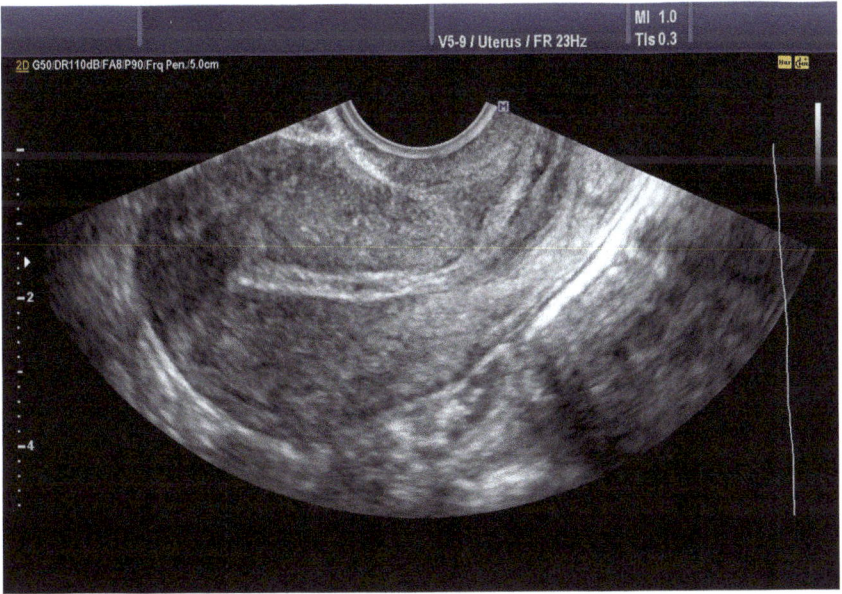

Fig. 5.1.2: This endometrium seen in the menstrual phase

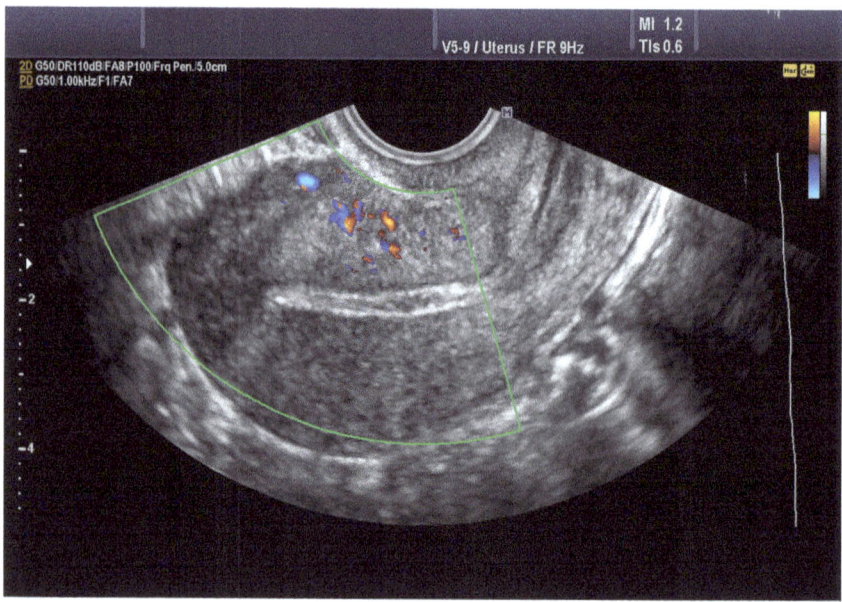

Fig. 5.1.3: Vascularity of the endometrium and subendometrial layer

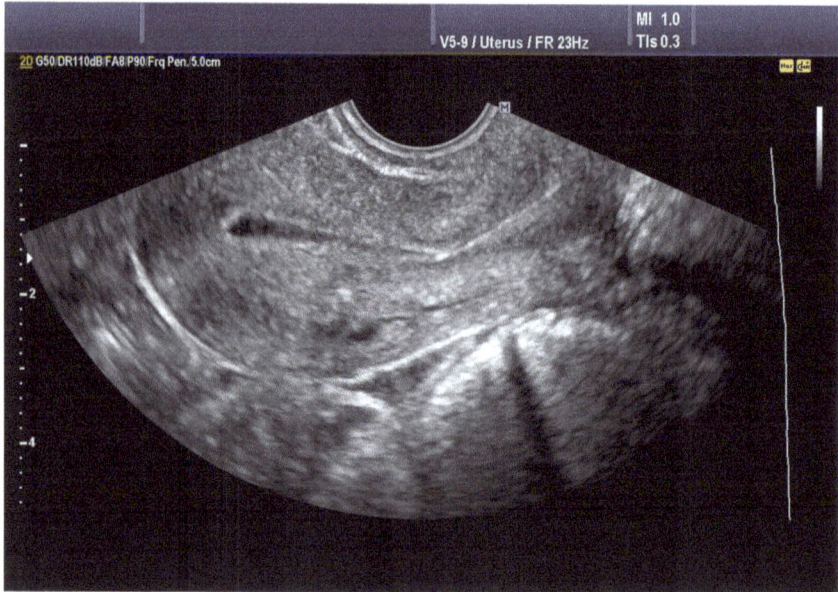

Fig. 5.1.4: Endometrial fluid collection

5.1. Normal Endometrium

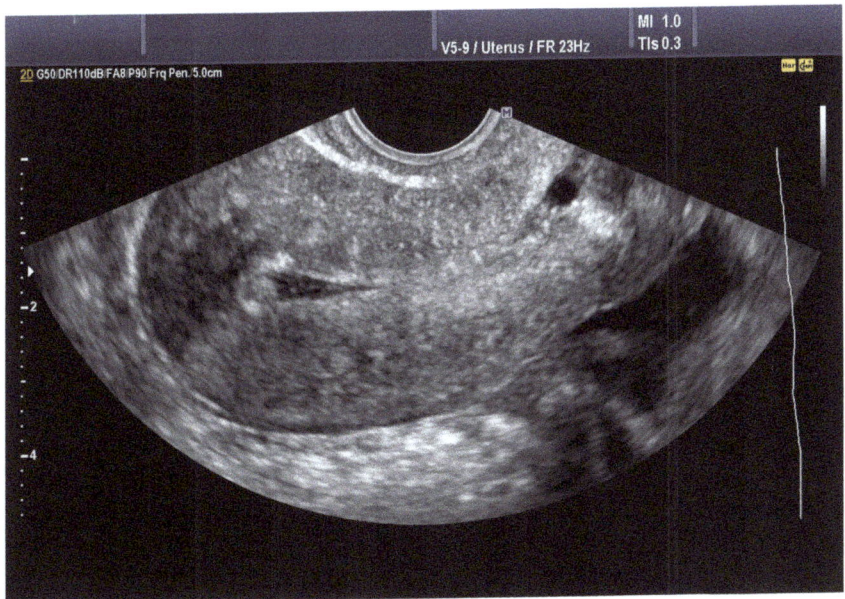

Fig. 5.1.5: Menstrual endometrium

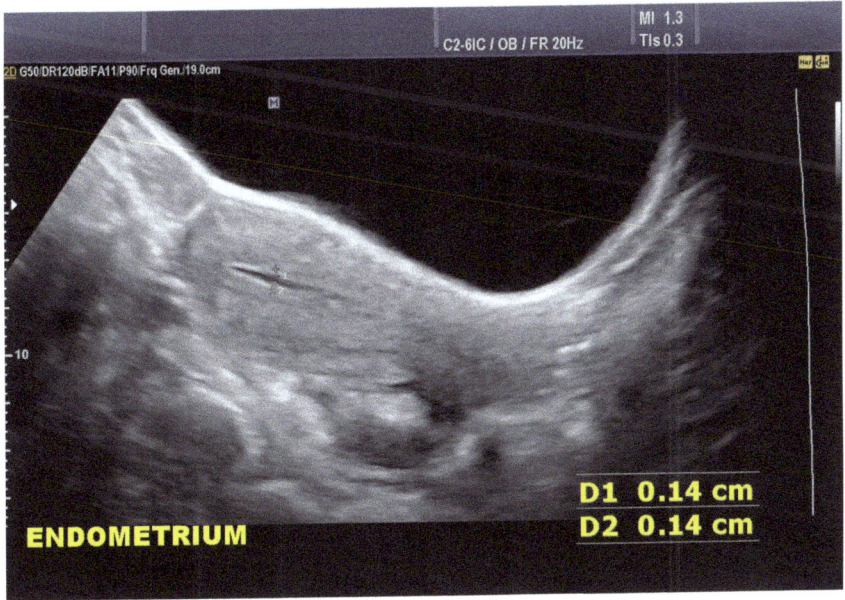

Fig. 5.1.6: Endometrial fluid collection as seen on TAS

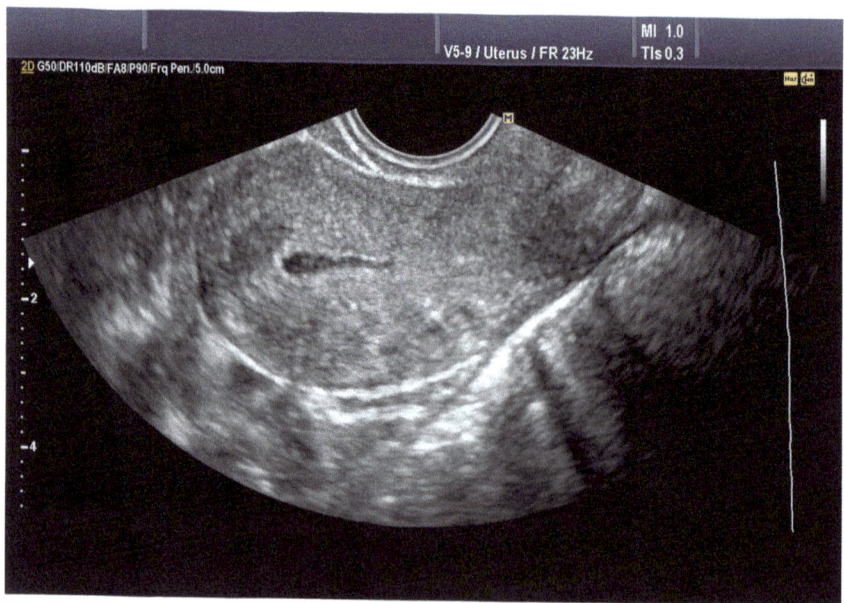

Fig. 5.1.7: TVS can be done on D2-D3 of the cycle

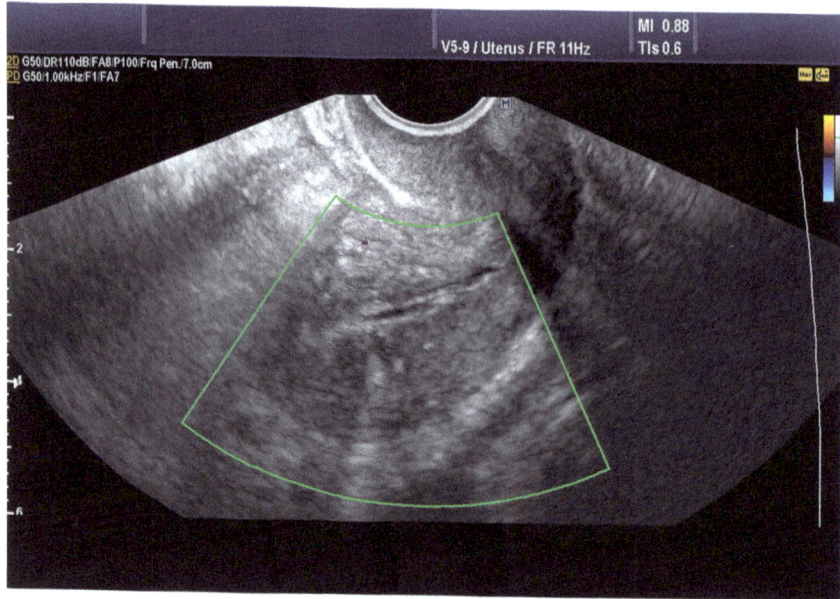

Fig. 5.1.8: Color flow mapping of the uterus D2-D3

5.1. Normal Endometrium

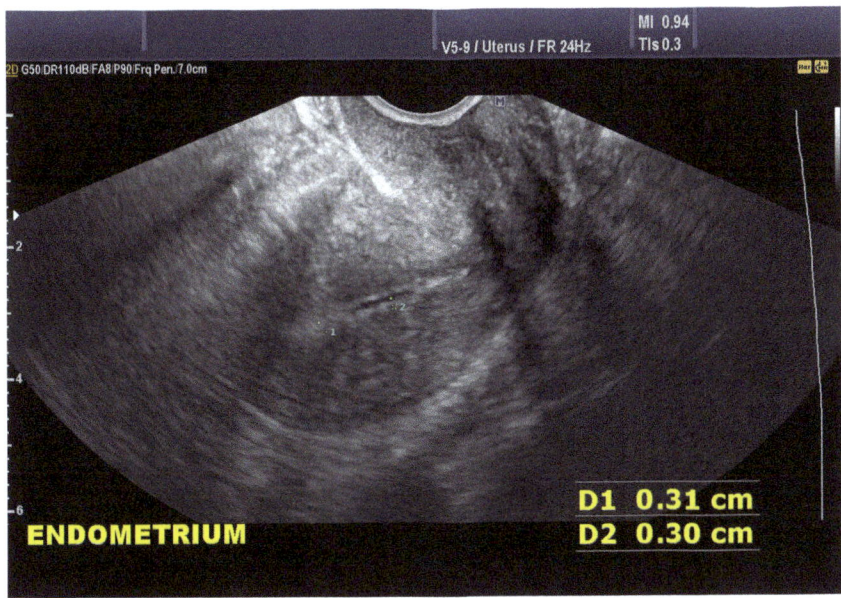

Fig. 5.1.9: For measurement of the endometrium, exclude the fluid collection from the measurements

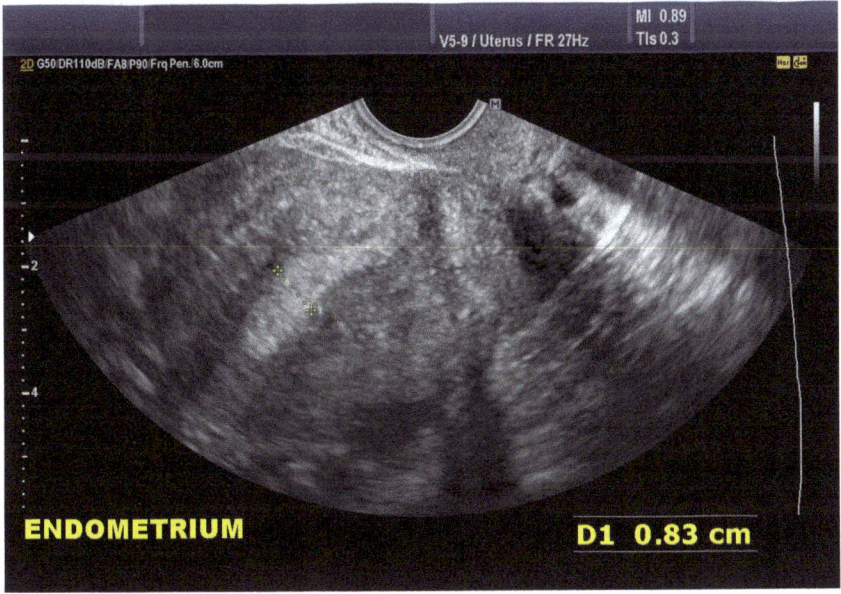

Fig. 5.1.10: Endometrium on 2D

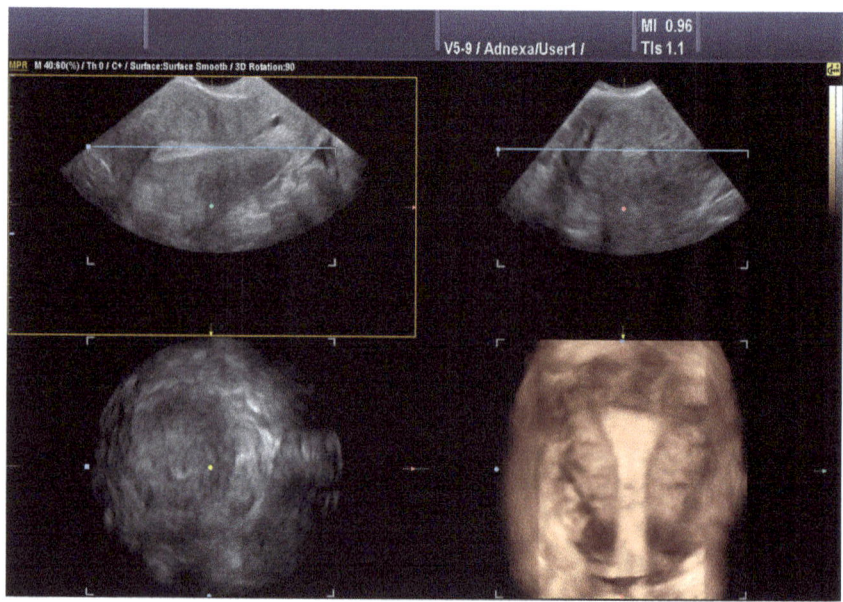

Fig. 5.1.11: Endometrium on MPR. The coronal plane improves evaluation of the uterine shape and endometrium

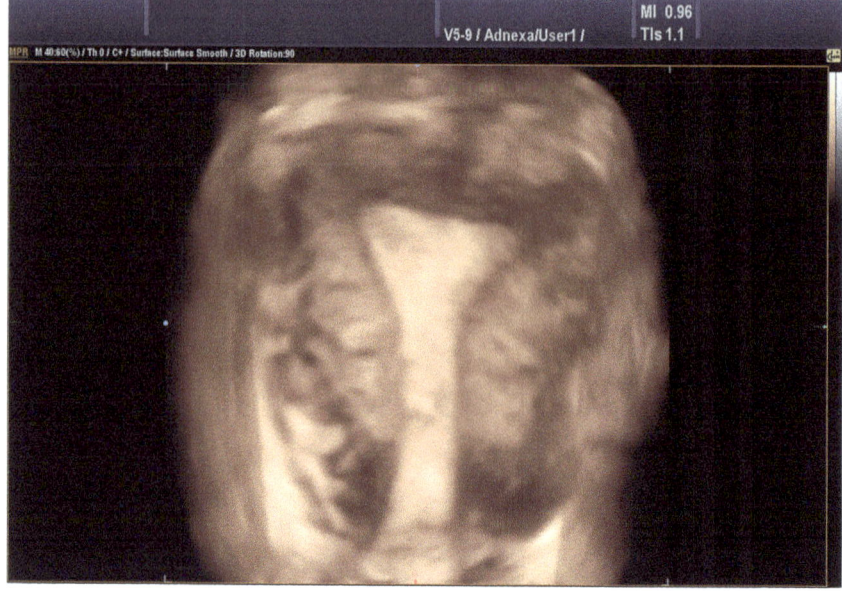

Fig. 5.1.12: Endometrium as seen on 3D. Congenital abnormalities of the uterus can be diagnosed more confidently

5.1. Normal Endometrium

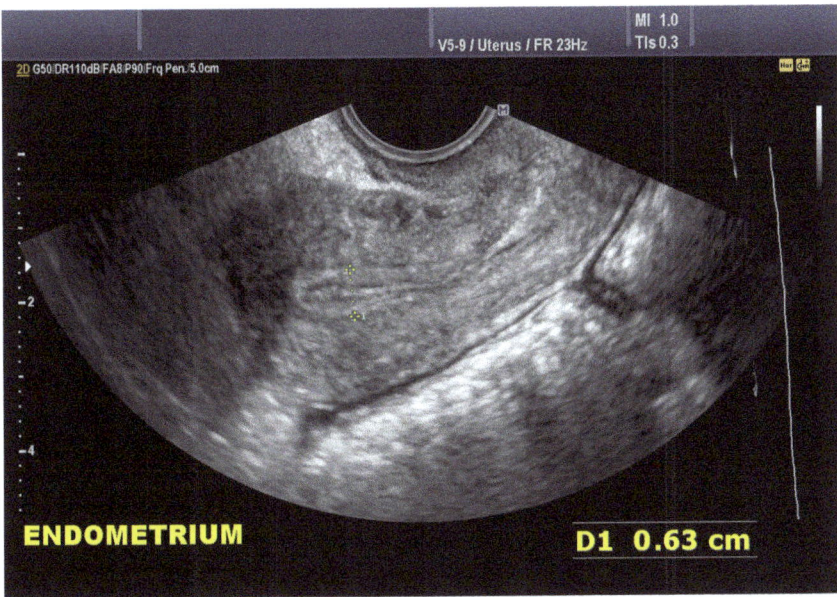

Fig. 5.1.13: Evaluate the endometrium carefully in respect to patients's symtoms and phase of cycle

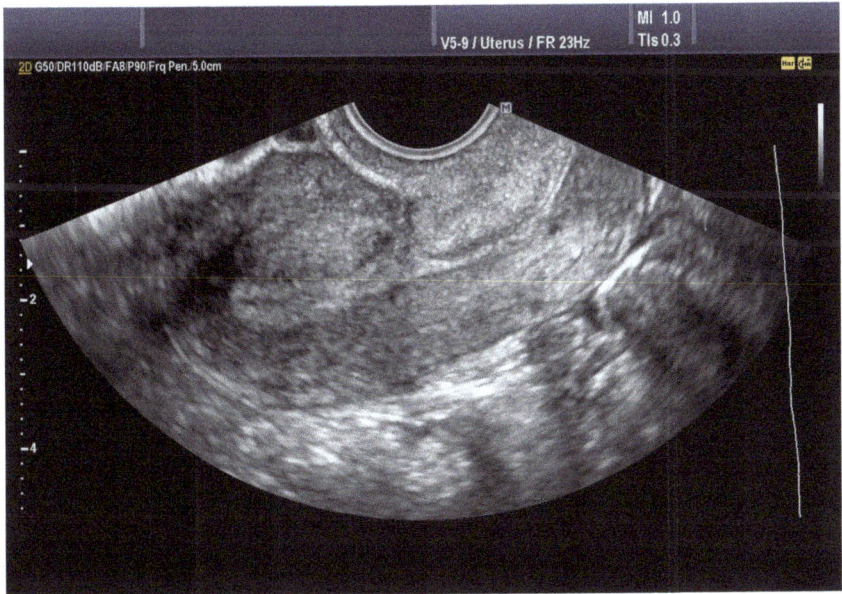

Fig. 5.1.14: Endometrium seen on day 6. Assess endometrial thickness and morphology

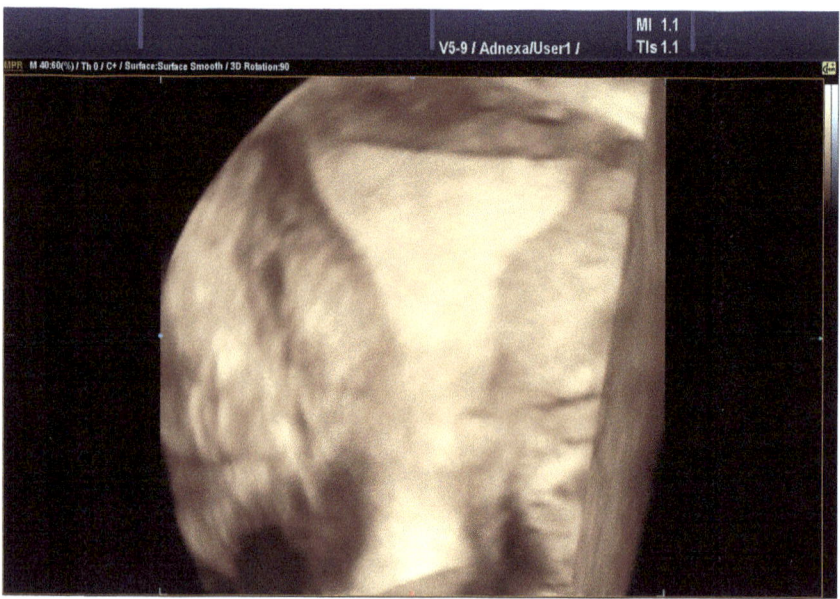

Fig. 5.1.15: Endometrium on 3D, endometrial polyp can be visualized more easily on 3D

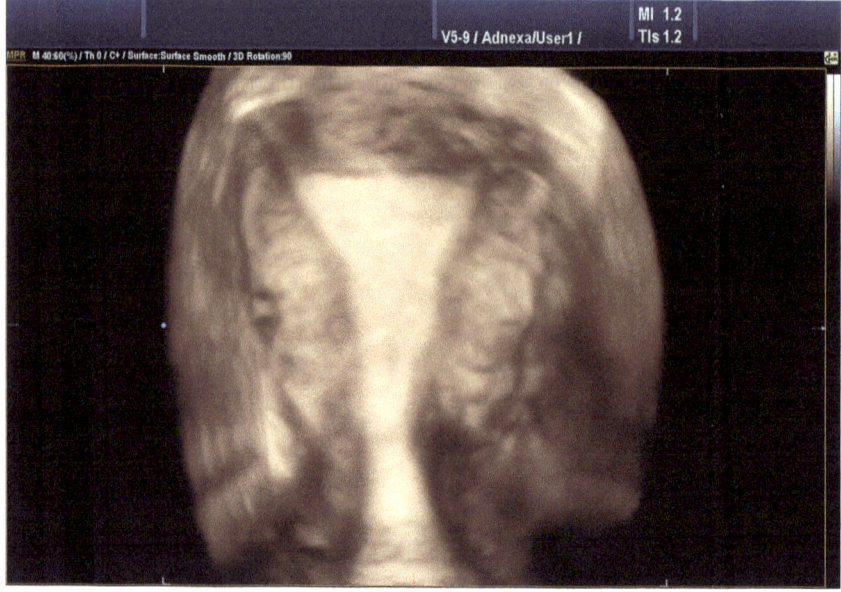

Fig 5.1.16: Normal endometrium, seen on 3D

5.1. Normal Endometrium

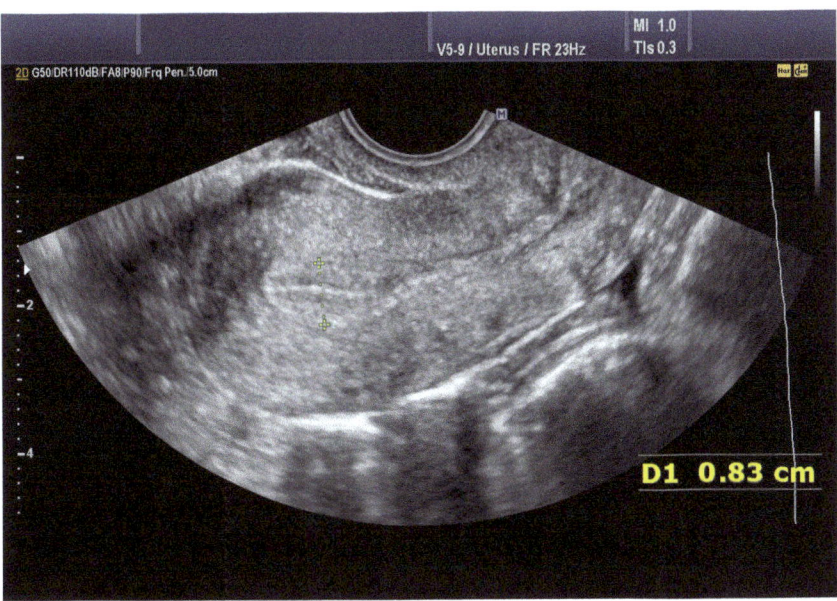

Fig. 5.1.17: Triple layered endometrium seen on day 9

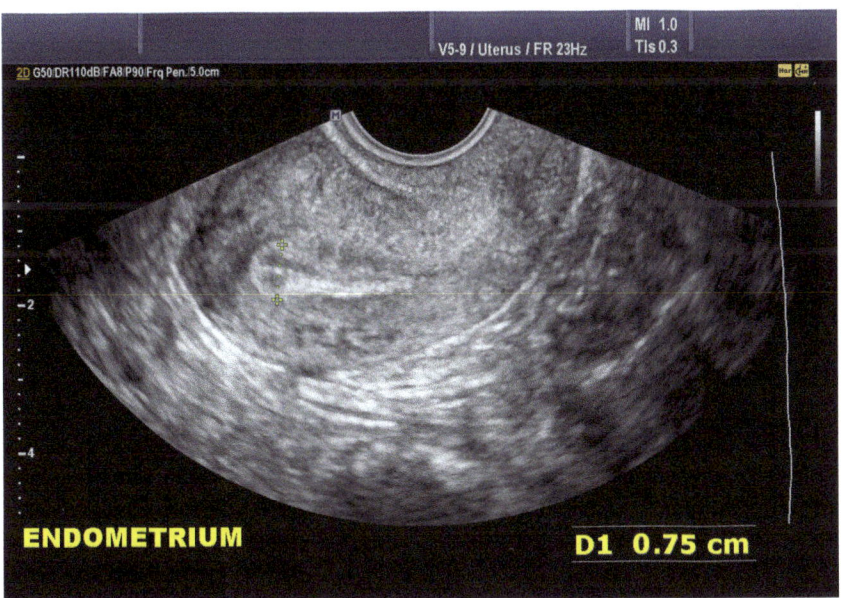

Fig. 5.1.18: Triple layered endometrium <10 mm premenopausal, <4 mm postmenopause or <6 mm HRT in postmenopause

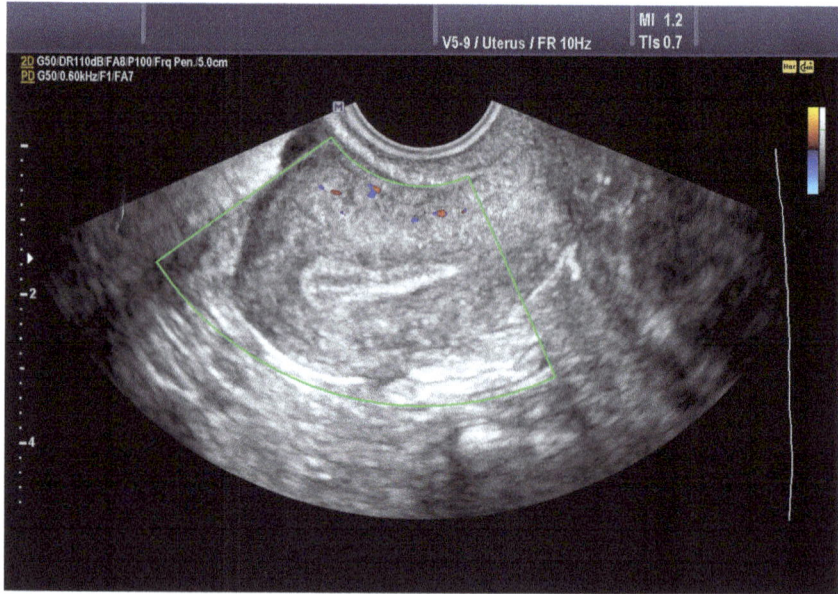

Fig. 5.1.19: Vascularity of the endometrium

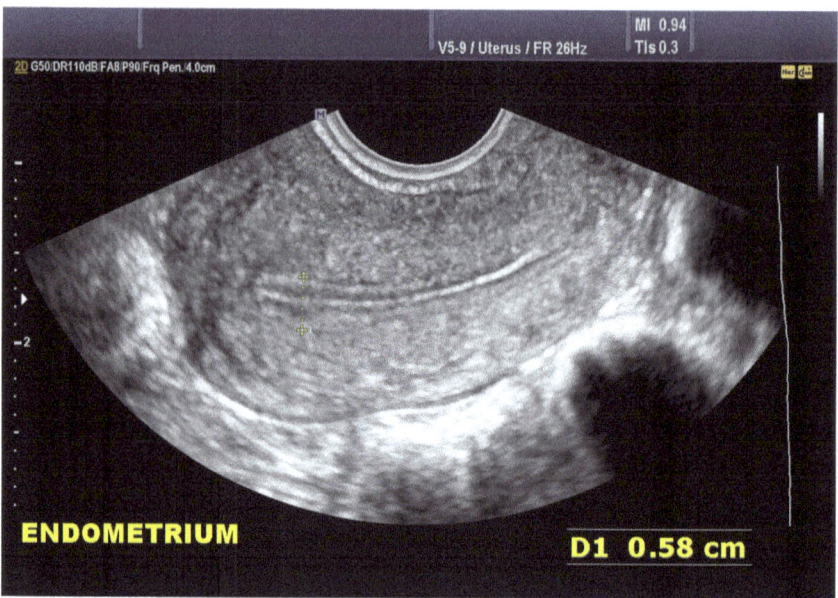

Fig. 5.1.20: Complete evaluation of the endometrium is mandatory from fundus till cervix

5.1. Normal Endometrium

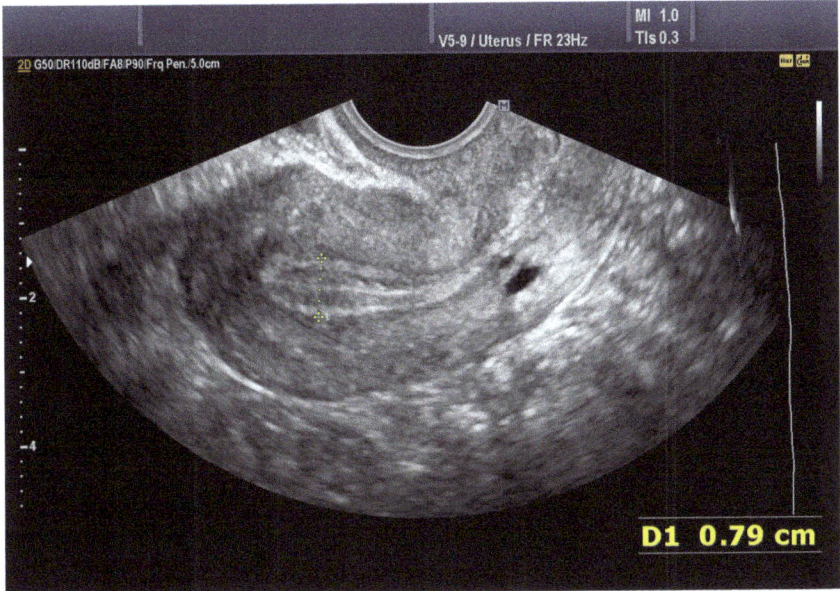

Fig. 5.1.21: Triple layered endometrium with no focal thickening or lesion

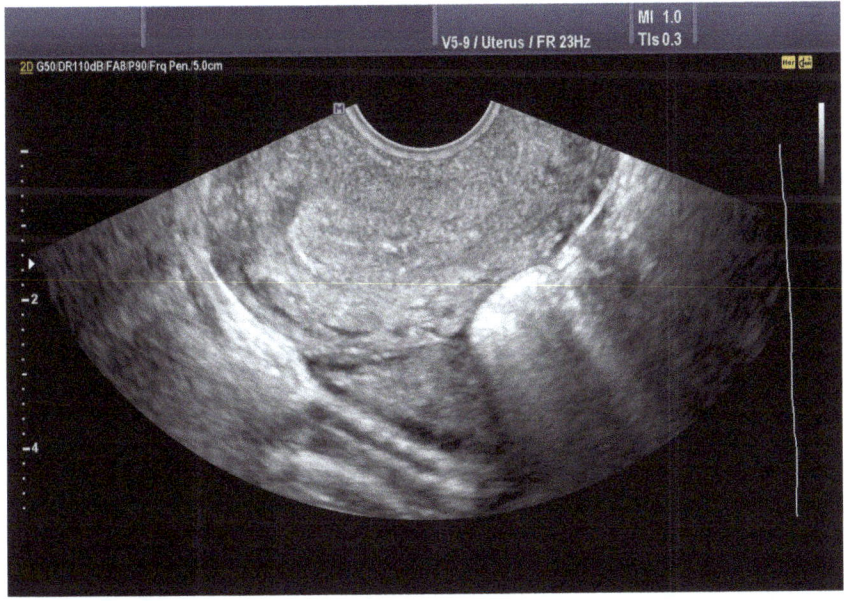

Fig. 5.1.22: Endometrium as seen on D12 of the cycle

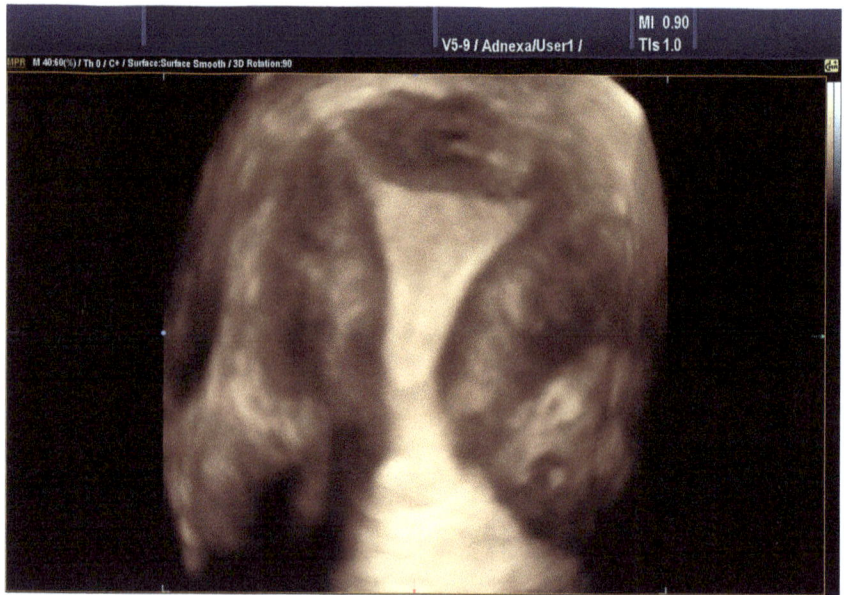

Fig. 5.1.23: Endometrium as seen on 3D

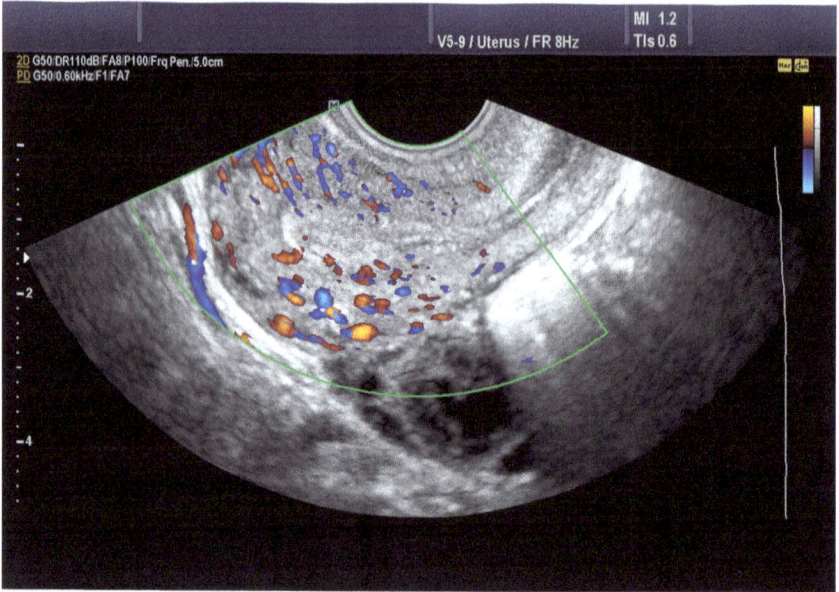

Fig. 5.1.24: Endometrial vascularity seen on D12 of the cycle

5.1. Normal Endometrium

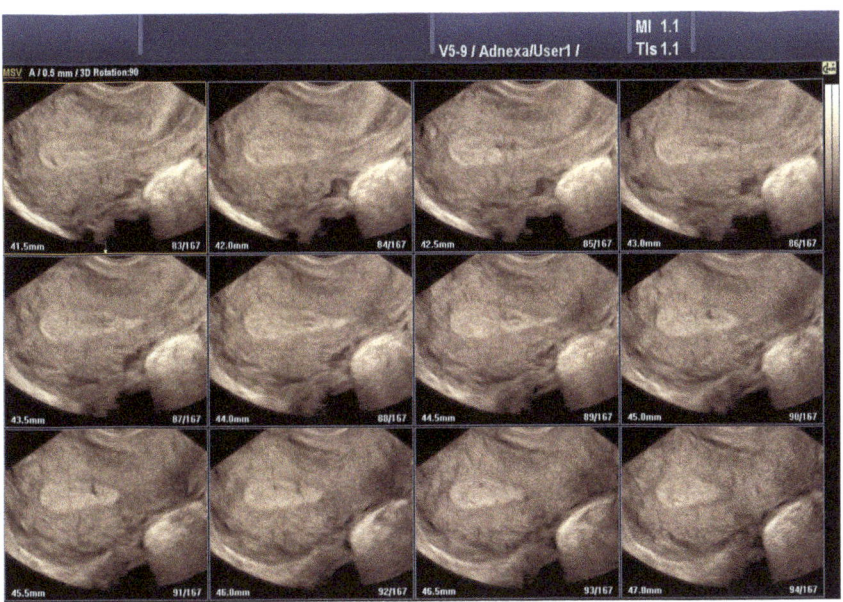

Fig. 5.1.25: Endometrium as seen on MSV

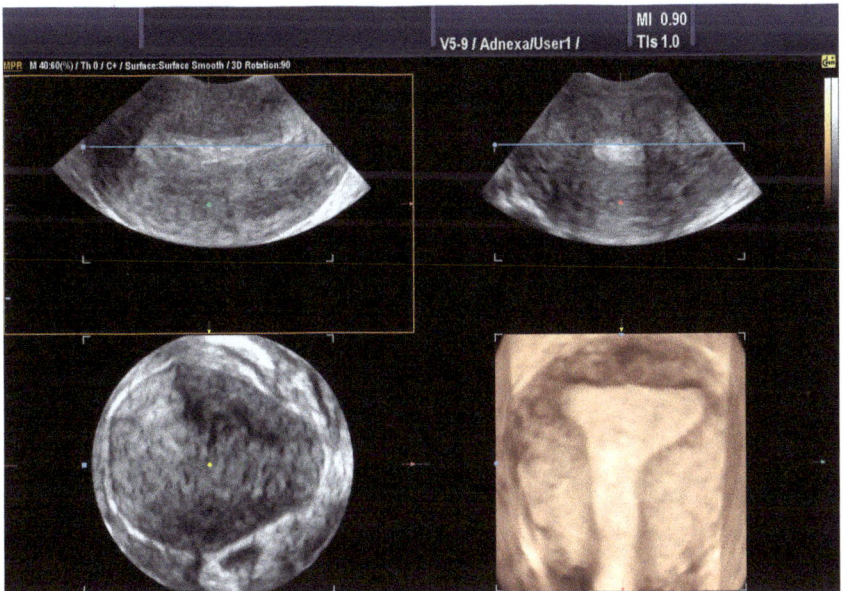

Fig. 5.1.26: Endometrium on MPR

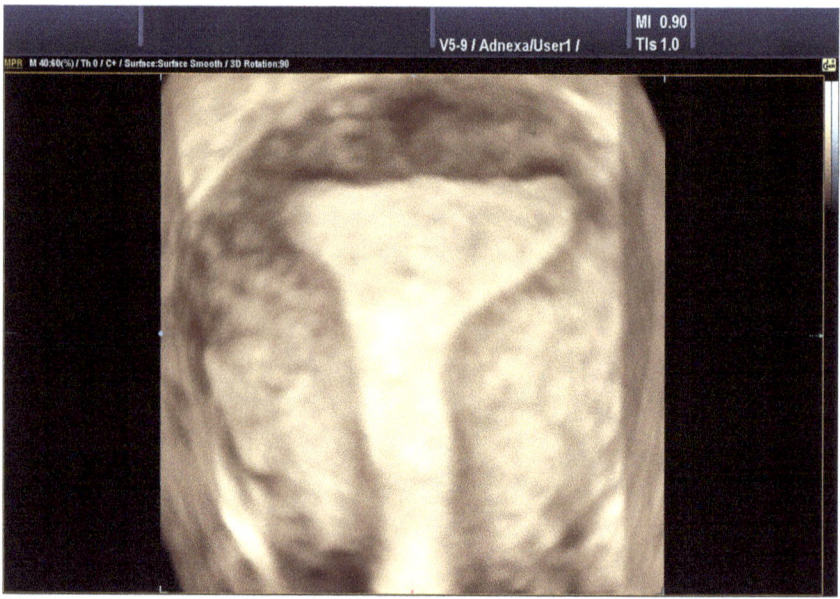

Fig. 5.1.27: Endometrium on 3D

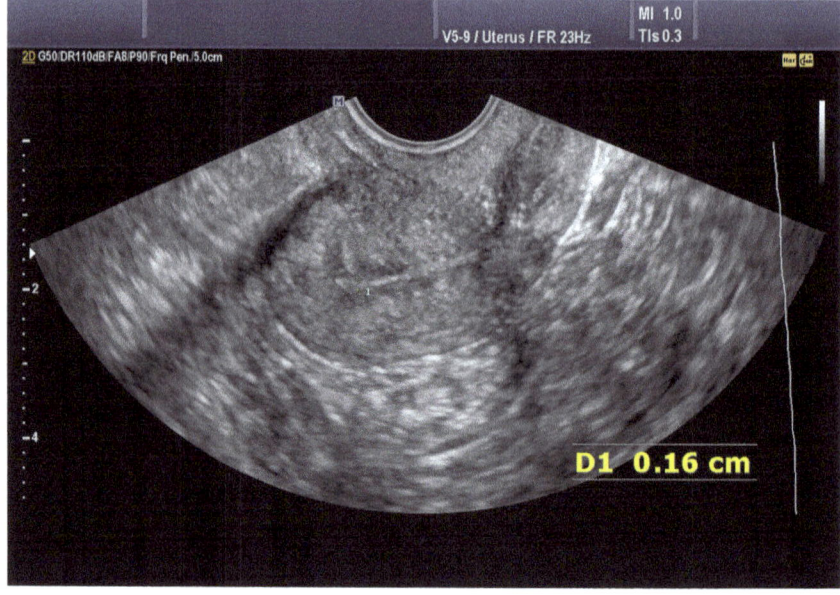

Fig. 5.1.28: Thin homogeneous endometrium seen in a postmenopausal patient

5.1. Normal Endometrium

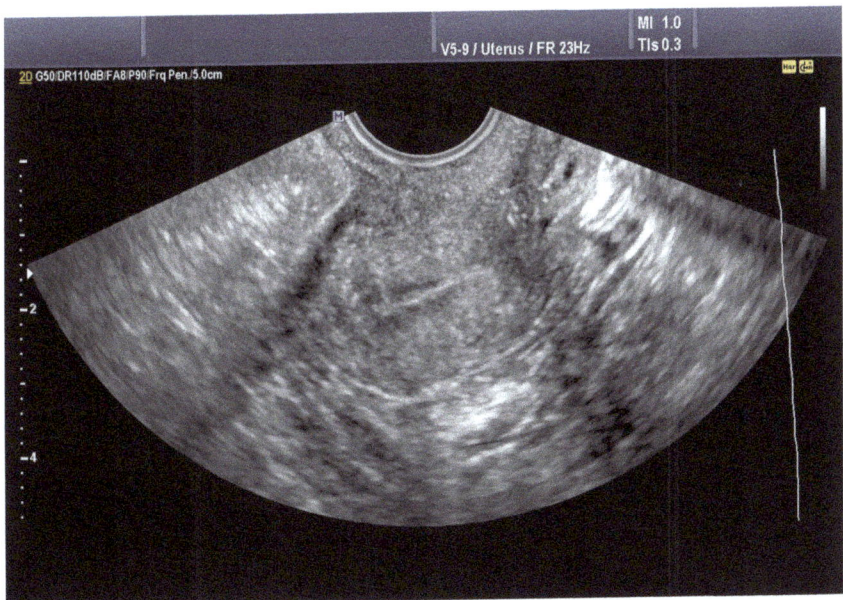

Fig. 5.1.29: No focal thickening, focal or diffuse inhomogeneity is seen. Likely to be an atrophic endometrium

5.2. NORMAL MYOMETRIUM

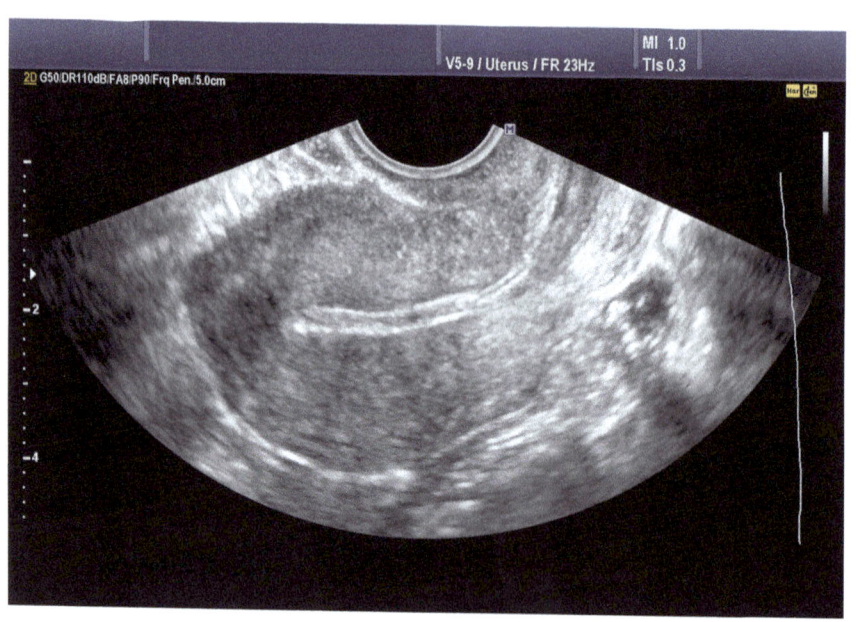

5.2. Normal Myometrium

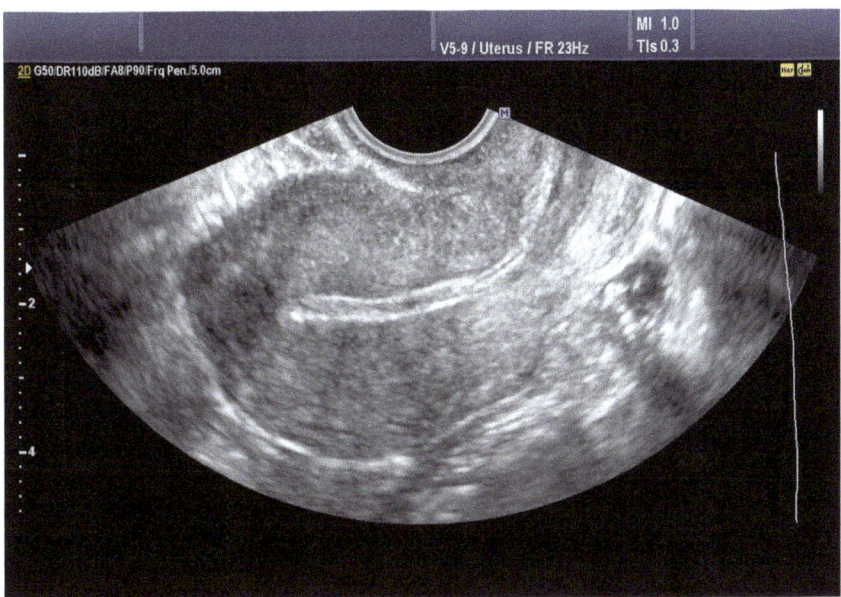

Fig. 5.2.1: Look for myometrium carefully for masses or changes in echo pattern

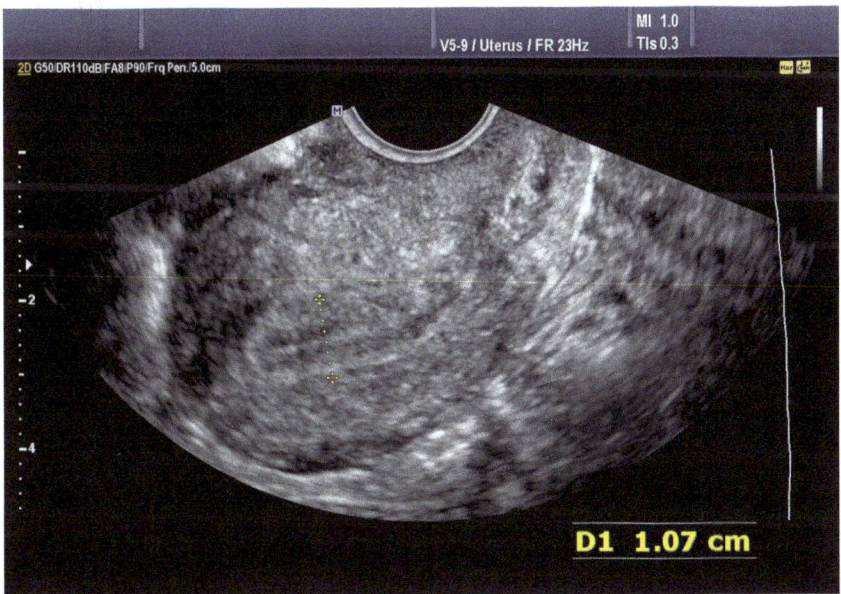

Fig. 5.2.2: Homogeneous myometrium as seen on 2D, any pathology must be measured in two planes

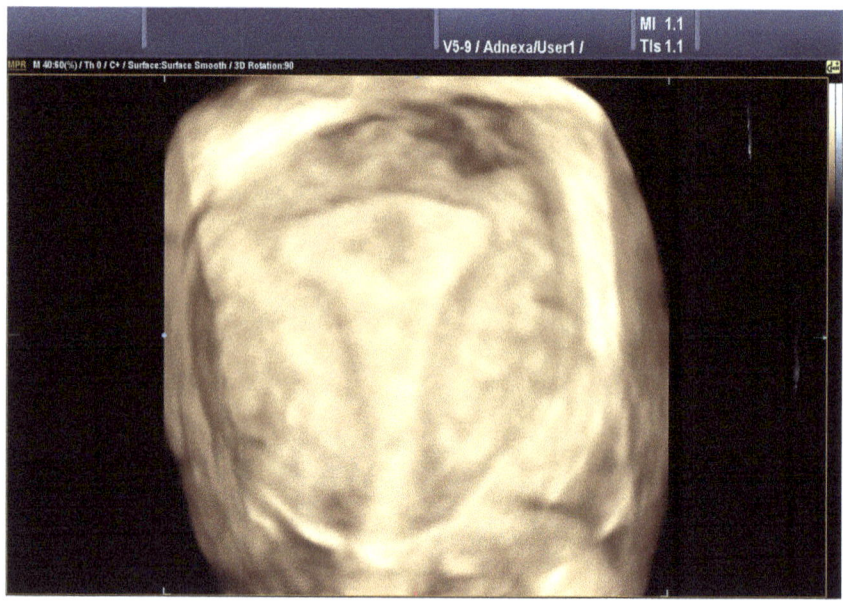

Fig. 5.2.3: Normal myometrium as seen on 3D

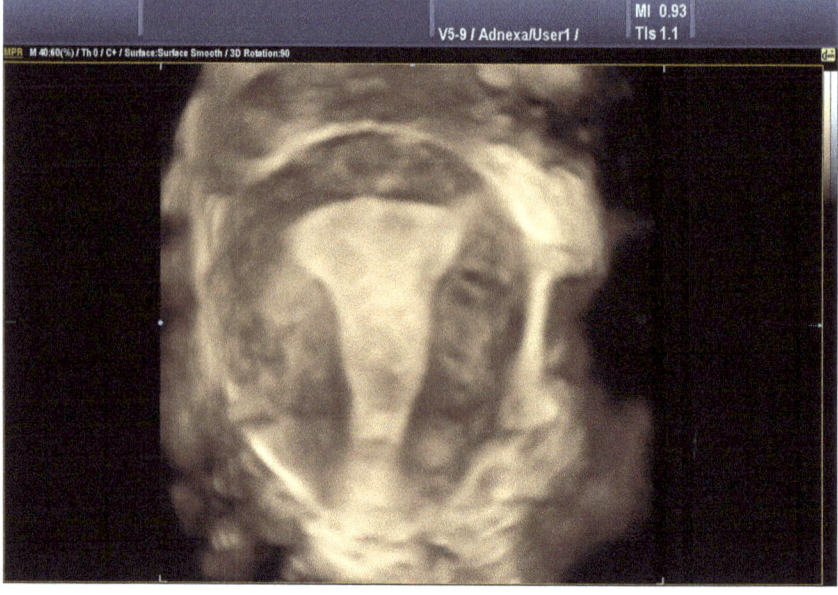

Fig. 5.2.4: Normal myometrium as seen on 3D

5.3. NORMAL CAVITY

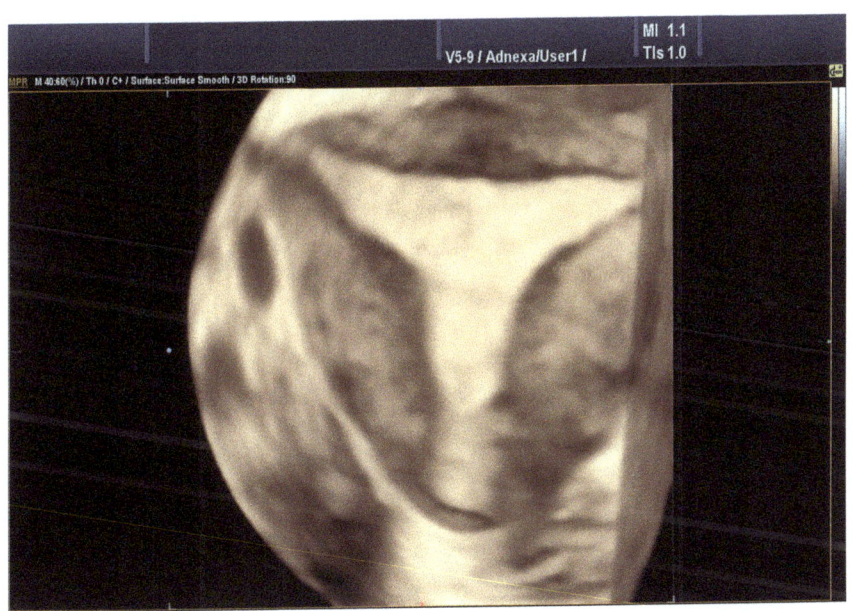

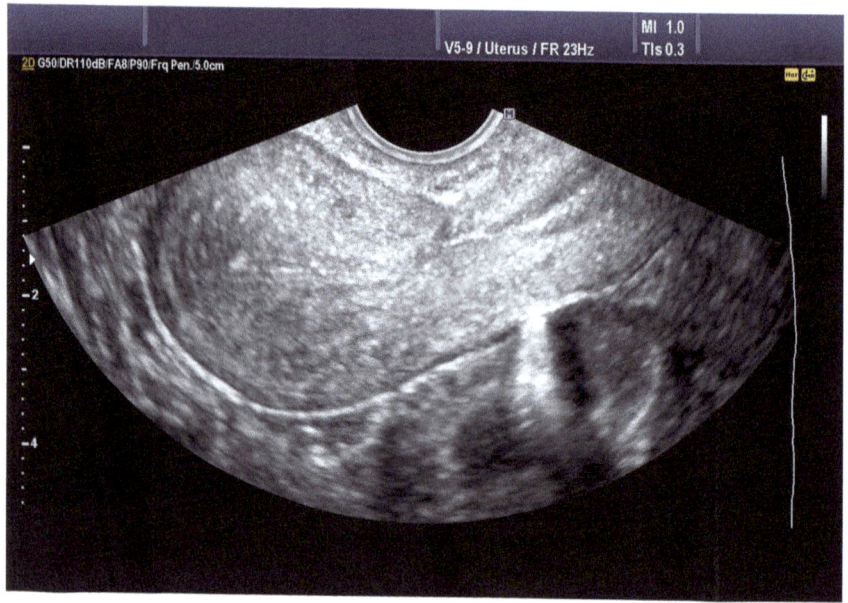

Fig. 5.3.1: Uterine cavity as seen on 2D

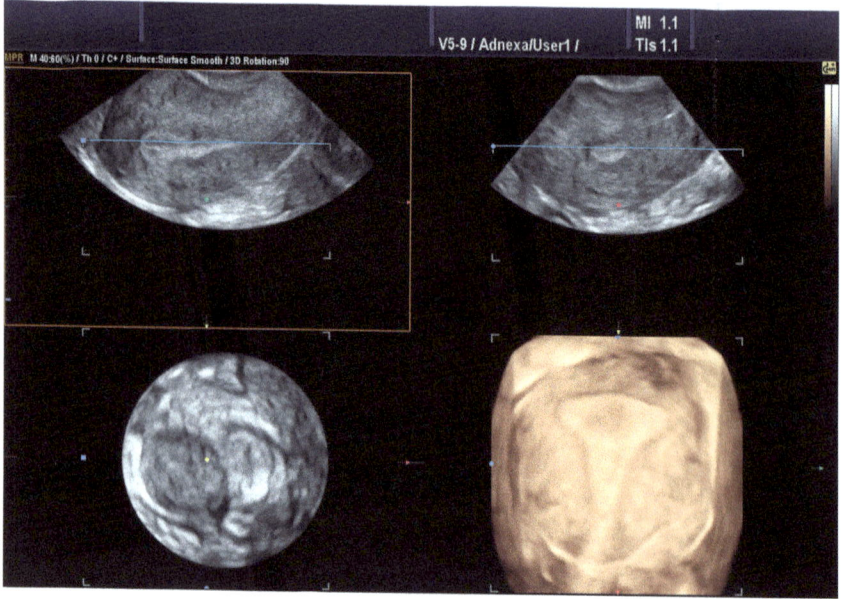

Fig. 5.3.2: Cavity on MPR

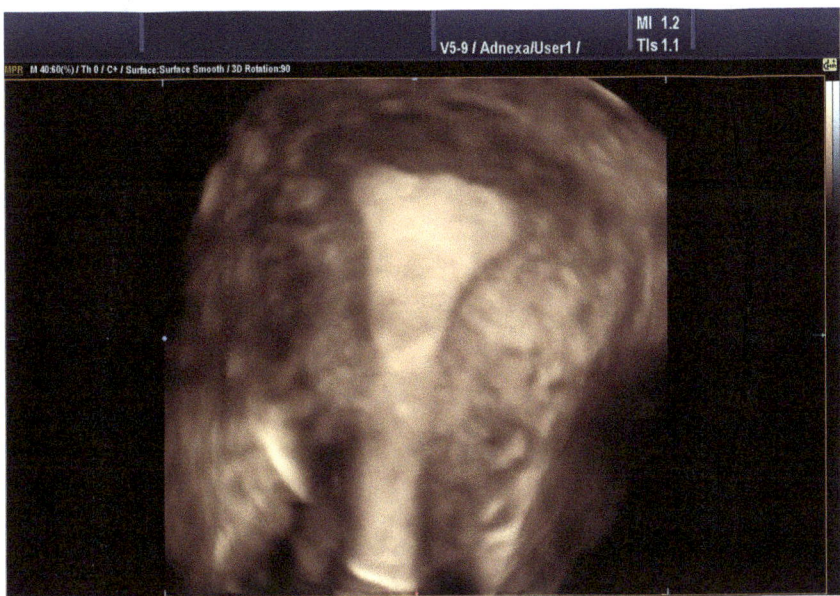

Fig. 5.3.3: Normal shape of cavity nicely demonstrated on 3D

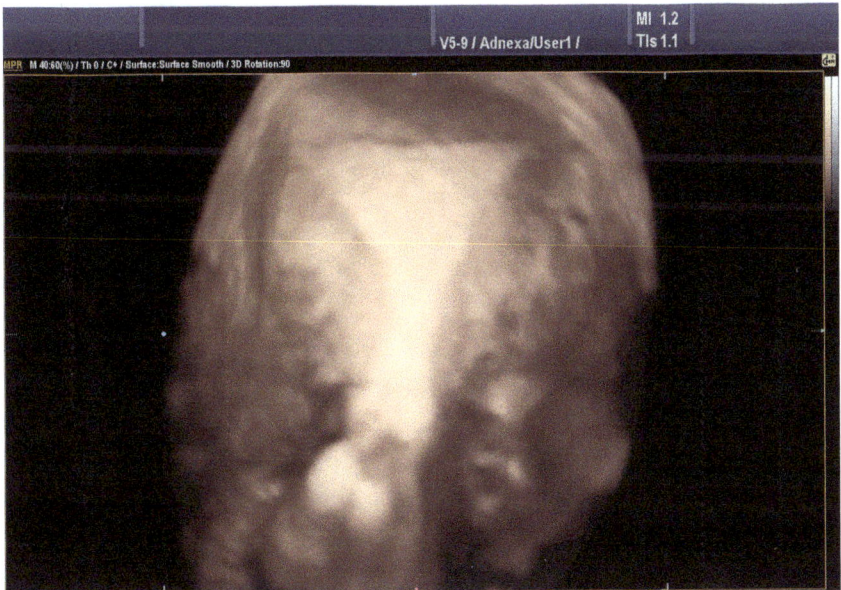

Fig. 5.3.4: Uterine cavity on 3D

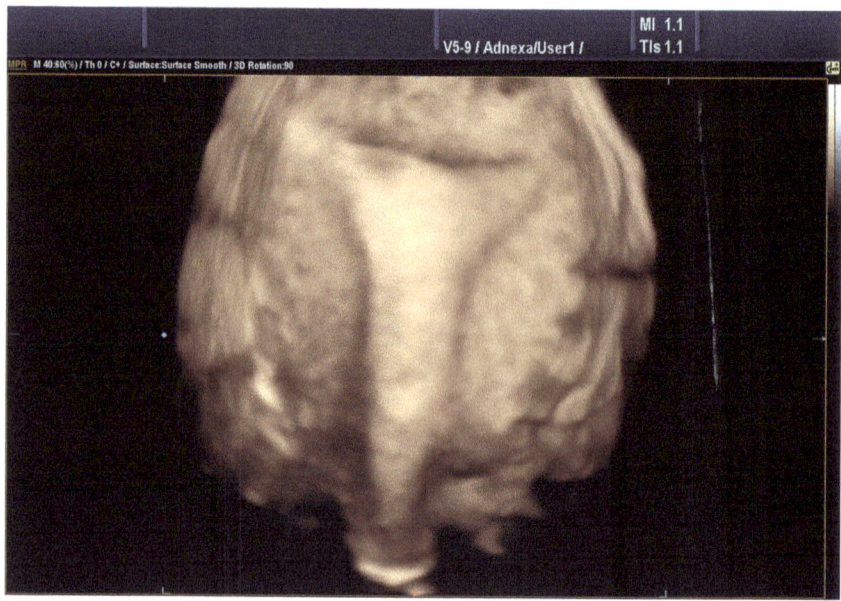

Fig. 5.3.5: Uterine cavity seen on 3D

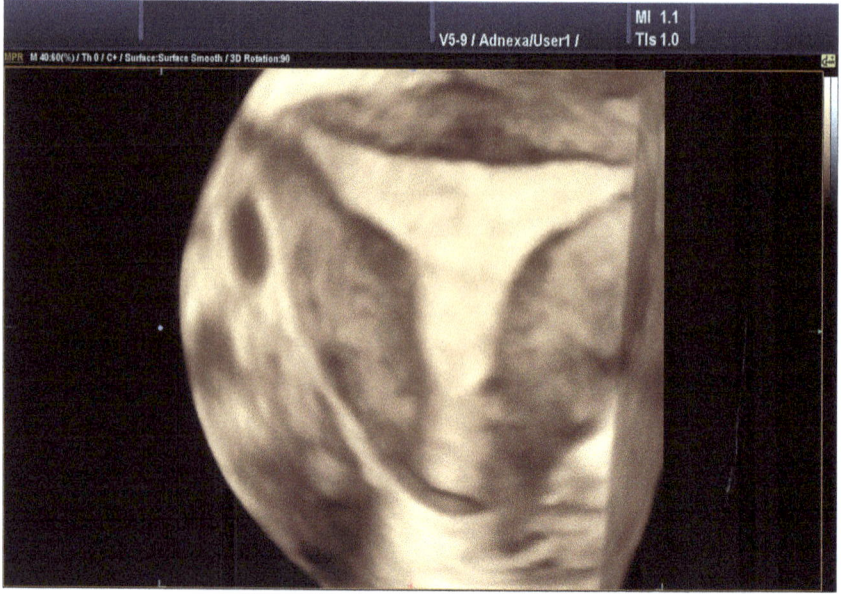

Fig. 5.3.6: Complete uterine cavity as seen on 3D

5.4. NORMAL CONTOUR

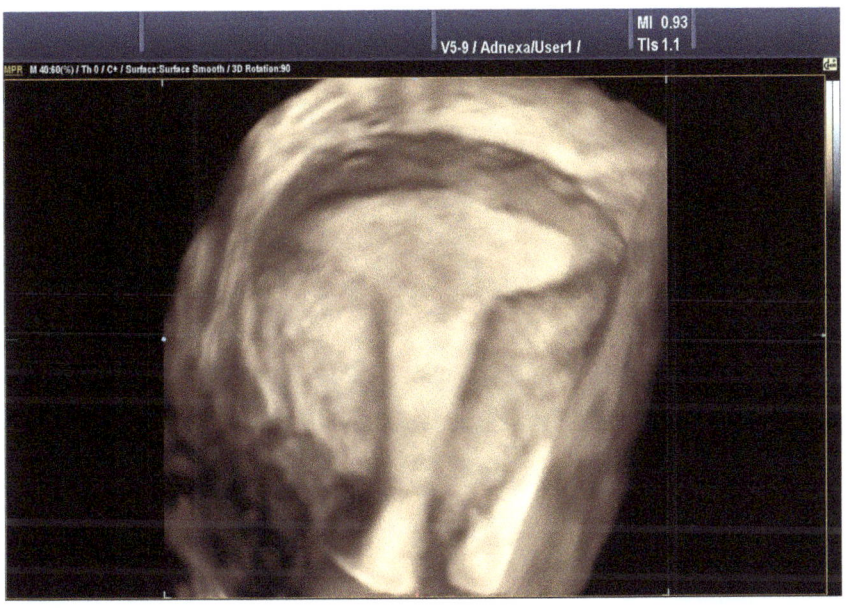

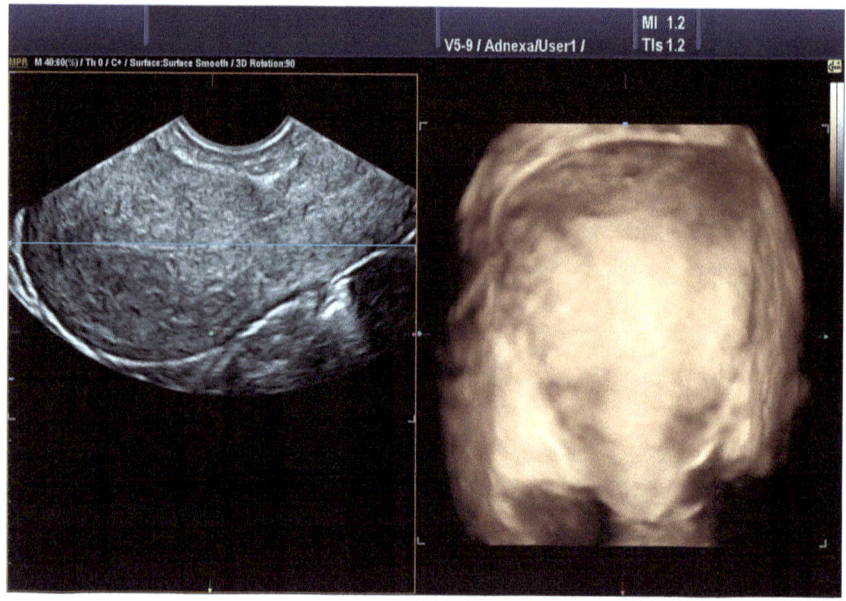

Fig. 5.4.1: Uterine contour as seen on 2D and 3D

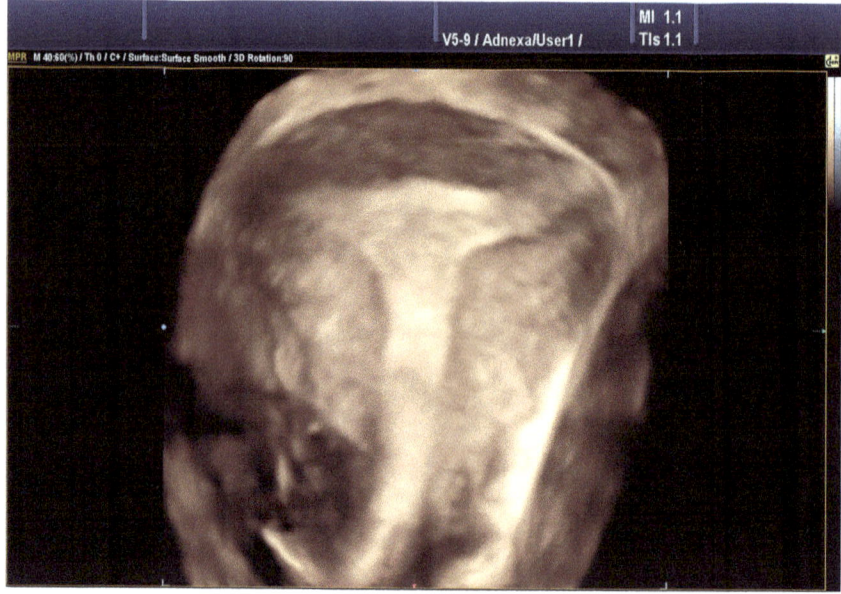

Fig. 5.4.2: Cavity and contour as seen on 3D

5.4. Normal Contour

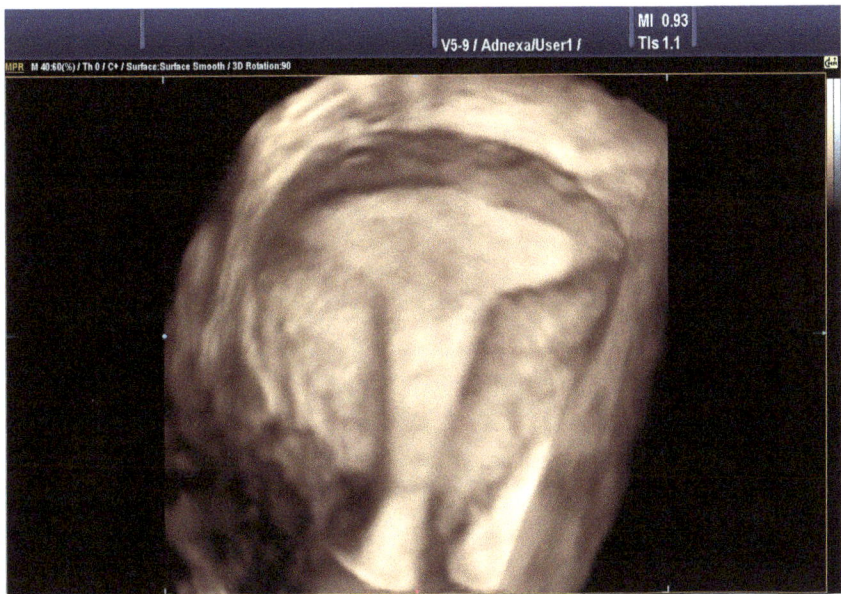

Fig. 5.4.3: Contour of the uterus nicely visualized on 3D. Any change in contour should be mentioned

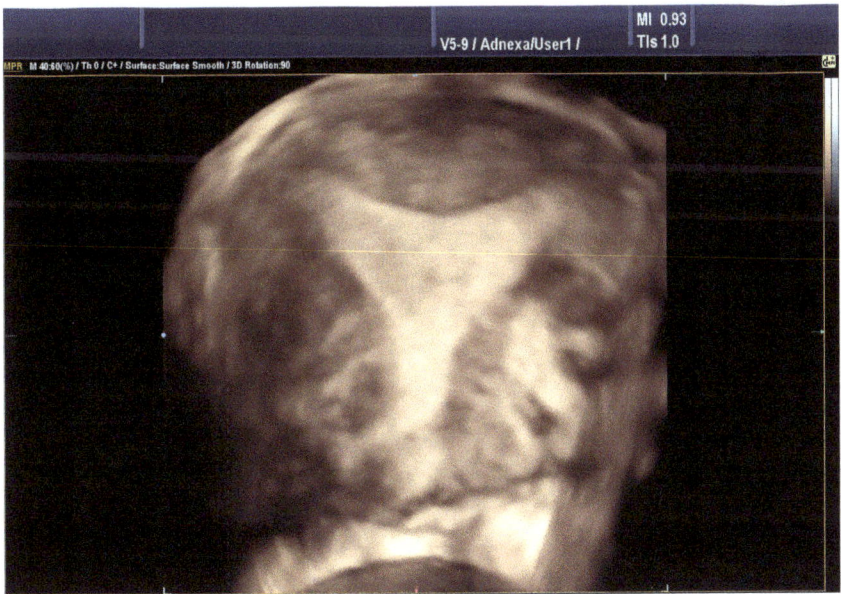

Fig. 5.4.4: Uterine cavity and contour nicely demonstrated on 3D

5.5. NORMAL INTRAUTERINE CONTRACEPTIVE DEVICE

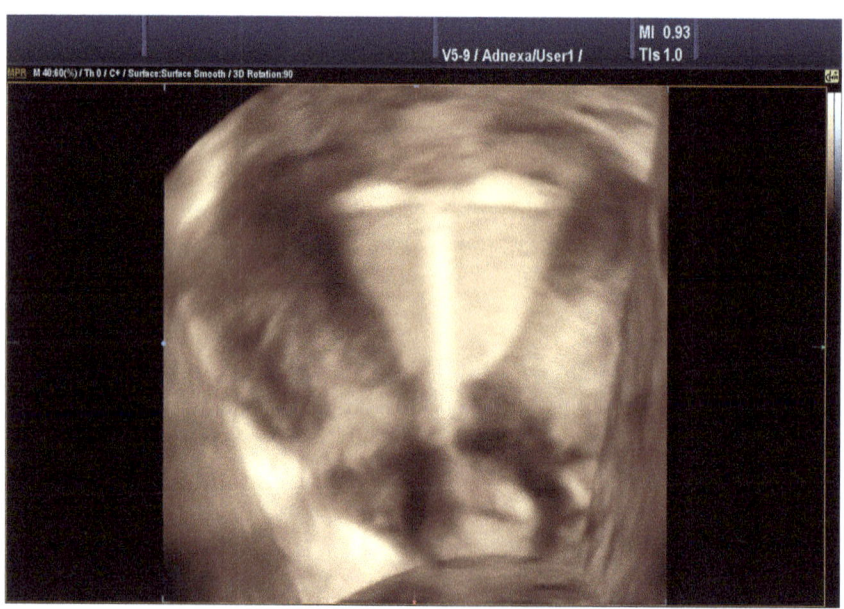

5.5. Normal Intrauterine Contraceptive Device

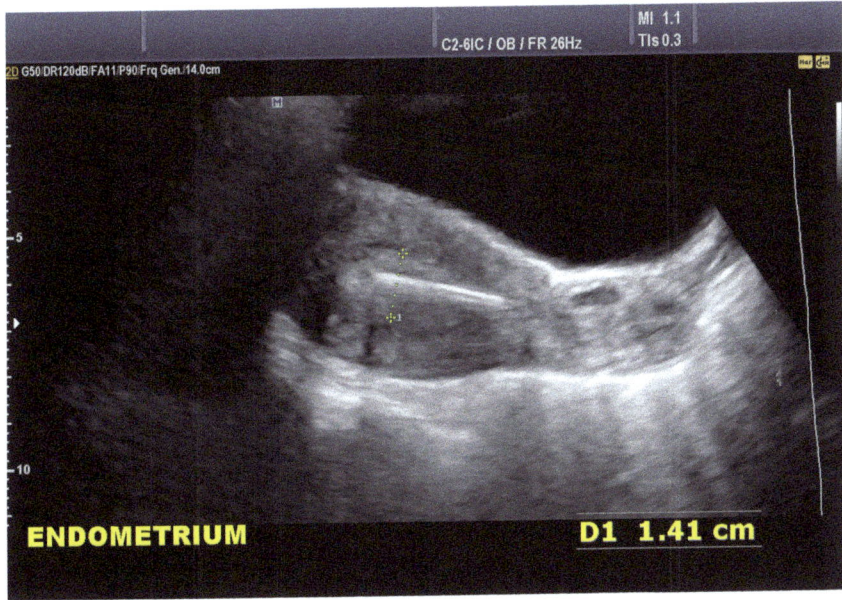

Fig. 5.5.1: Ultrasound is used routinely to check the position of IUCD on 2D on TAS

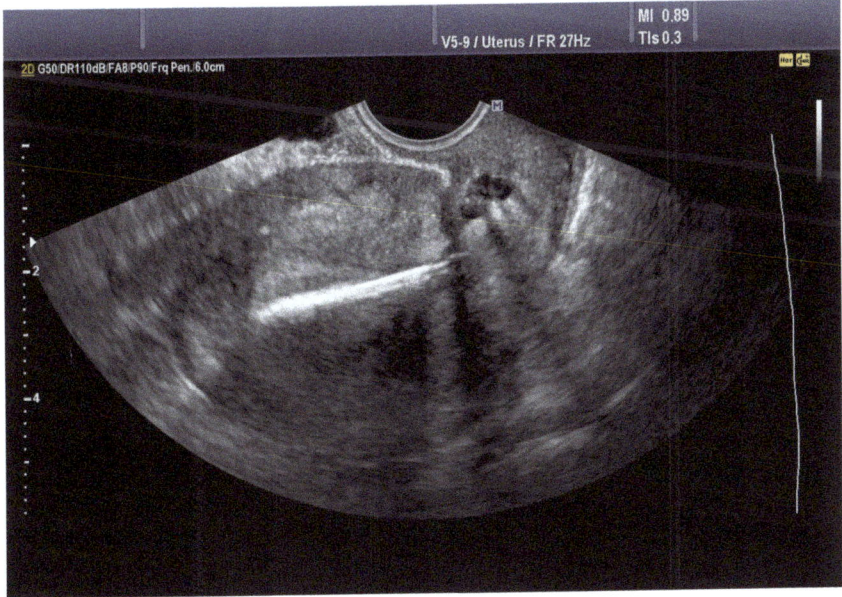

Fig. 5.5.2: IUCD in place in the uterine cavity

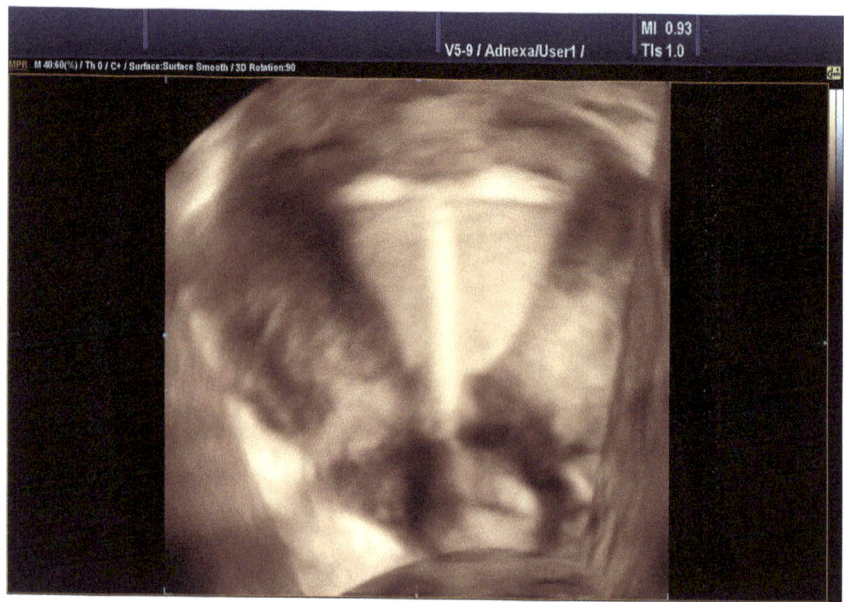

Fig. 5.5.3: Complete CuT seen on 3D, coronal 3D image shows accurate location of shaft and cross bars in the body and fundus of uterus

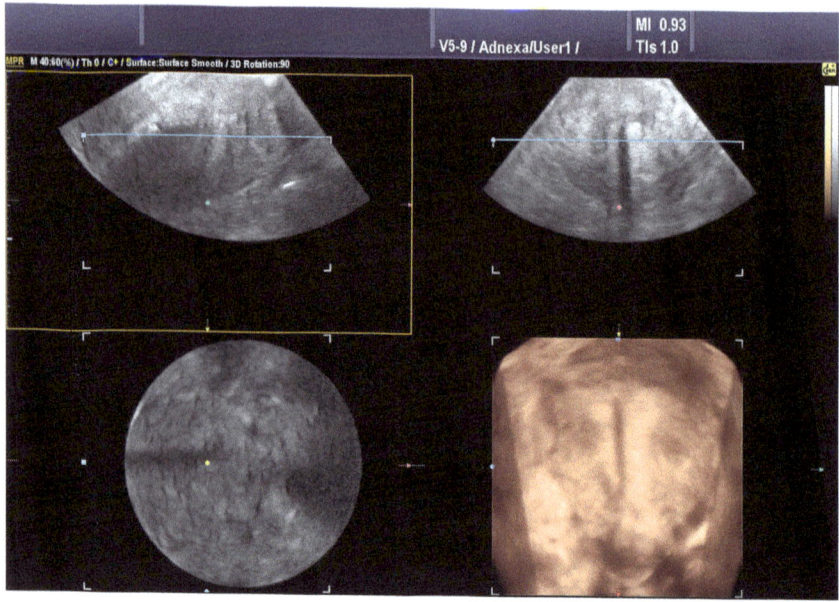

Fig. 5.5.4: IUCD seen on MPR

5.5. Normal Intrauterine Contraceptive Device

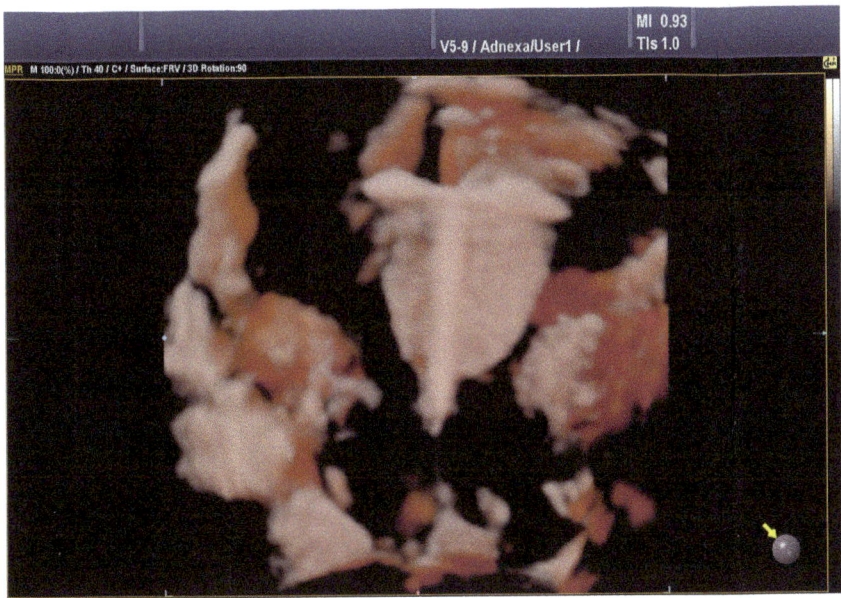

Fig. 5.5.5: On 3D you can see the endometrium as well as the IUCD

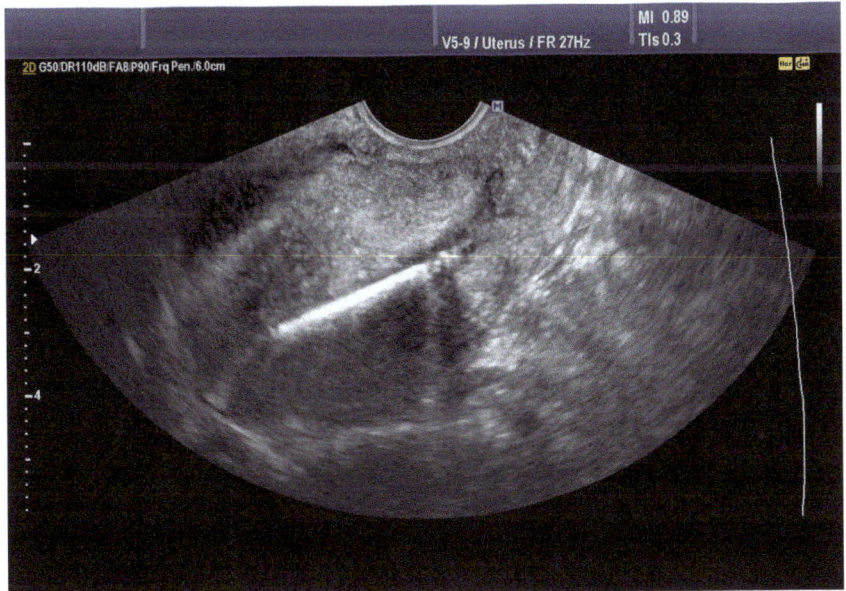

Fig. 5.5.6: IUCD in the uterus

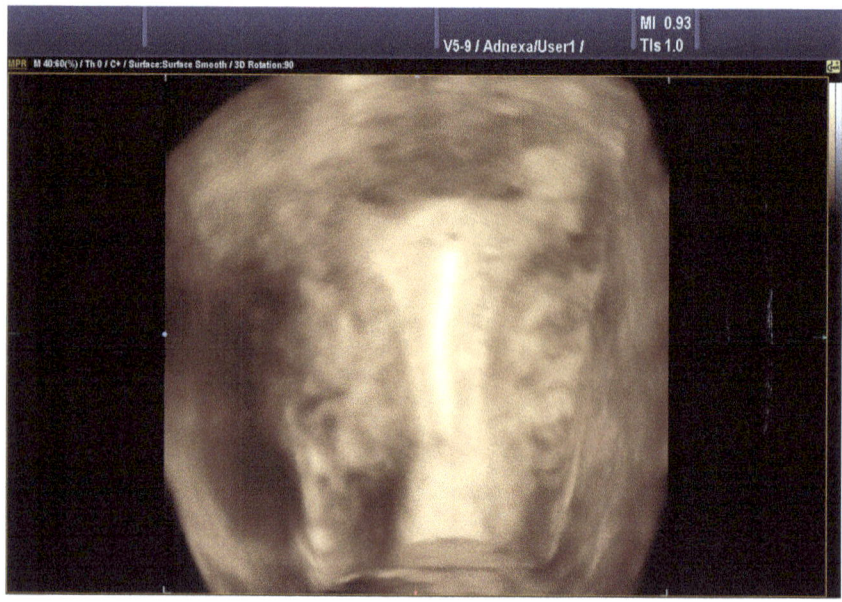

Fig. 5.5.7: As seen on 3D

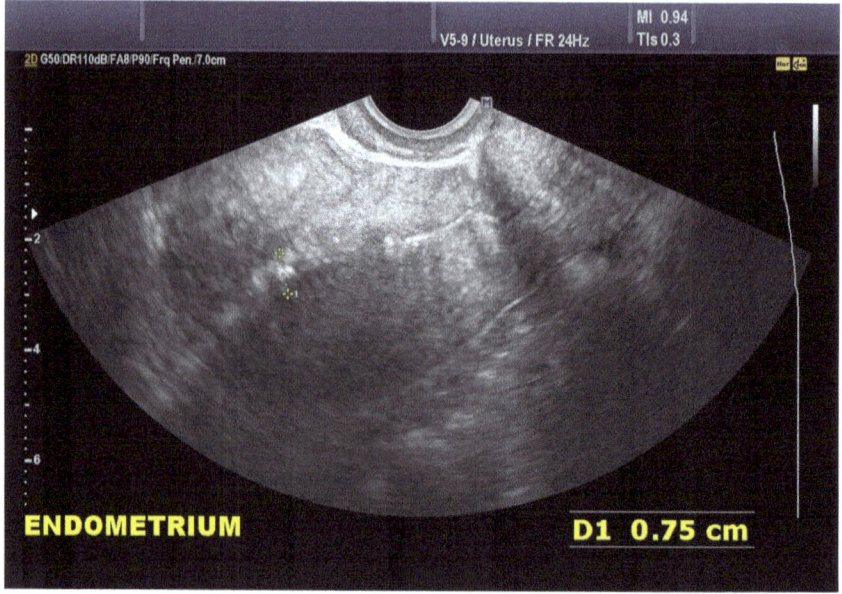

Fig. 5.5.8: Different types of IUCD give a different appearance on 2D

5.5. Normal Intrauterine Contraceptive Device

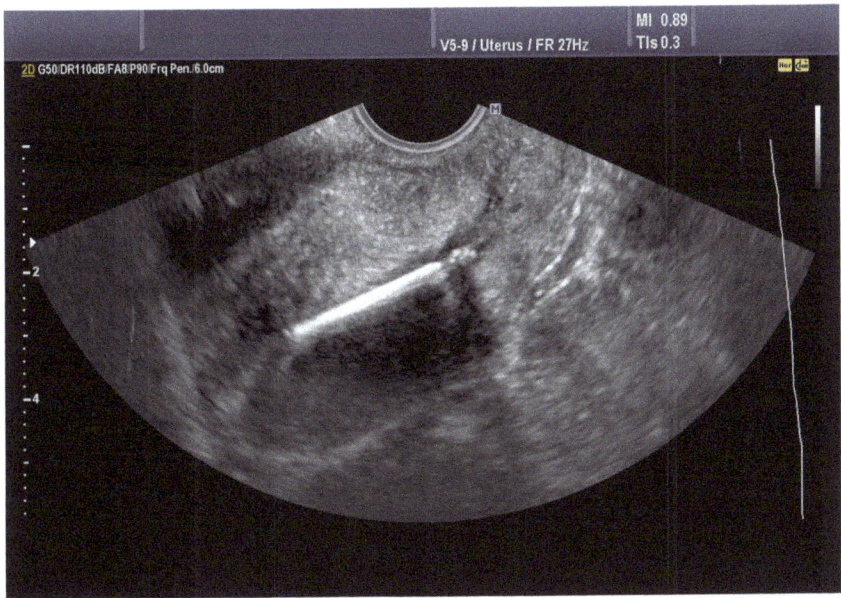

Fig. 5.5.9: IUCD on 2D

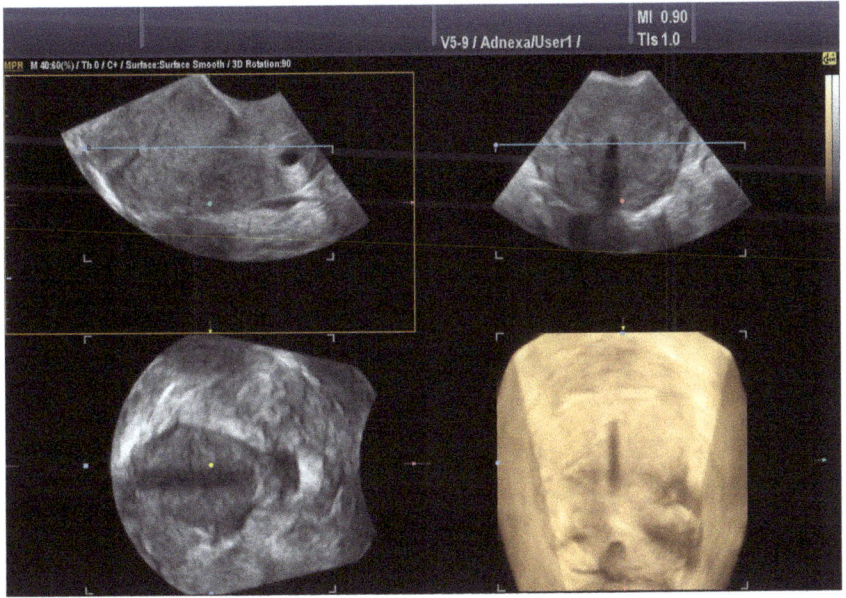

Fig. 5.5.10: IUCD as seen on MPR

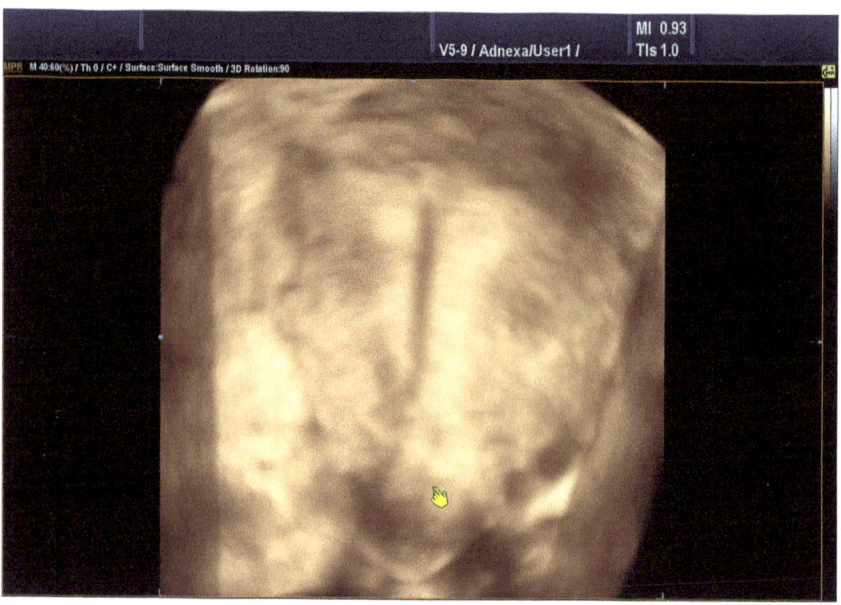

Fig. 5.5.11: IUCD seen on 3D. The vertical limb can appear hypoechoic

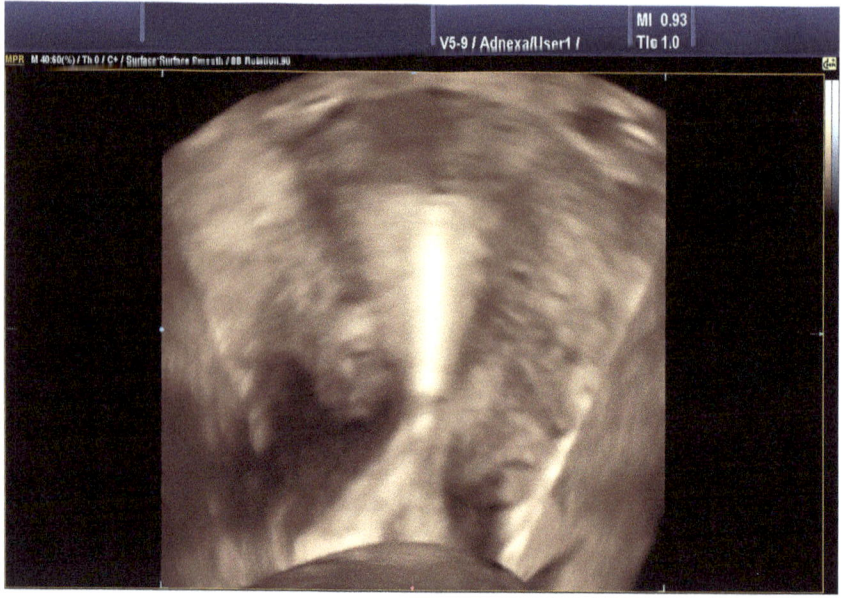

Fig. 5.5.12: Vertical limb appearing hyperechoic

5.6. NORMAL VAGINAL VAULT

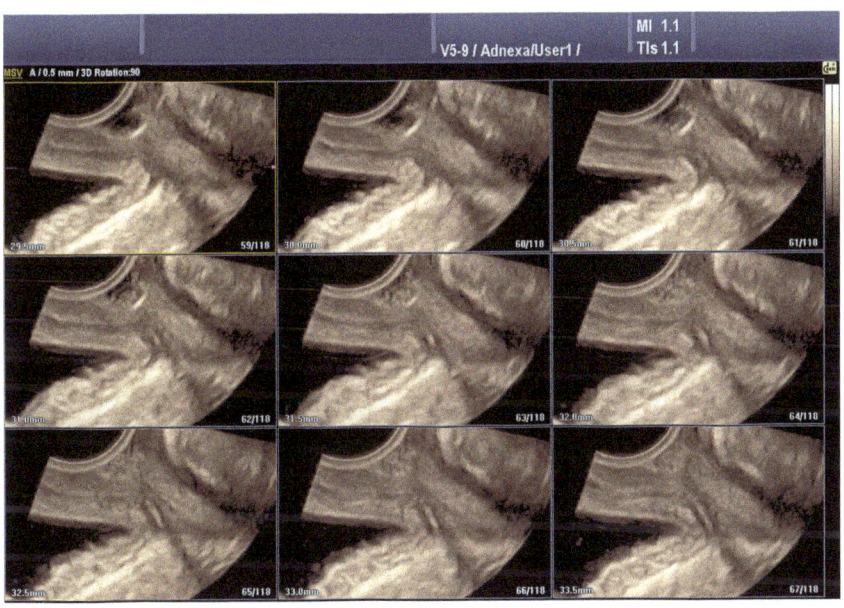

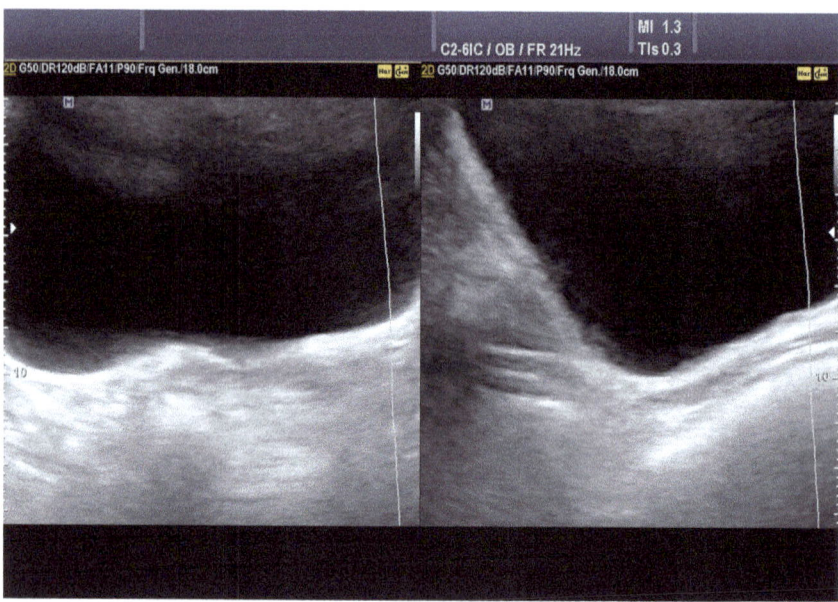

Fig. 5.6.1: Posthysterectomy—vaginal vault as seen in TAS

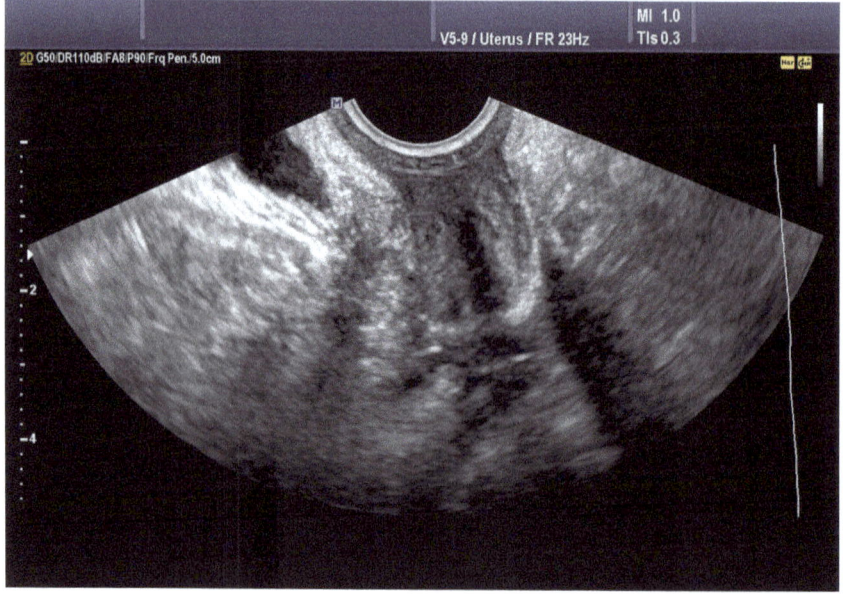

Fig. 5.6.2: Vaginal vault as seen on TVS

5.6. Normal Vaginal Vault

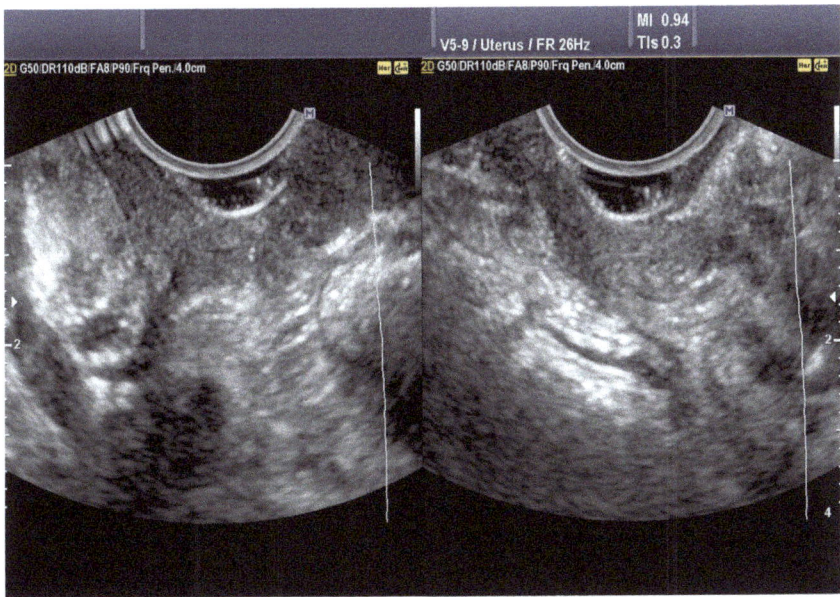

Fig. 5.6.3: Vaginal vault as seen on TVS

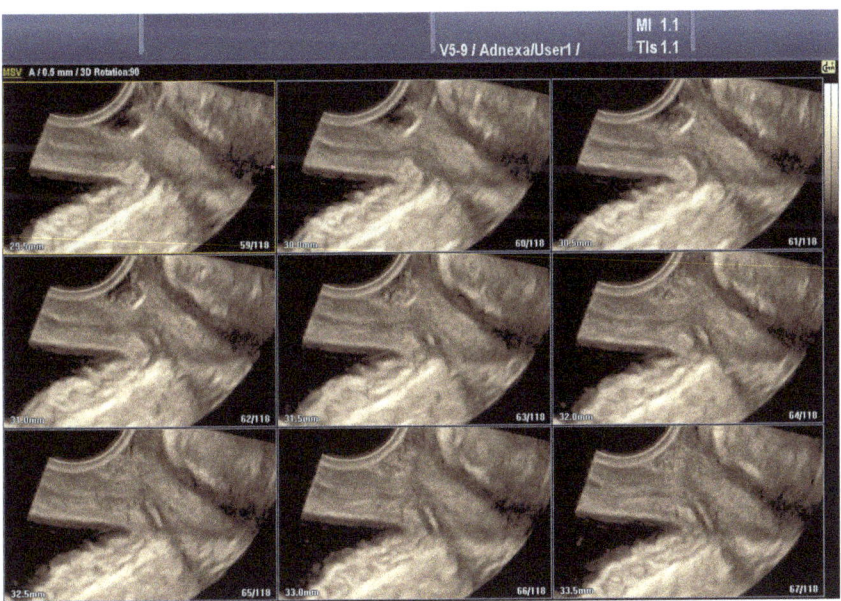

Fig. 5.6.4: As seen on MSV

5.7. NORMAL ADNEXA

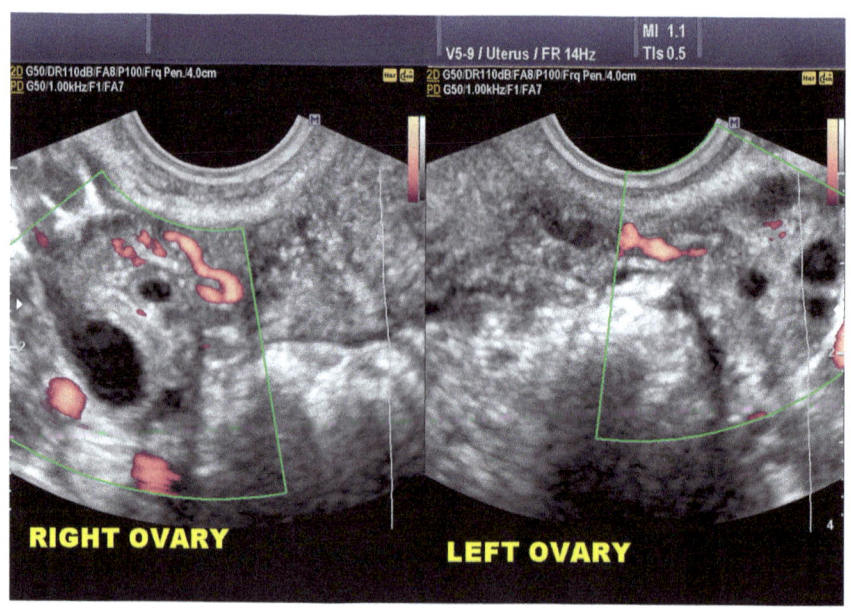

5.7. Normal Adnexa

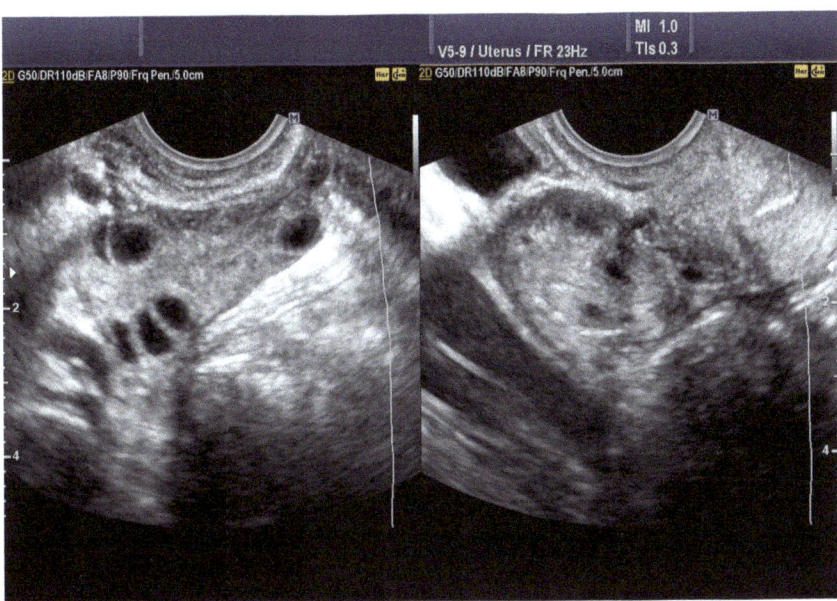

Fig. 5.7.1: With a TVS assess, the ovary for diameter and volume and to assess antral follicles. Measure the ovary in all three dimensions by rotating the probe

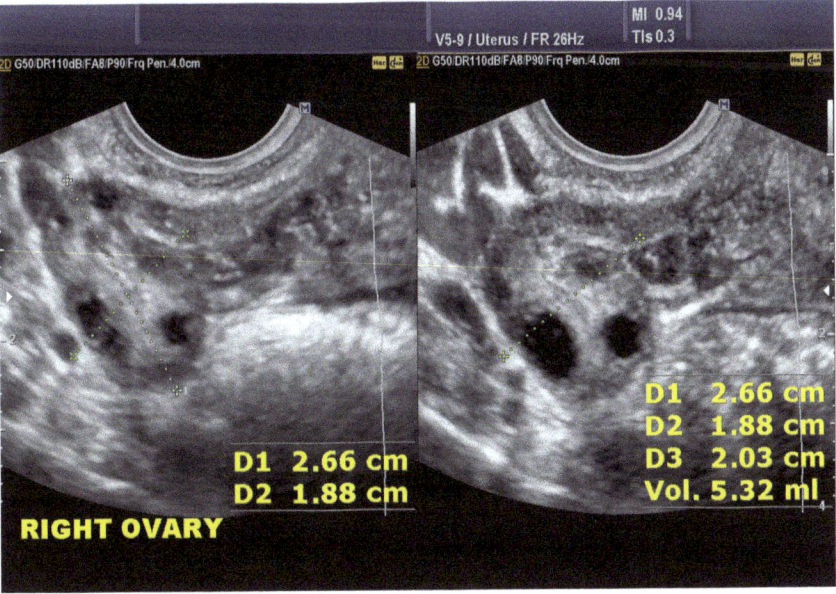

Fig. 5.7.2: In a baseline scan look at the ovaries to see whether they are normal/small/polycystic

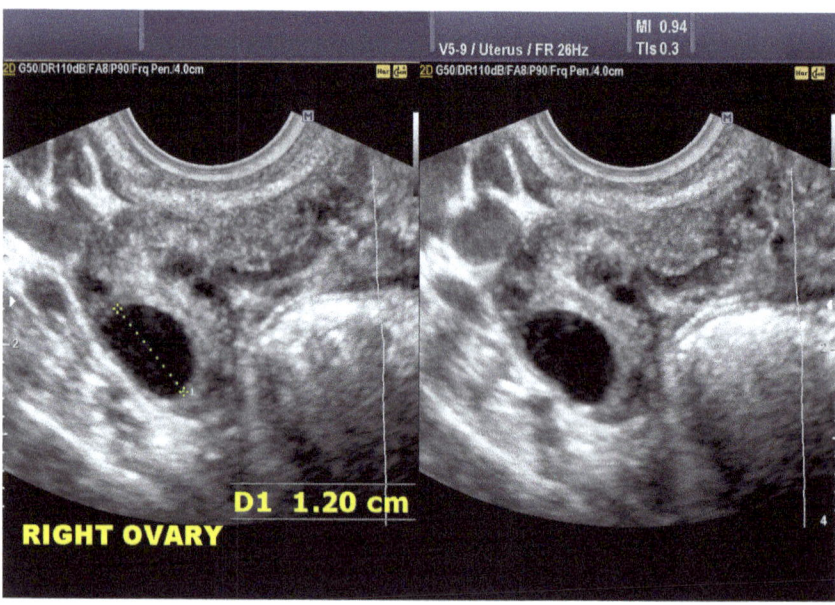

Fig. 5.7.3: Evaluate the ovary with phase of the cycle. A cyclical change should not be misinterpreted as cyst

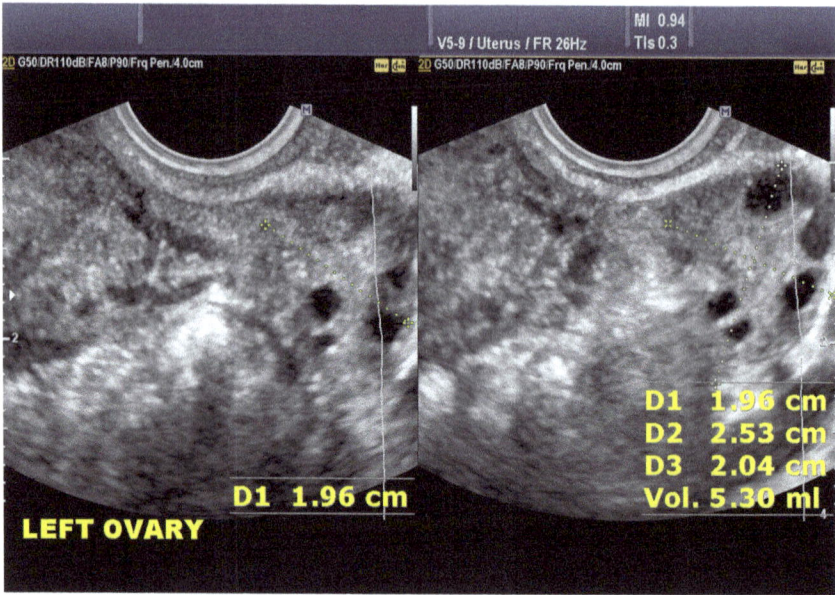

Fig. 5.7.4: Stromal echogenecity to be evaluated in respect to the myometrium. Ovarian stroma is hypoechoic or isoechoic to the myometrium

5.7. Normal Adnexa

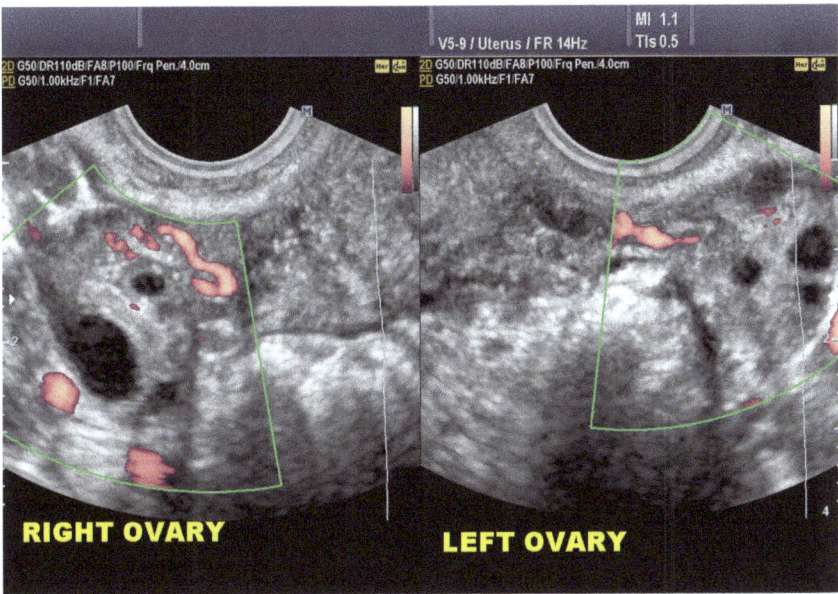

Fig. 5.7.5: On color flow mapping and power angio studies evaluate the ovarian stroma

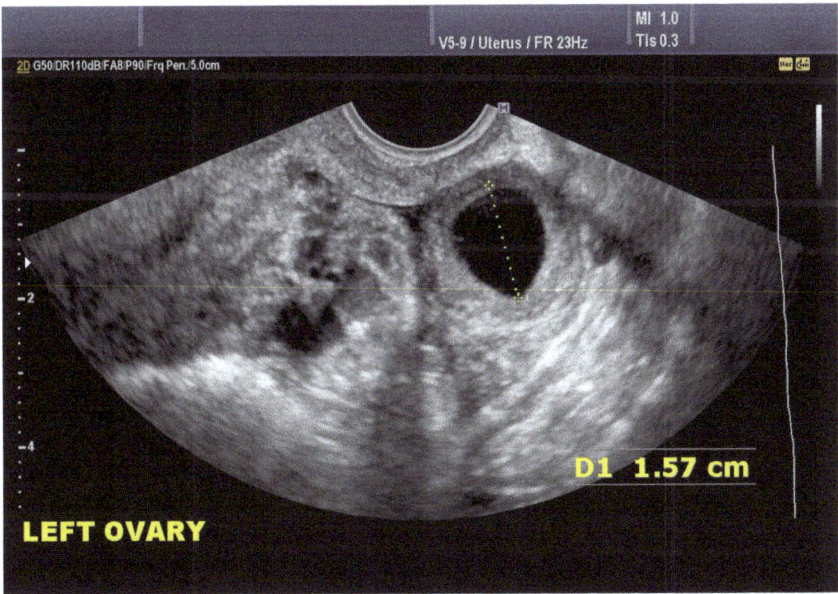

Fig. 5.7.6: In the luteal phase evaluate the ovary and see for corpus luteum

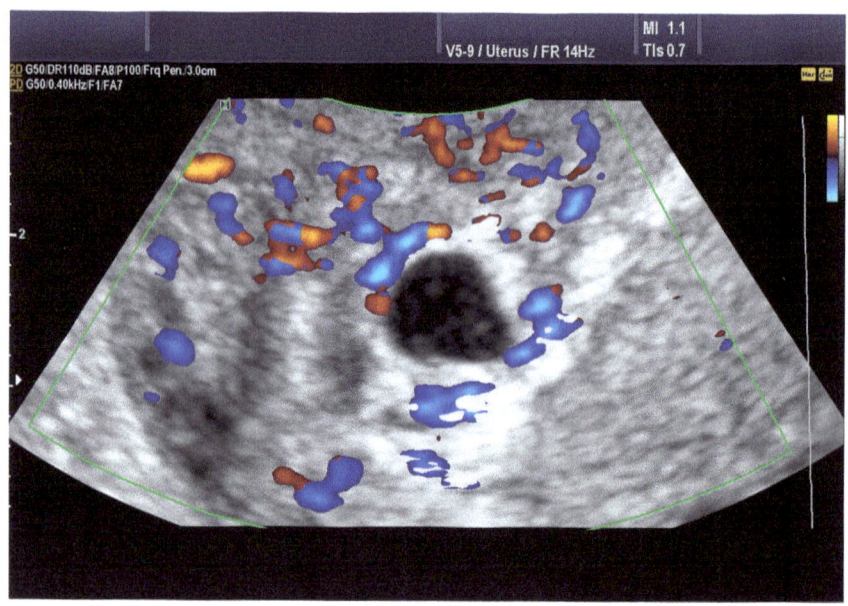

Fig. 5.7.7: Vascularity seen around the corpus luteum

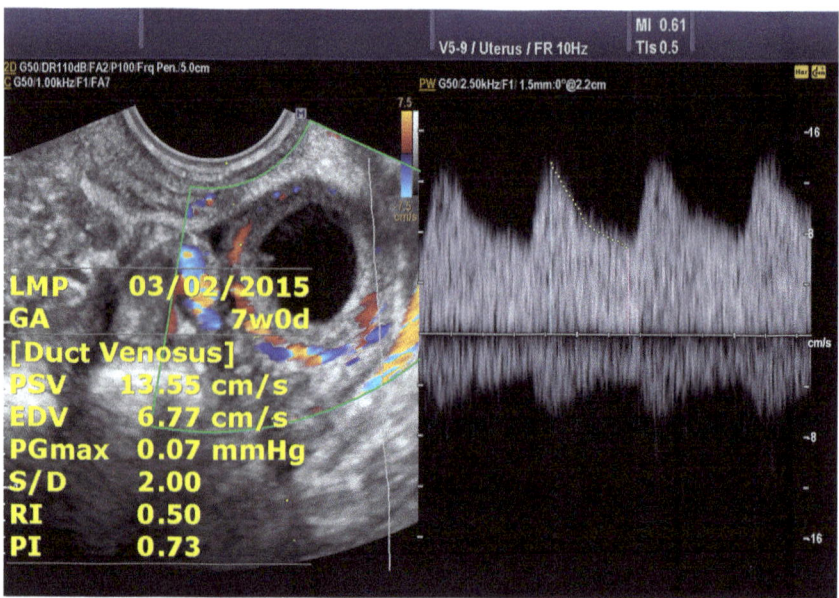

Fig. 5.7.8: On duplex Doppler evaluation low impedance flow with a resistive index of 0.50 is seen

5.7. Normal Adnexa

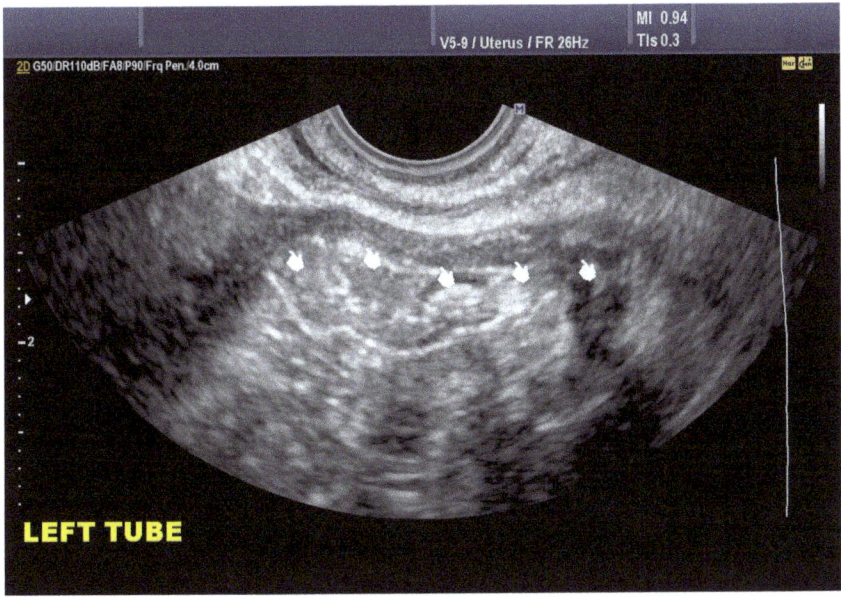

Fig. 5.7.9: Tube is seldom seen and evaluate it for any thickening or fluid collection

CHAPTER 6

UTEROCERVICAL ABNORMALITIES

6.1. Congenital Uterine Defects
6.2. Fibroids
6.3. Fibroid Polyp
6.4. Adenomyosis
6.5. Asherman's Syndrome
6.6. Endometrial Polyp
6.7. Endometrium: Abnormal Thickness and Echo Pattern
6.8. Cervical Polyp
6.9. Cervical Mass

6.1. CONGENITAL UTERINE DEFECTS

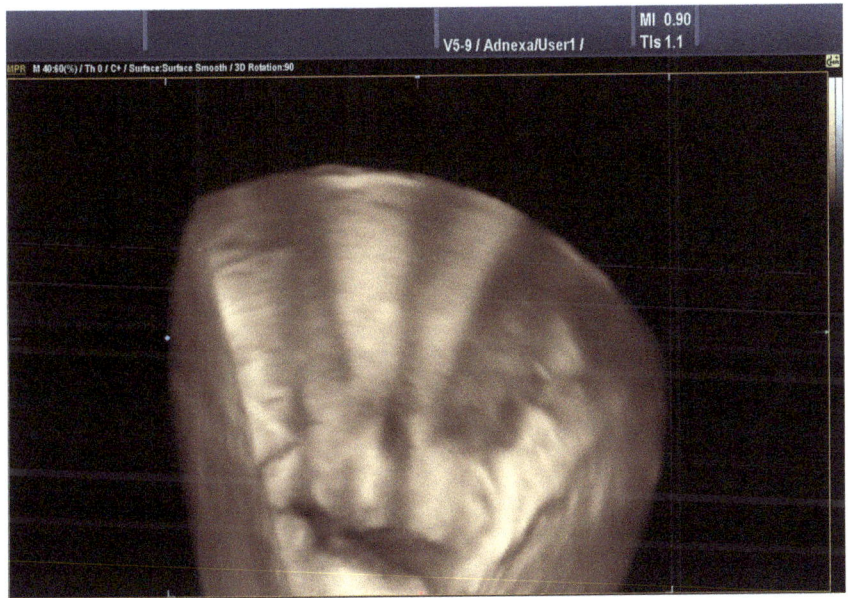

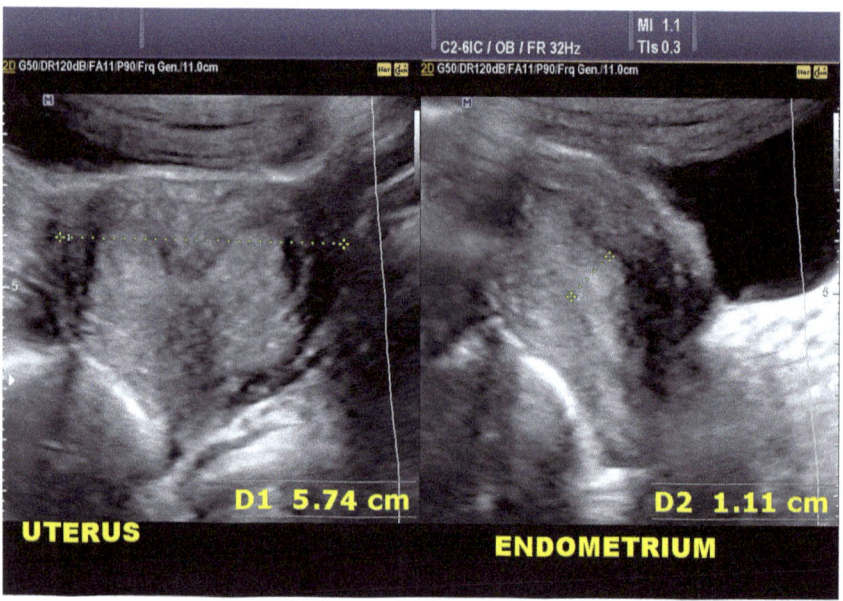

Fig. 6.1.1: With 2D ultrasound one can suspect a congenital uterine defect

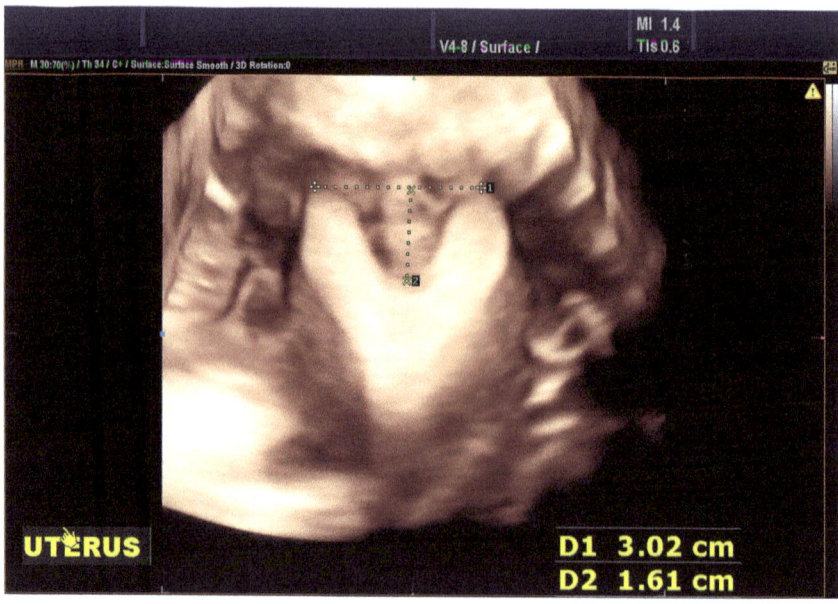

Fig. 6.1.2: Thick muscular septum seen on 3D

6.1. Congenital Uterine Defects

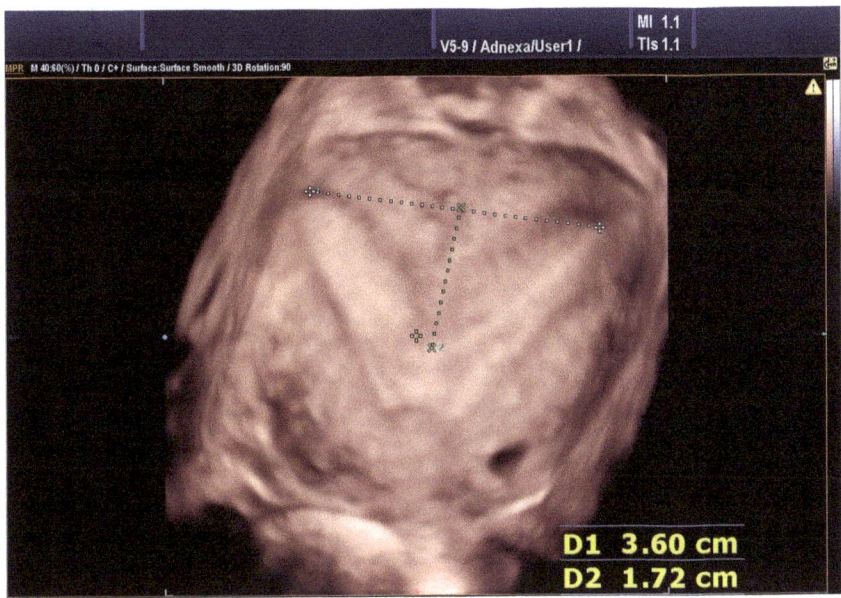

Fig. 6.1.3: Normal fundal contour with two uterine cavities in a septate uterus

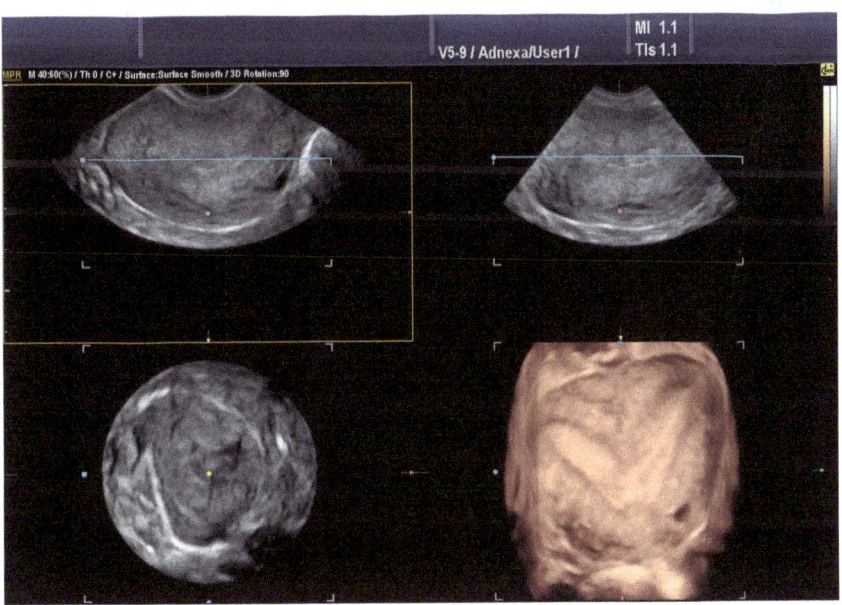

Fig. 6.1.4: Carefully look at uterine fundal contour

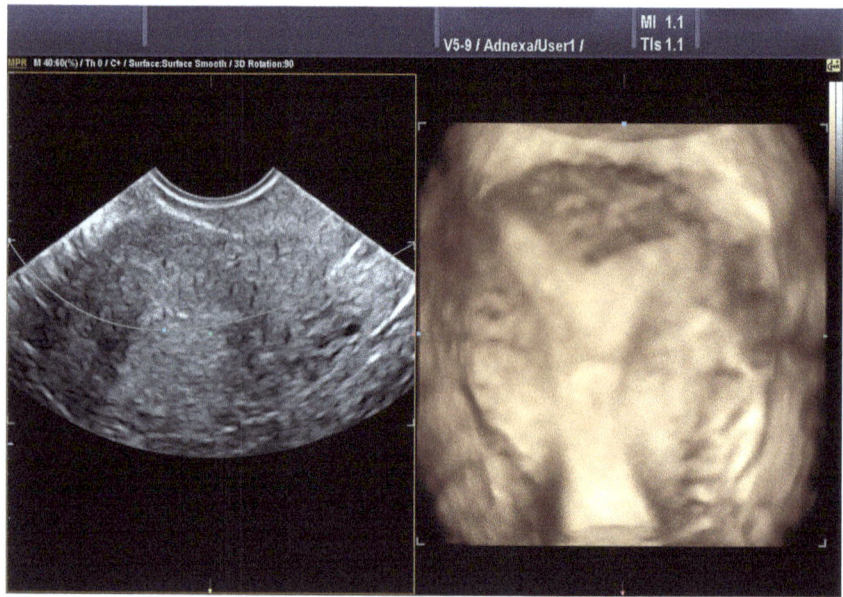

Fig. 6.1.5: Partial septate uterus

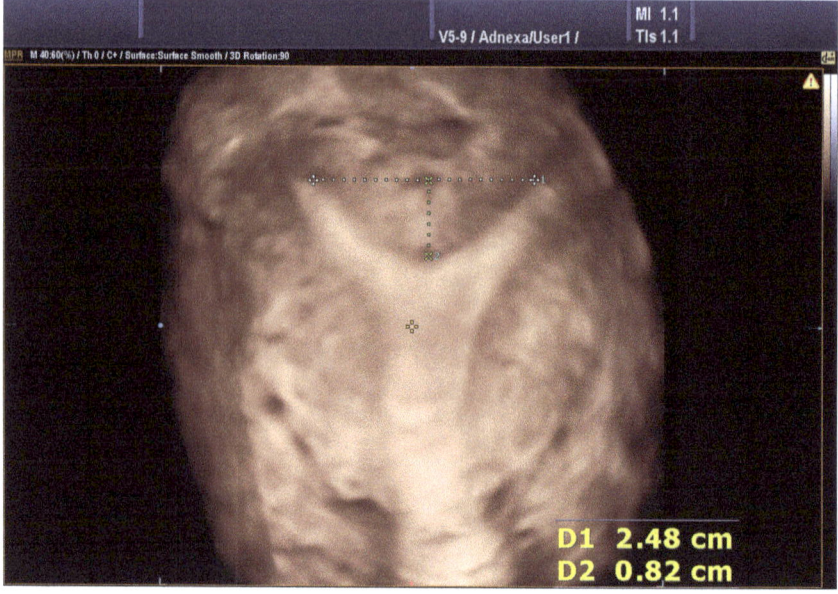

Fig. 6.1.6: Measurements taken to look at the septum in a case of recurrent early pregnancy losses

6.1. Congenital Uterine Defects

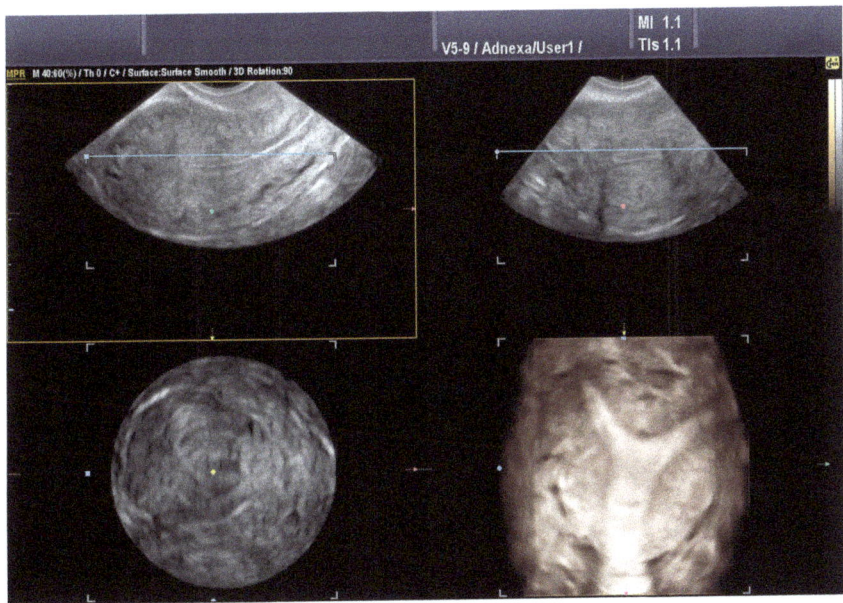

Fig. 6.1.7: Septate uterus as seen on MPR

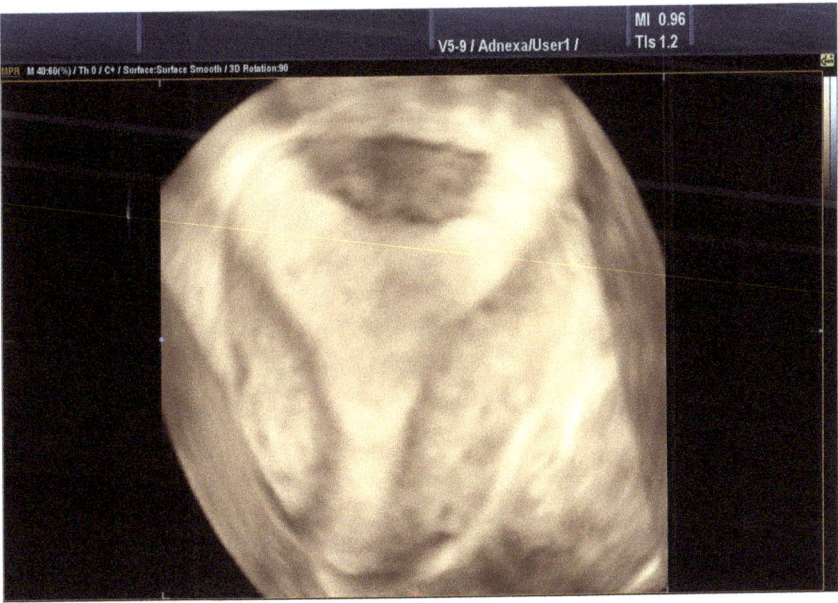

Fig. 6.1.8: Septate uterus on 3D

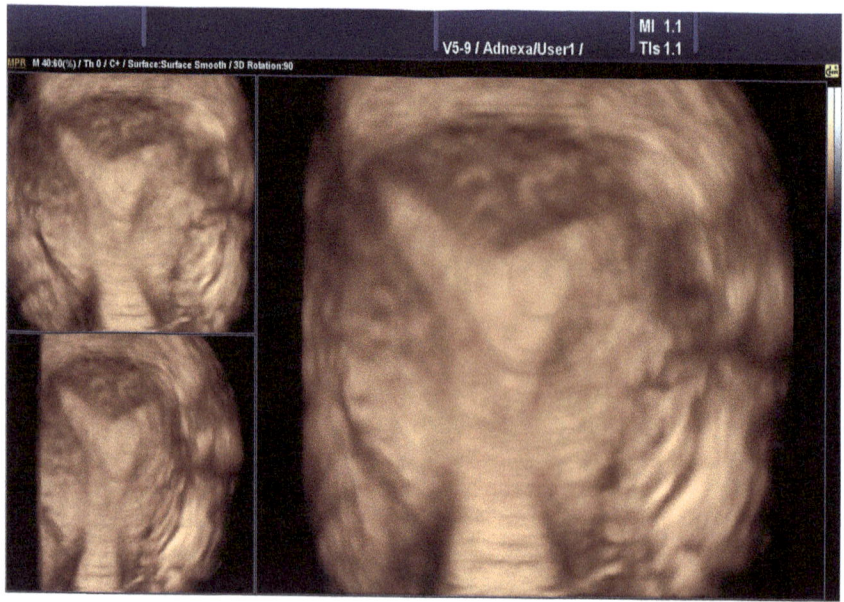

Fig. 6.1.9: Septate uterus with normal fundal contour

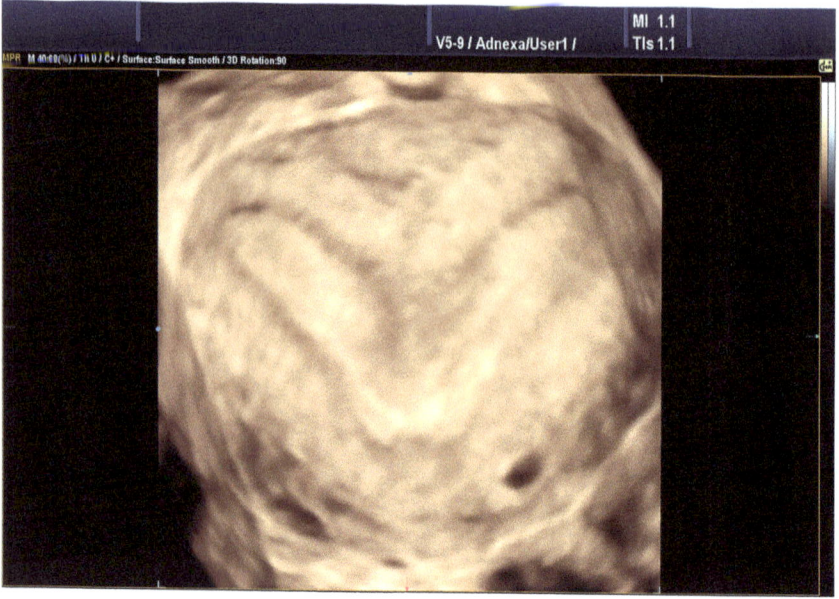

Fig. 6.1.10: 3D of a bicornuate uterus

6.1. Congenital Uterine Defects

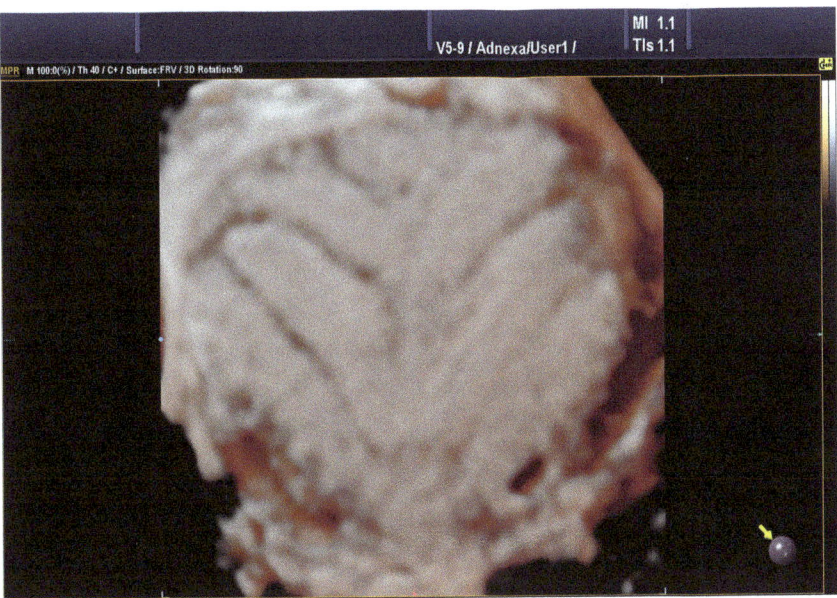

Fig. 6.1.11: Wide endometrial cavities seen in a case of bicornuate uterus

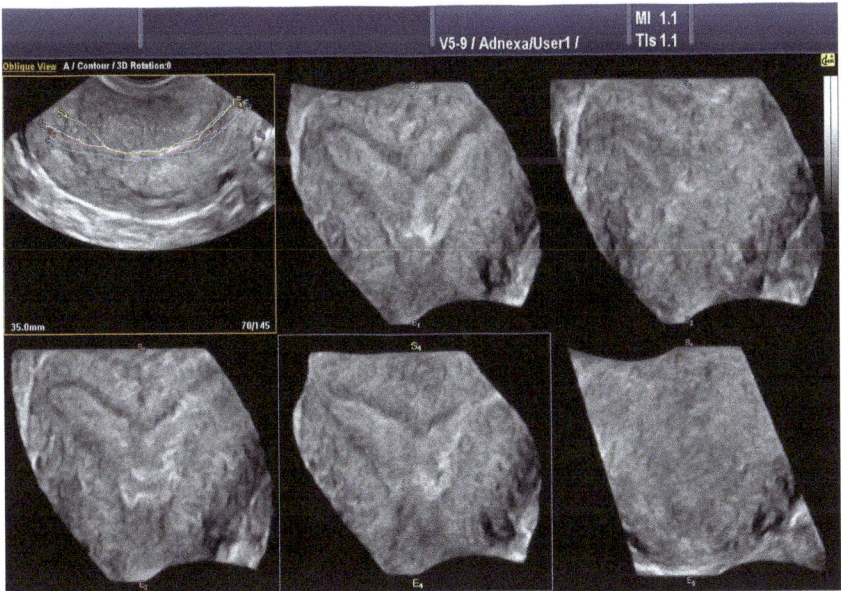

Fig. 6.1.12: Bicornuate uterus as seen on MSV

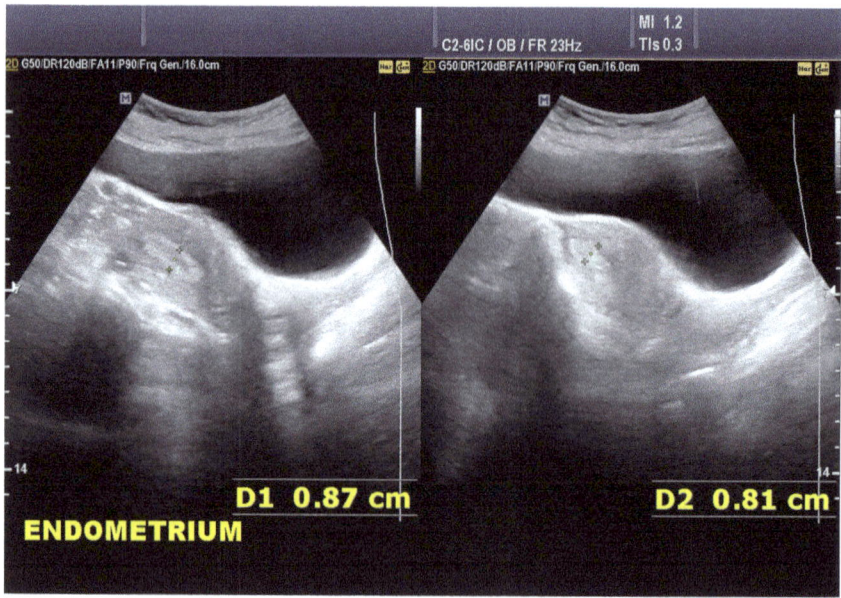

Fig. 6.1.13: Two uterine horn as seen on TAS

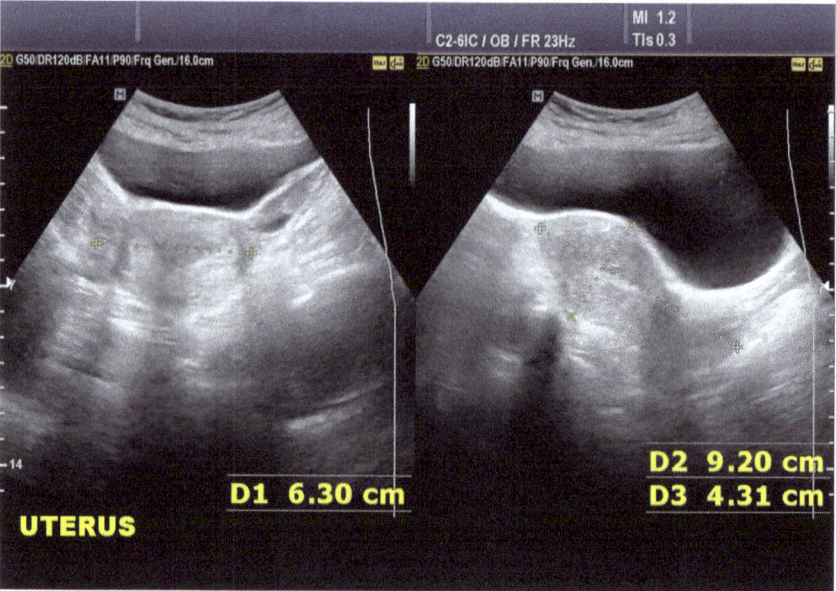

Fig. 6.1.14: On TAS suspect a uterine duality if you see a very wide transverse section measurement

6.1. Congenital Uterine Defects

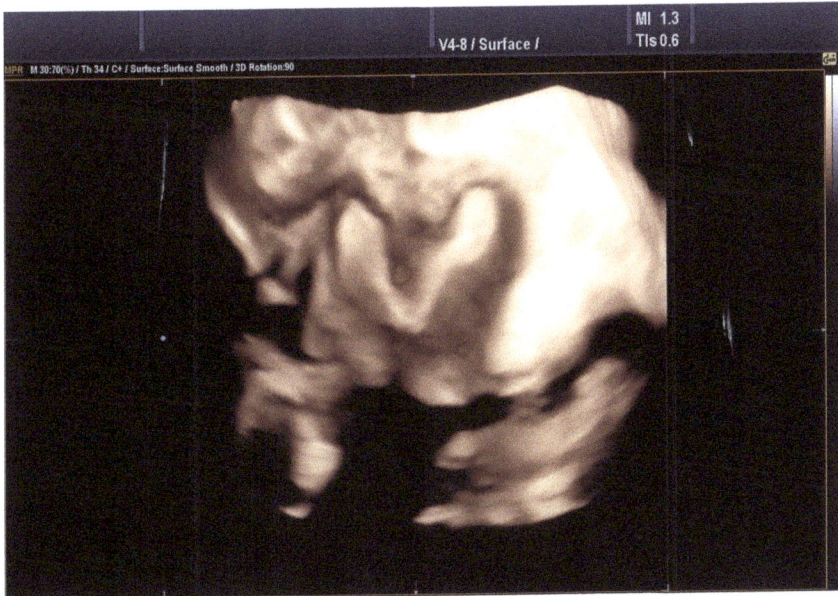

Fig. 6.1.15: Uterine cavities as seen on TAS 3D

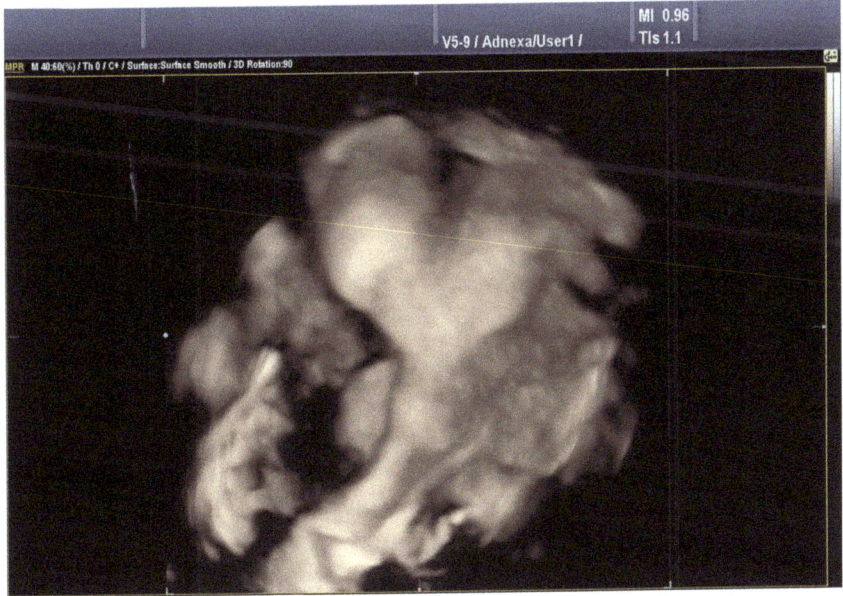

Fig. 6.1.16: TAS 3D of uterine duality

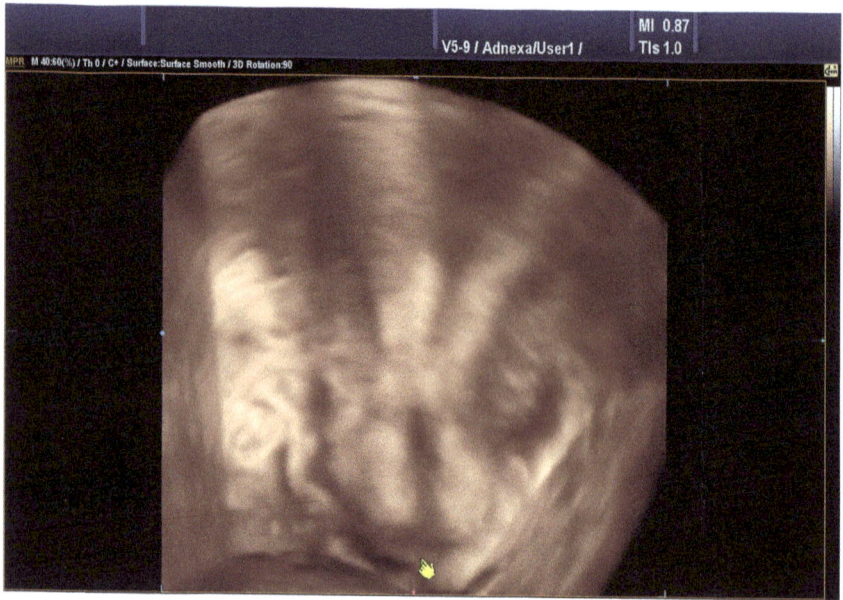

Fig. 6.1.17: Complete uterine and cervical cavities

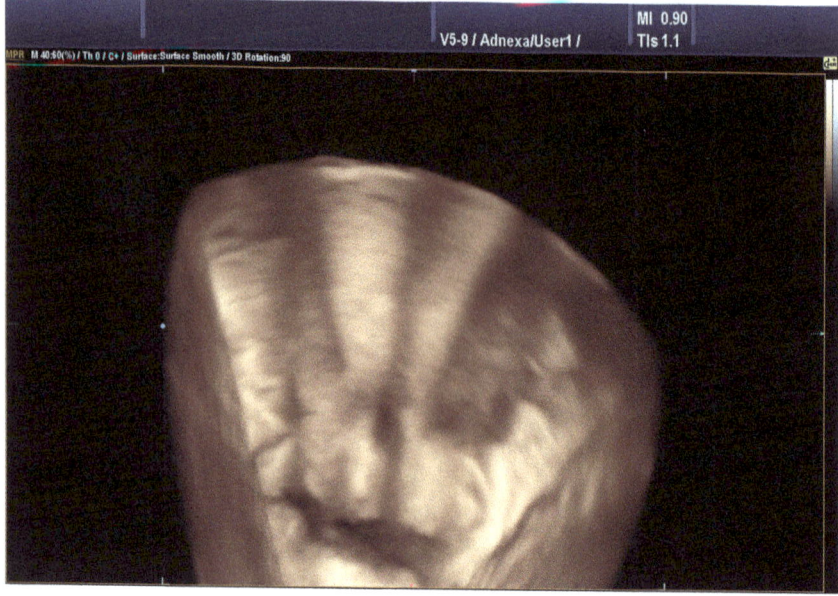

Fig. 6.1.18: Look in carefully for the endometrial canals

6.1. Congenital Uterine Defects

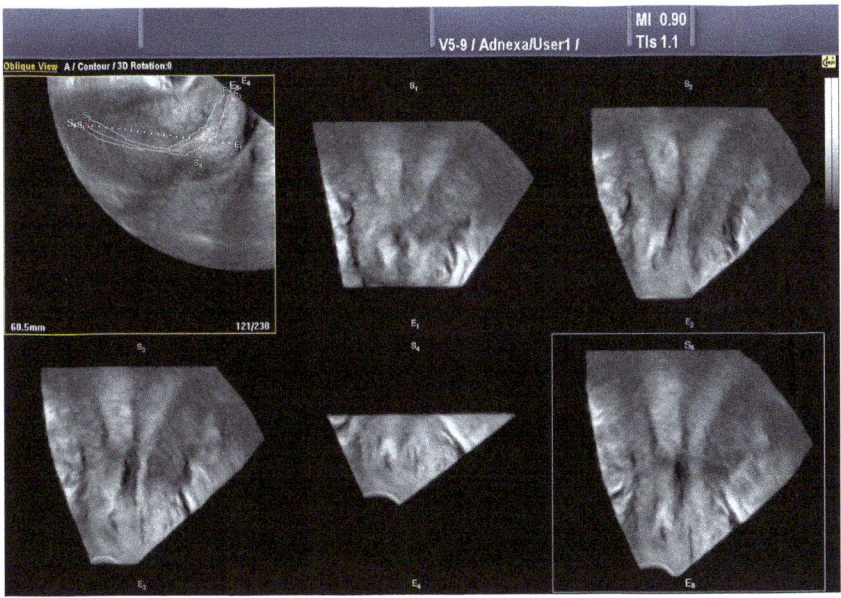

Fig. 6.1.19: Cavities seen in MSV

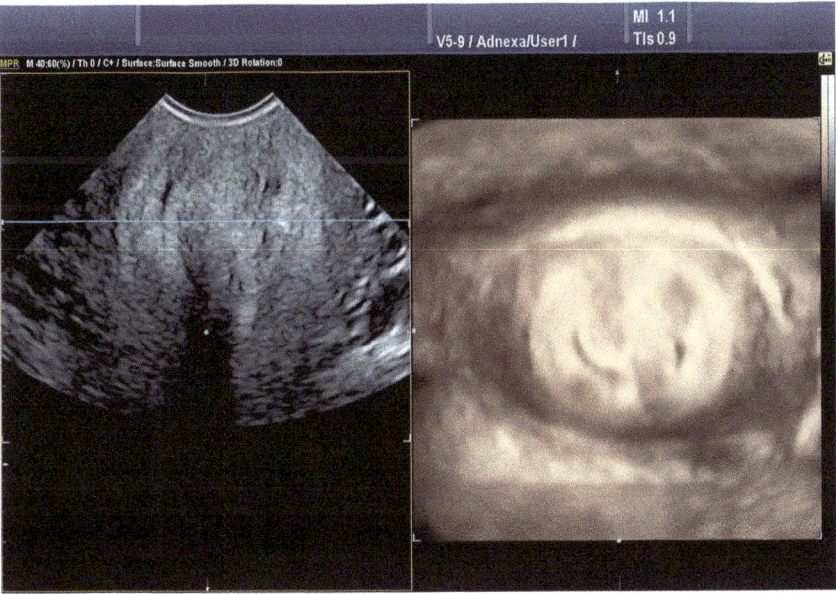

Fig. 6.1.20: Two cervical canals seen in a uterus didelphys

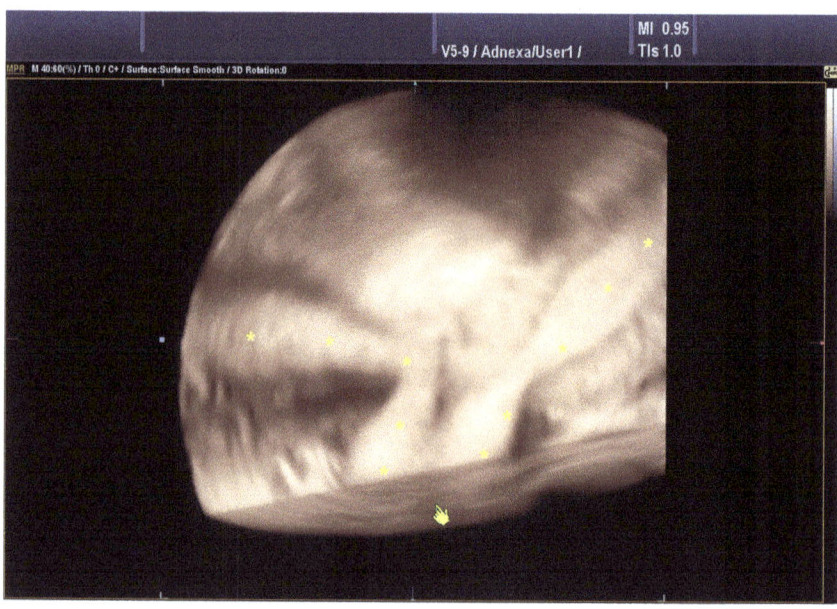

Fig. 6.1.21: Complete uterine and cervical cavities with both horns wide apart

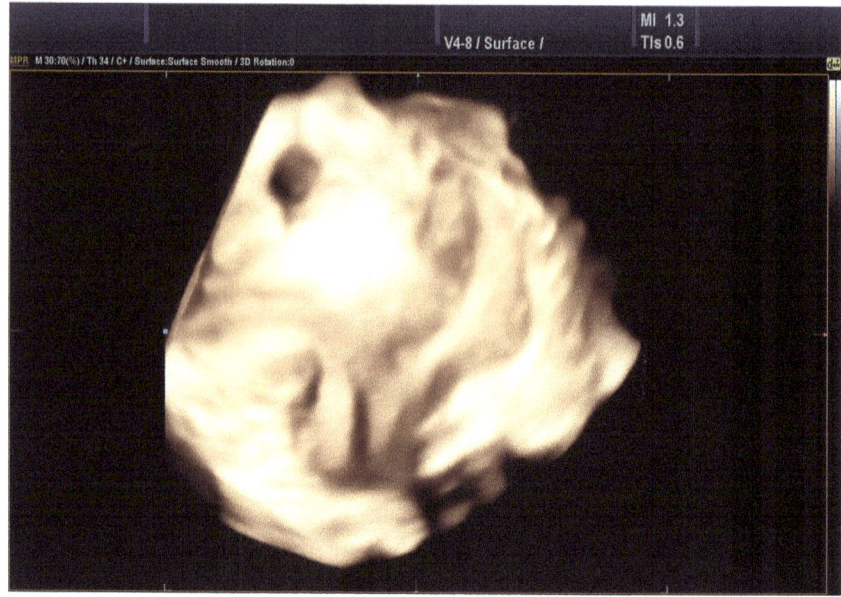

Fig. 6.1.22: Two uteri seen separately

6.1. Congenital Uterine Defects

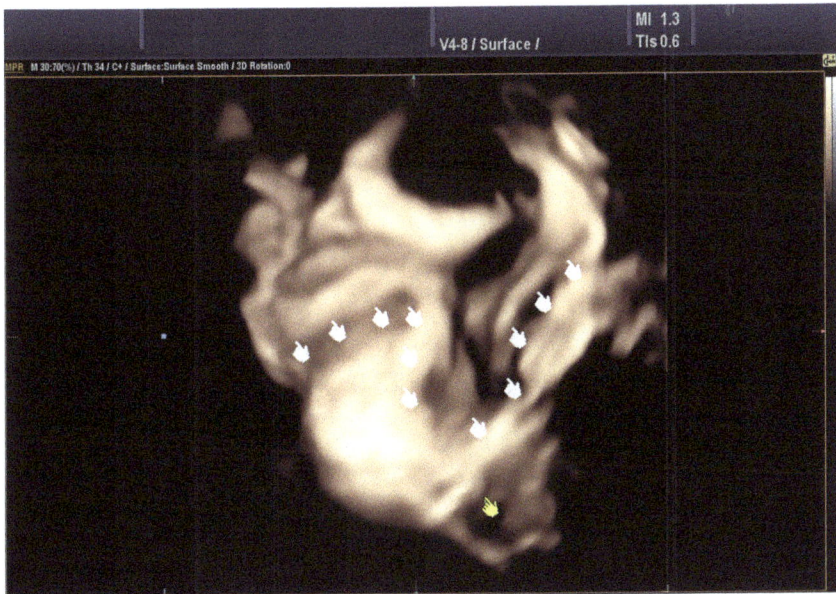

Fig. 6.1.23: Even in TAS we can trace the cavities

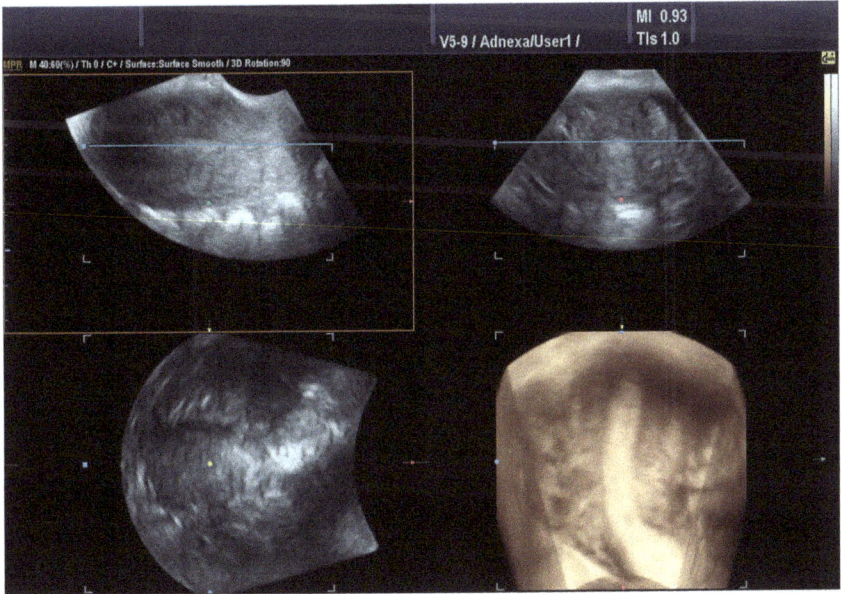

Fig. 6.1.24: Unicornuate uterus as seen on MPR

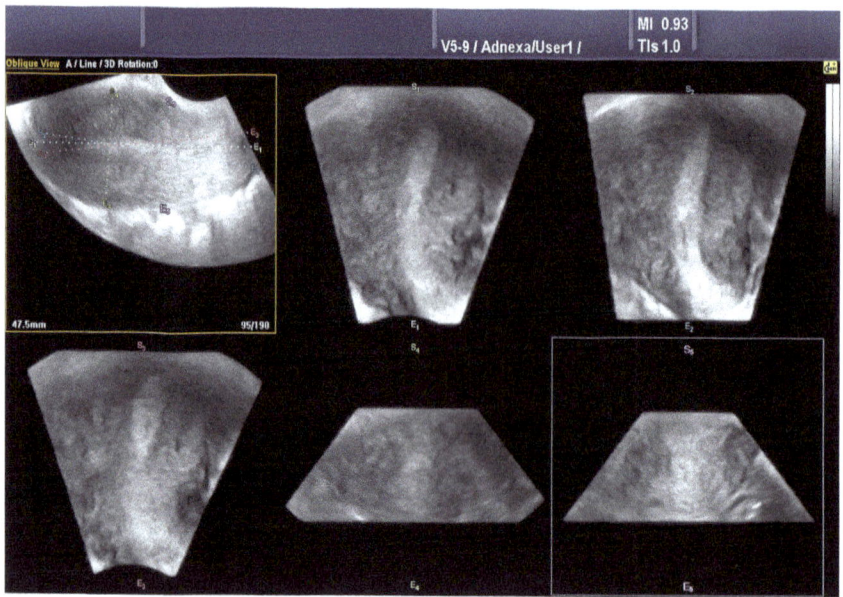

Fig. 6.1.25: Unicornuate uterus as seen on MSV

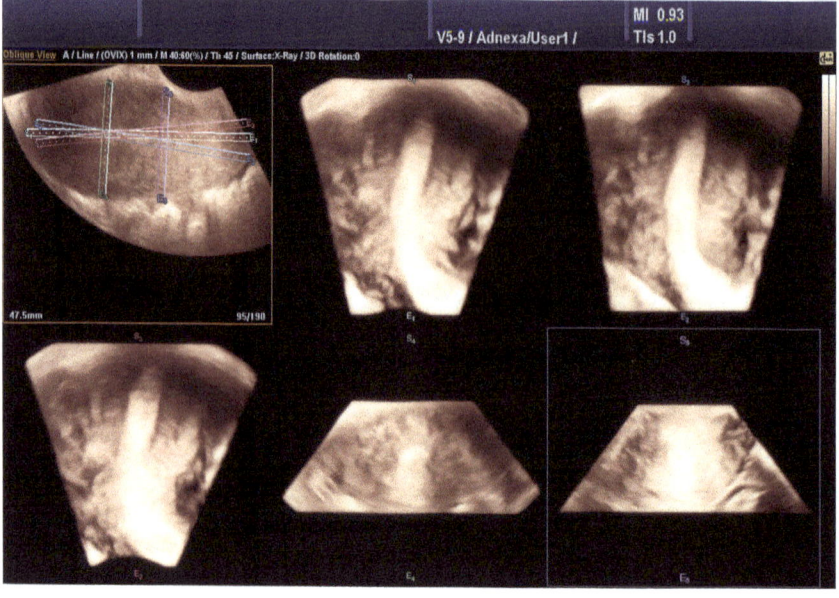

Fig. 6.1.26: Unicornuate uterus as seen on Ovix mode

6.1. Congenital Uterine Defects

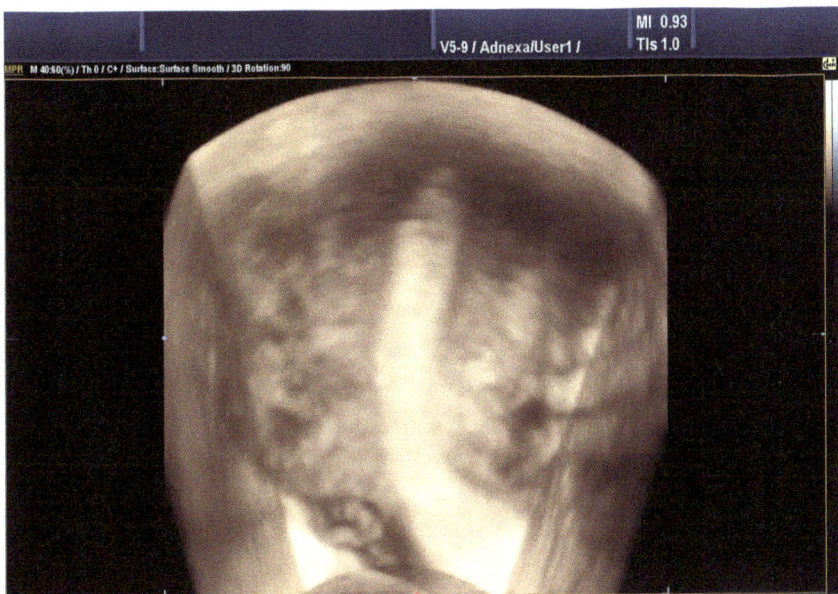

Fig. 6.1.27: Unicornuate uterus as seen on 3D

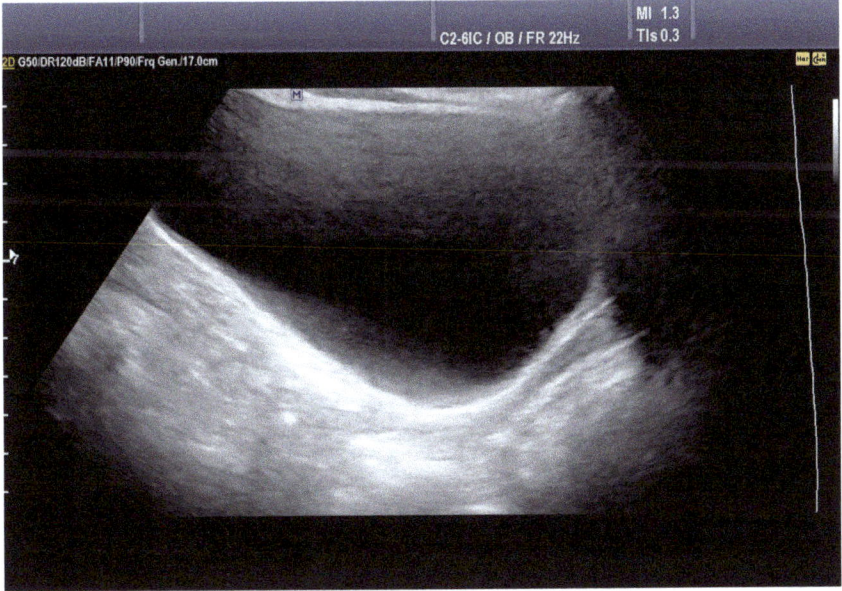

Fig. 6.1.28: Patient with primary amenorrhea with a very small uterus

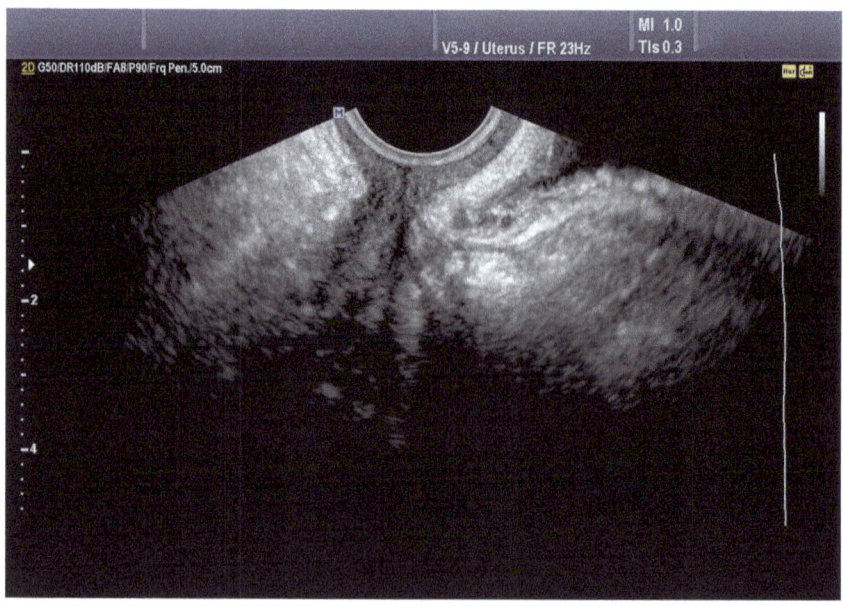

Fig. 6.1.29: Small uterus with no endometrial cavity with normal ovaries

6.2. FIBROIDS

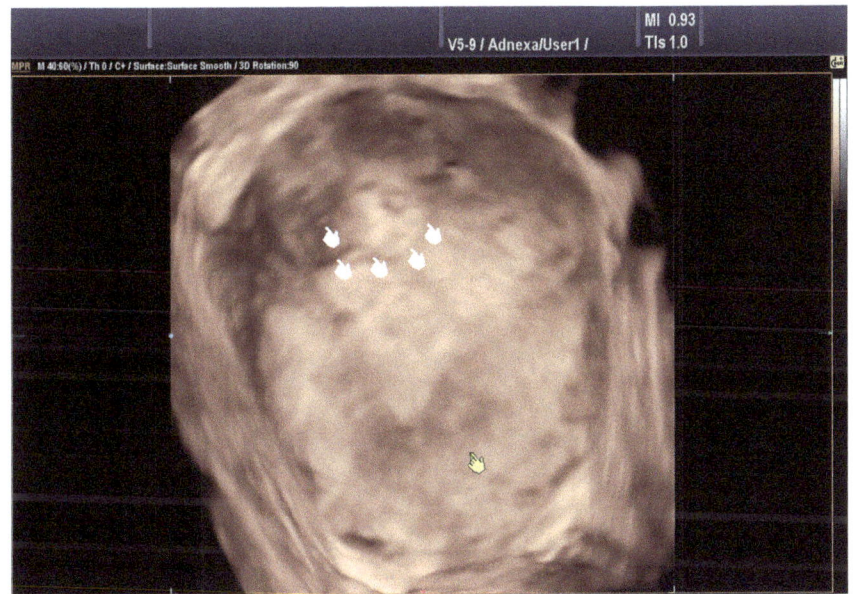

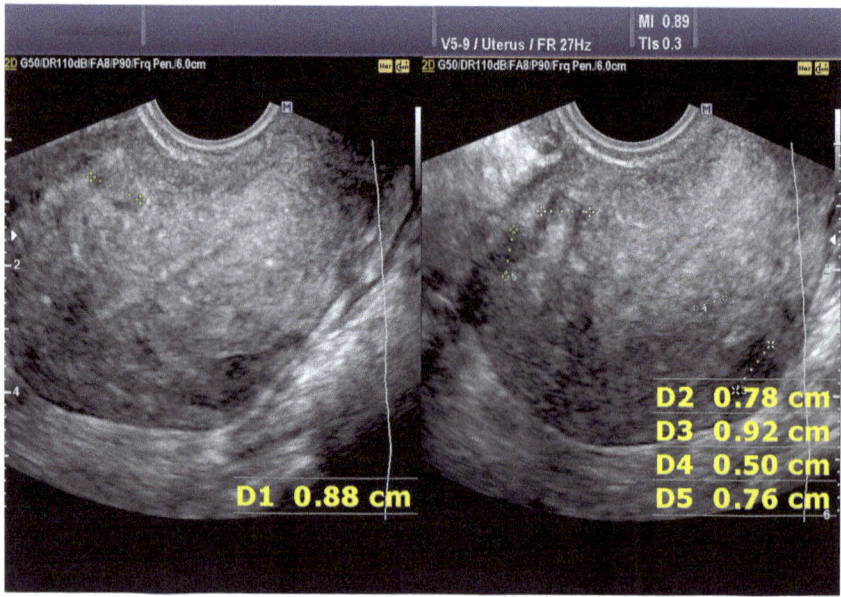

Fig. 6.2.1: Small interstitial fibroids

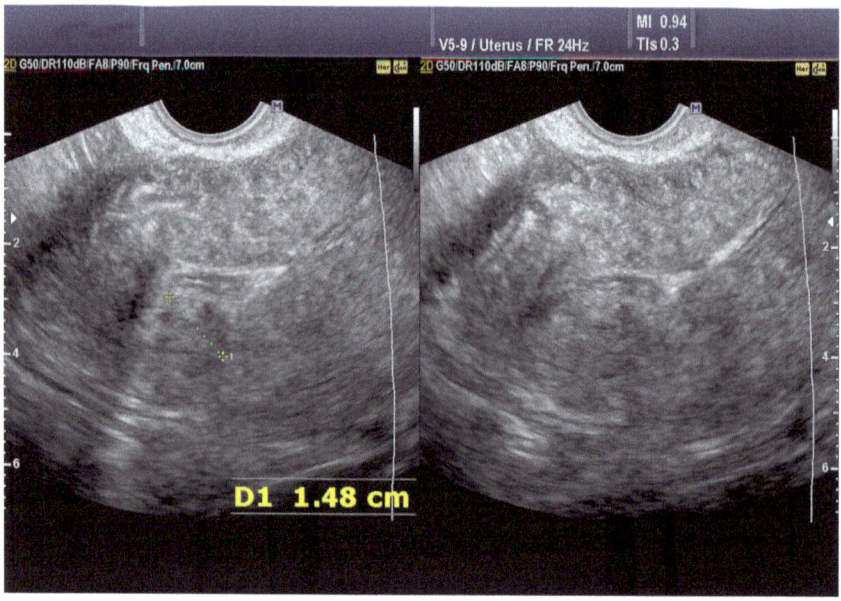

Fig. 6.2.2: Submucous fibroid just touching the cavity

6.2. Fibroids

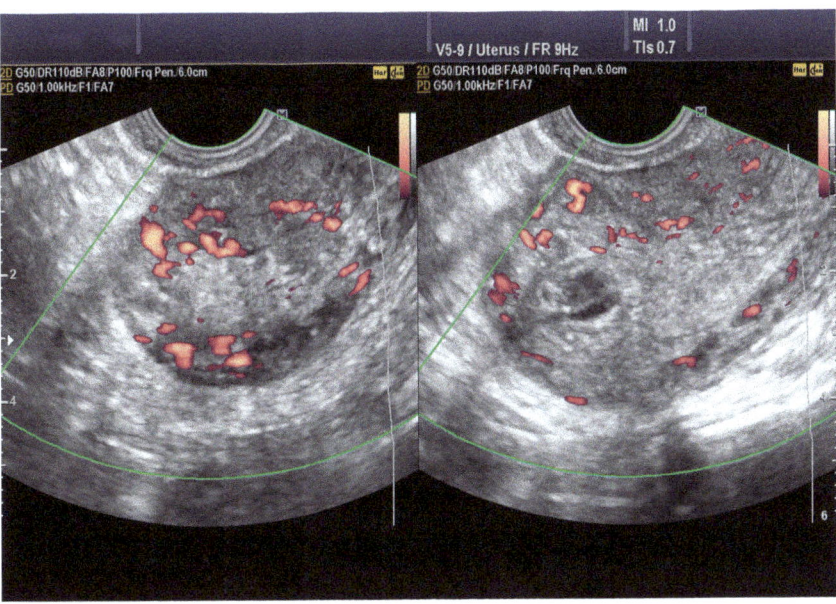

Fig. 6.2.3: Vascularity of the submucous fibroid

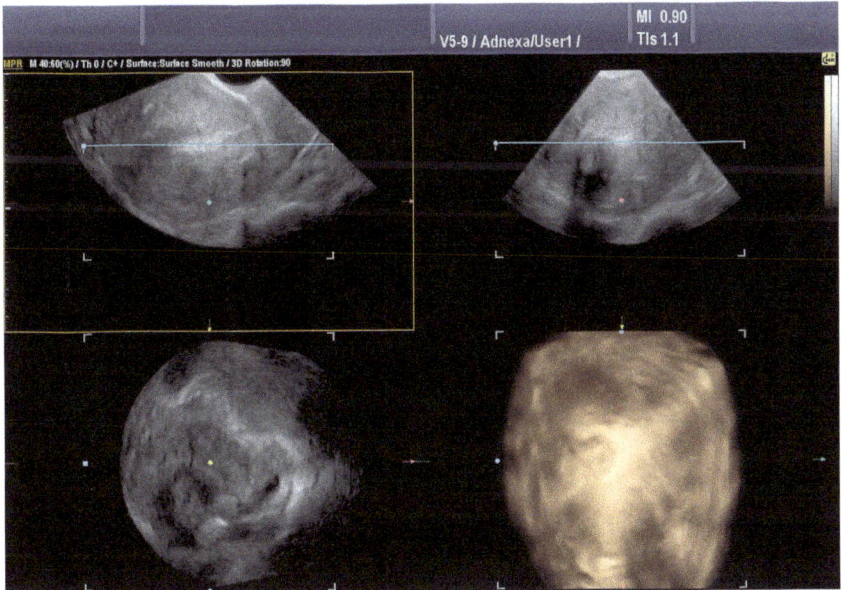

Fig. 6.2.4: Submucous fibroid on 3D

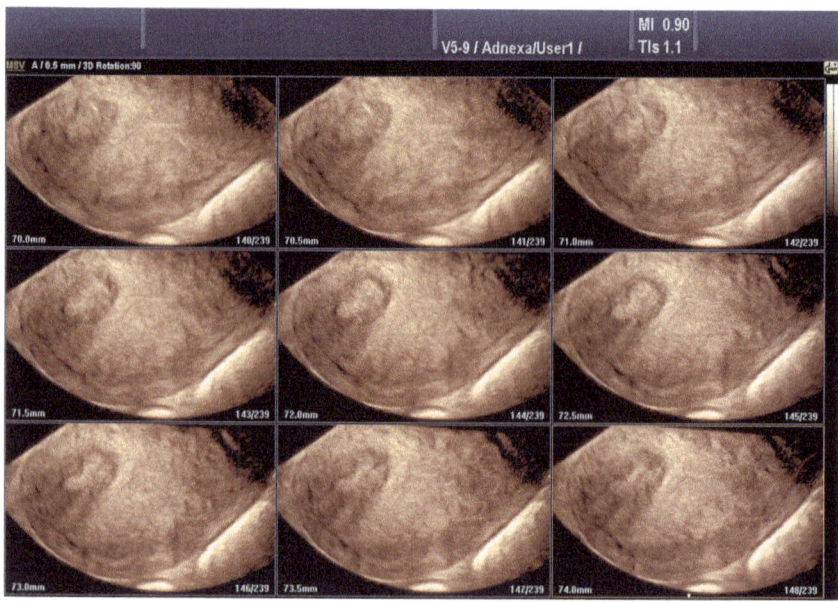

Fig. 6.2.5: Submucous fibroid on MSV

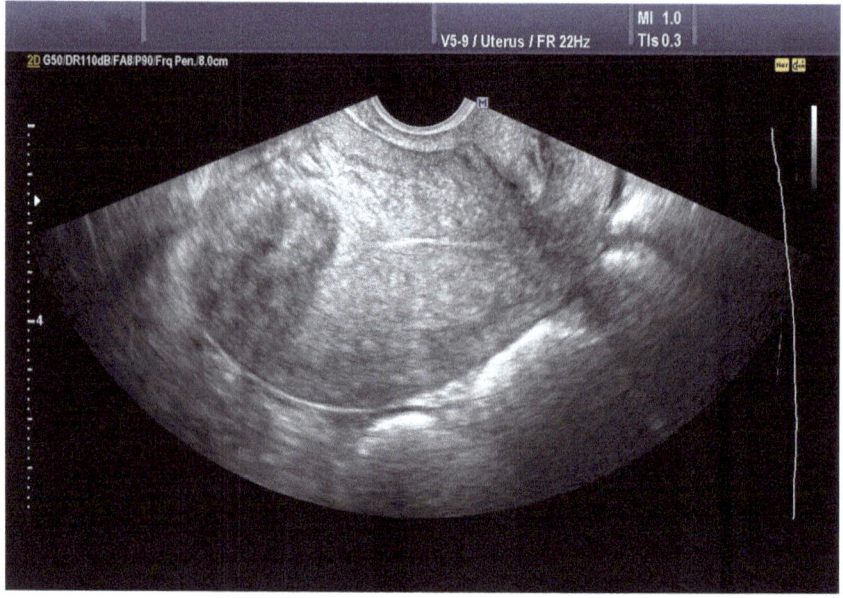

Fig. 6.2.6: Fundal submucous fibroid

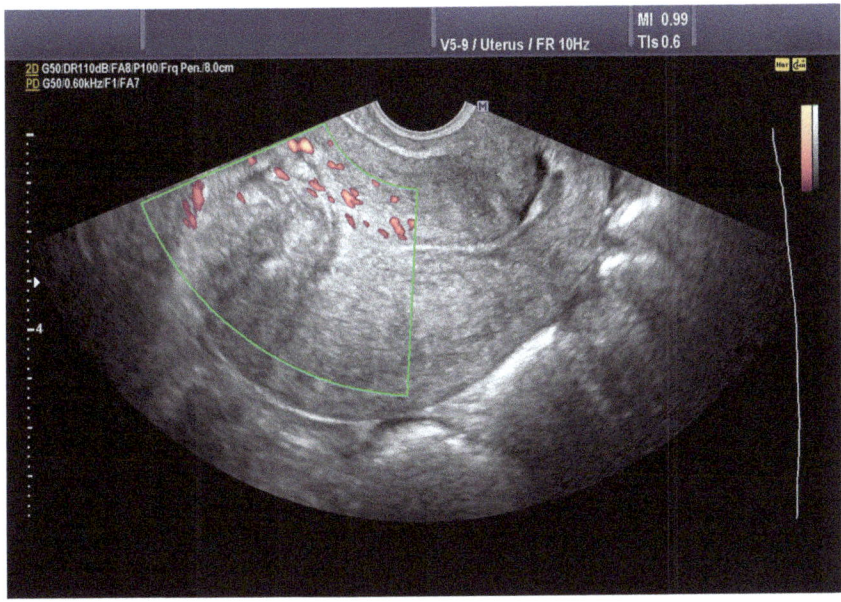

Fig. 6.2.7: Vascularity of submucous fibroid

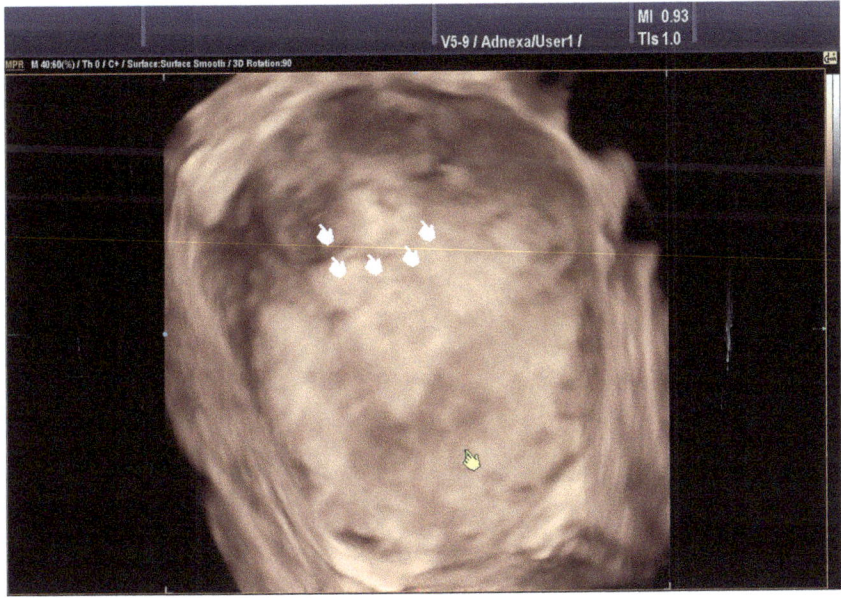

Fig. 6.2.8: Fundal submucous fibroid on 3D

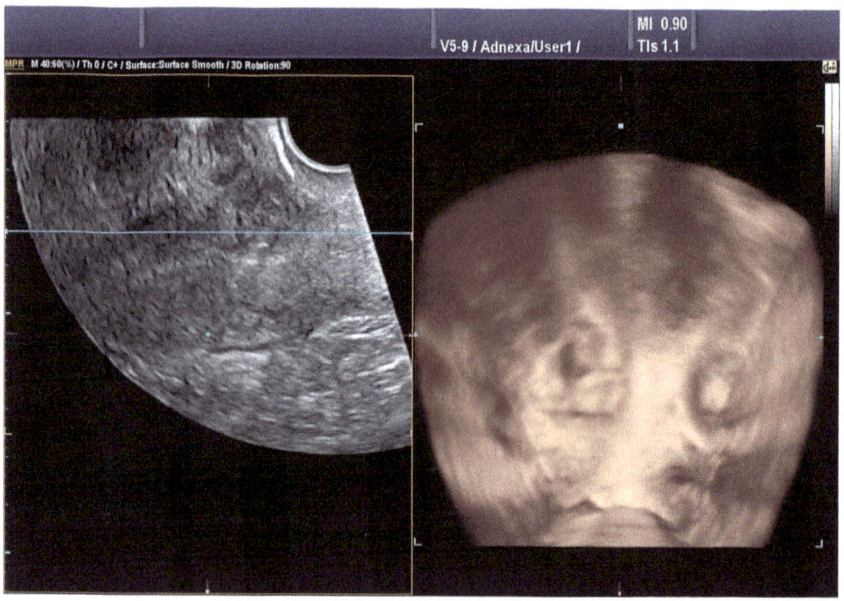

Fig. 6.2.9: Multiple submucous fibroids as seen on 3D

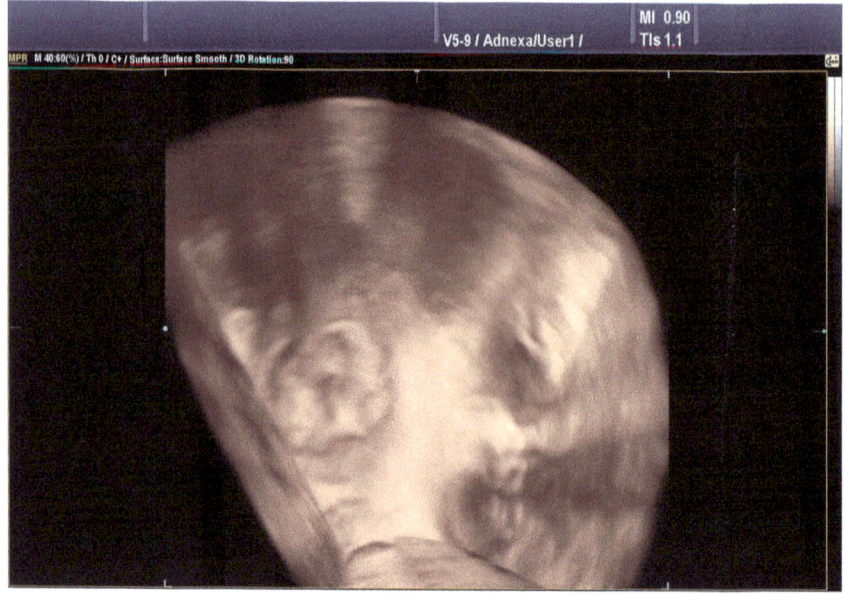

Fig. 6.2.10: Submucous fibroids

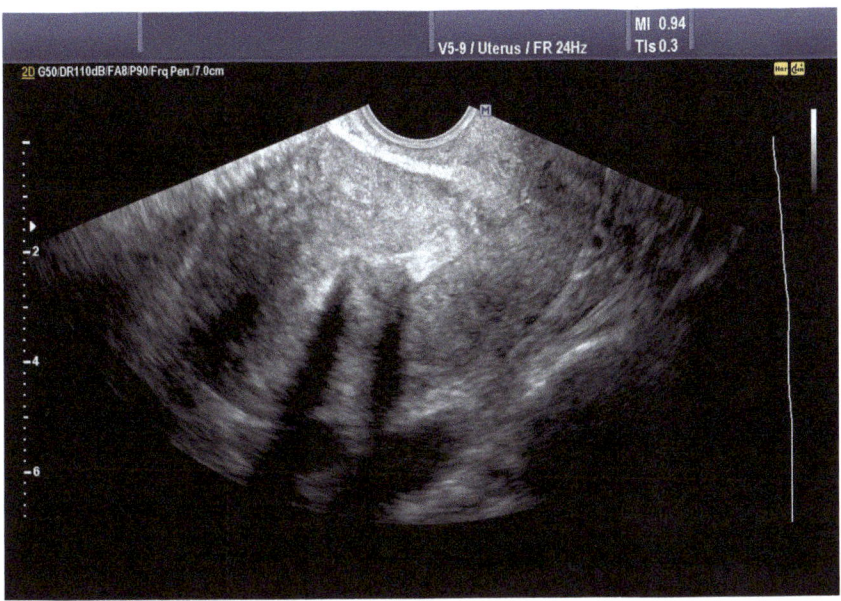

Fig. 6.2.11: Submucous fibroid in the posterior wall presenting as intermenstrual spotting

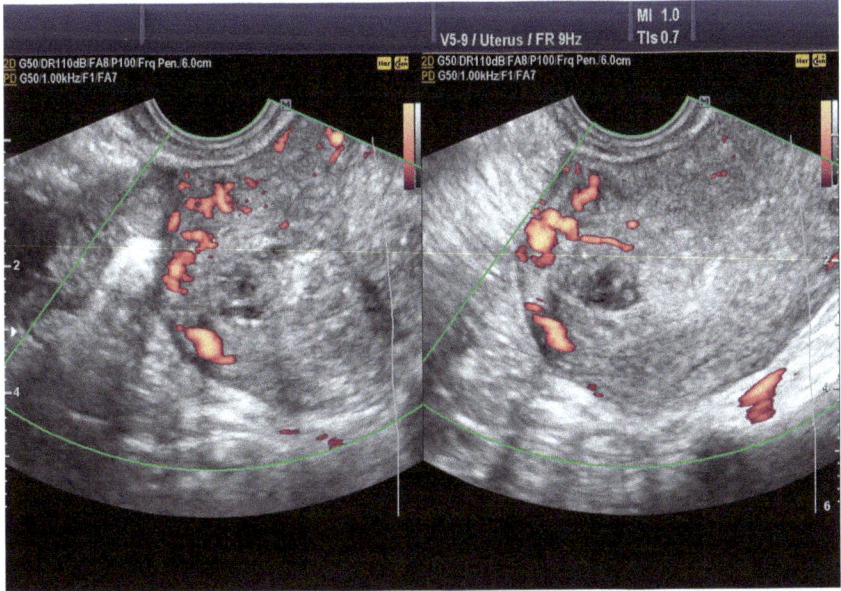

Fig. 6.2.12: Vascularity of submucous fibroid

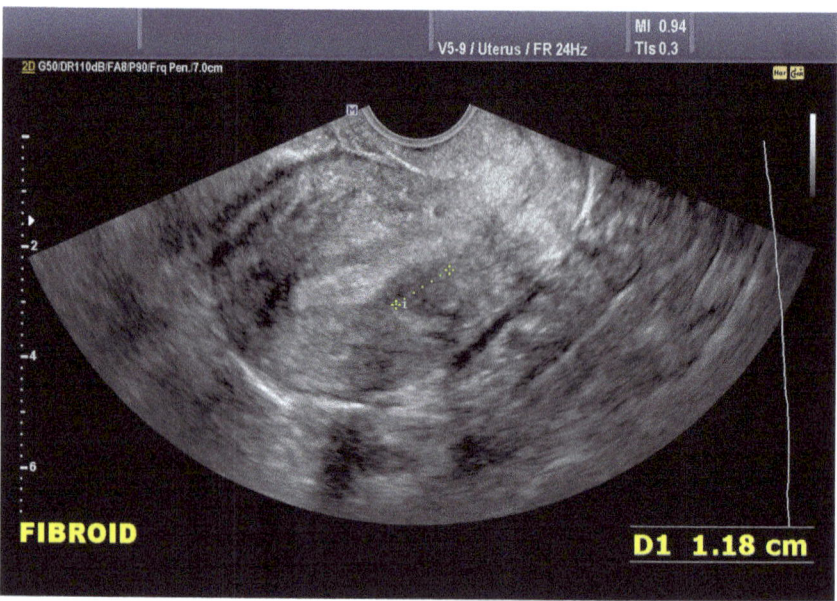

Fig. 6.2.13: Small submucous fibroid in an infertile patient

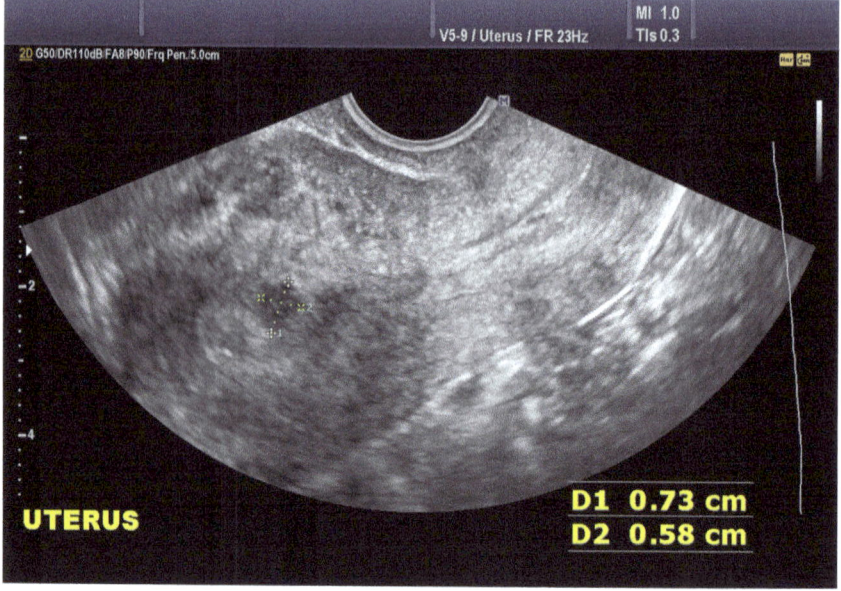

Fig. 6.2.14: Submucous fibroid >50% in the uterine cavity

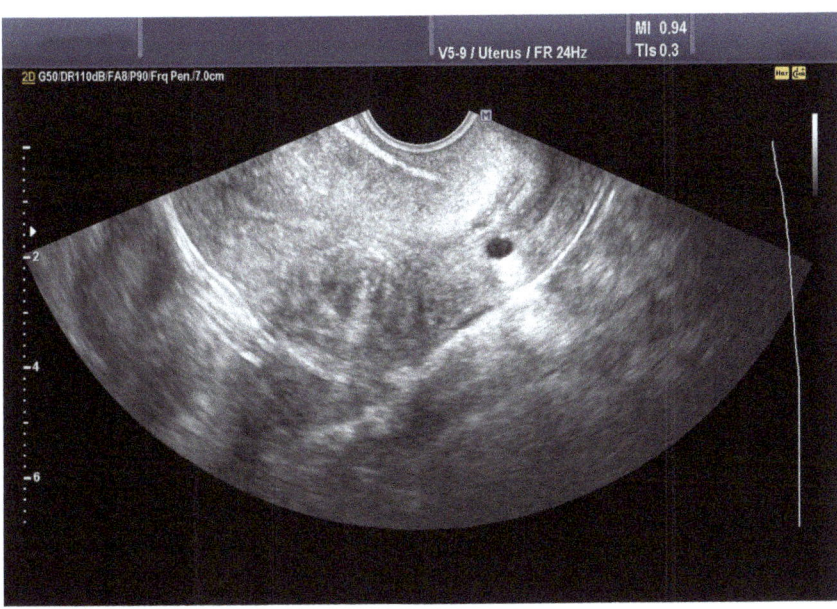

Fig. 6.2.15: Submucous fibroid just touching the endometrium

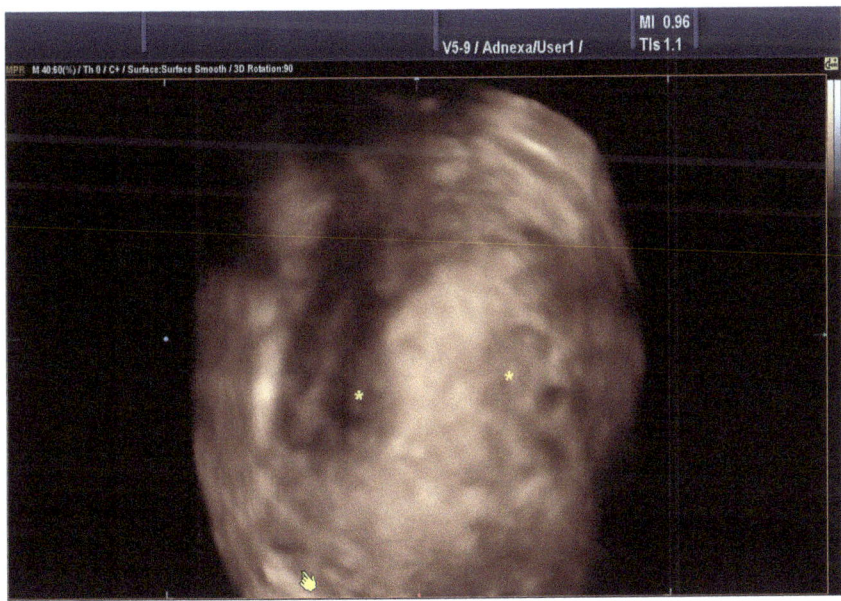

Fig. 6.2.16: Submucous fibroids as seen on 3D

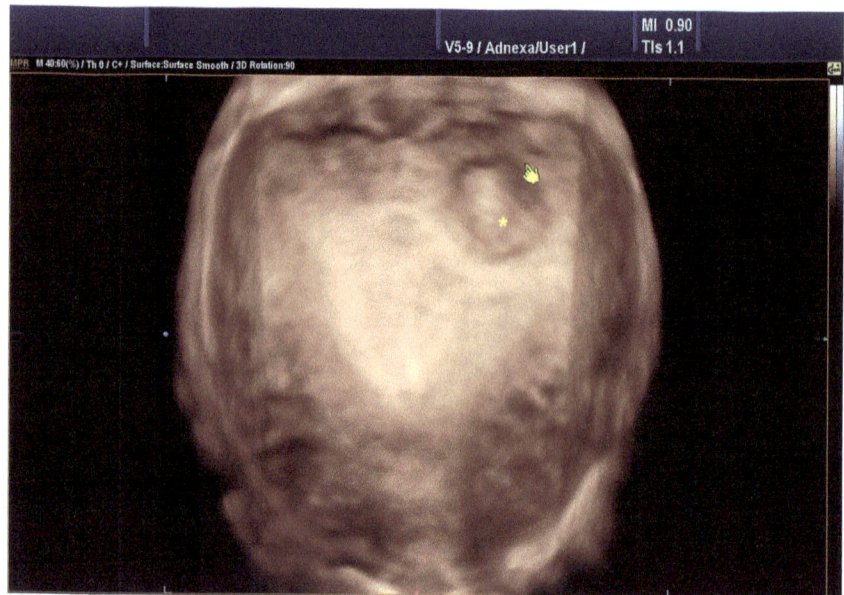

Fig. 6.2.17: Submucous fibroid as seen on 3D

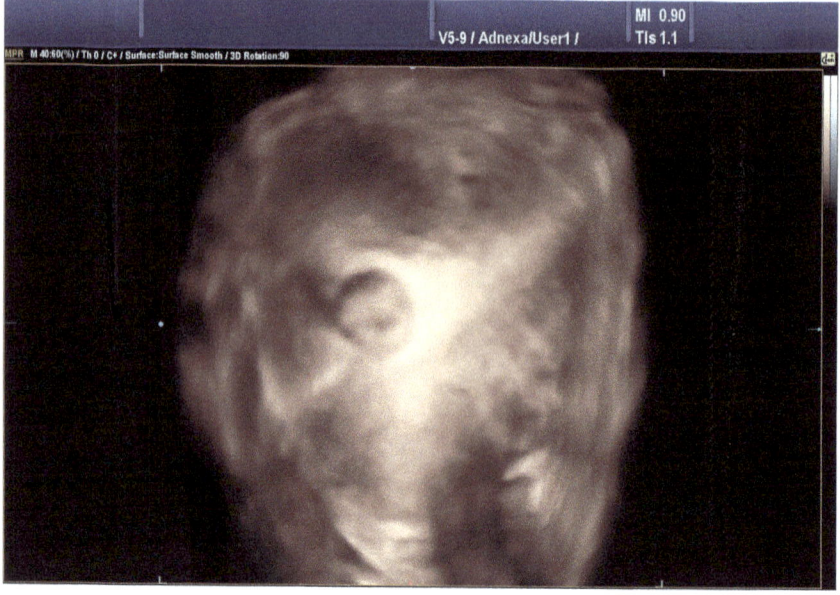

Fig. 6.2.18: Submucous fibroid as seen on 3D

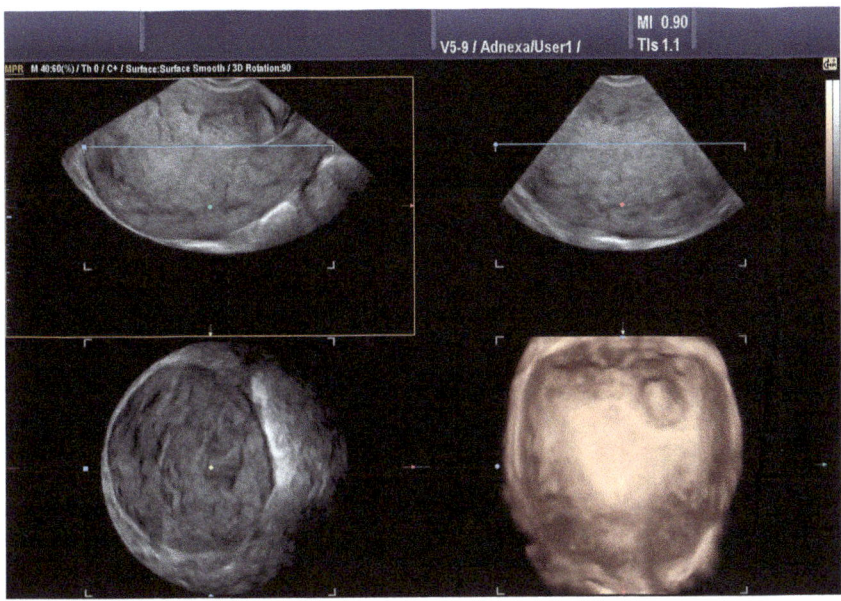

Fig. 6.2.19: Submucous fibroid as seen on MPR

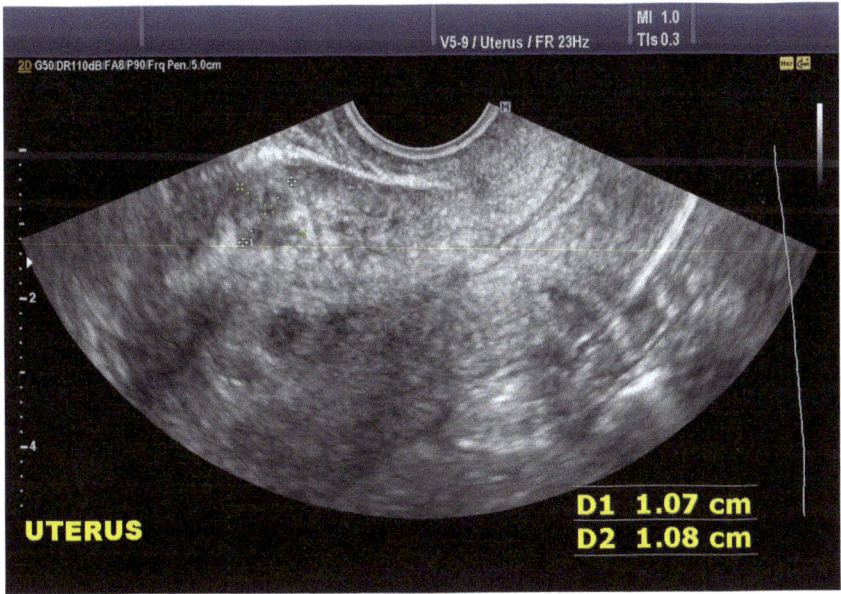

Fig. 6.2.20: Submucous fibroids, anterior and posterior wall

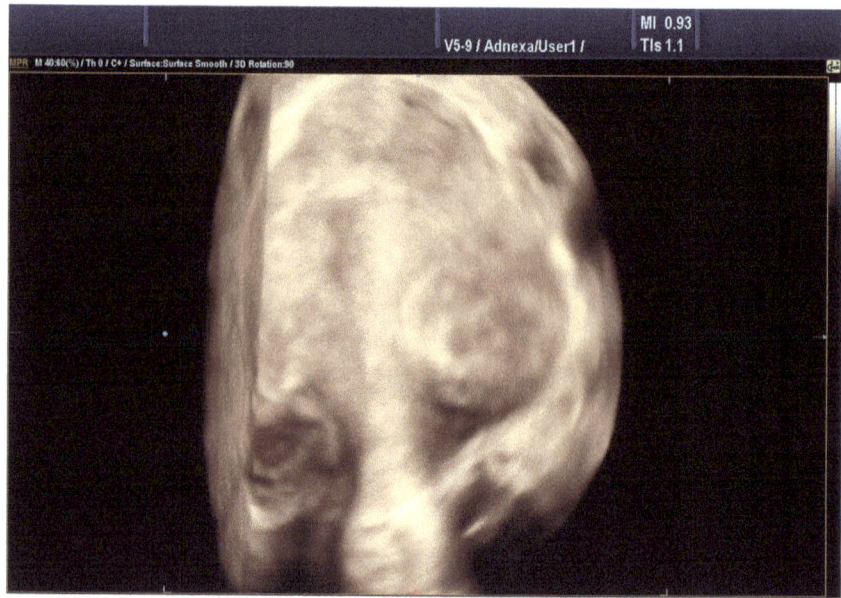

Fig. 6.2.21: Submucous fibroids as seen on 3D

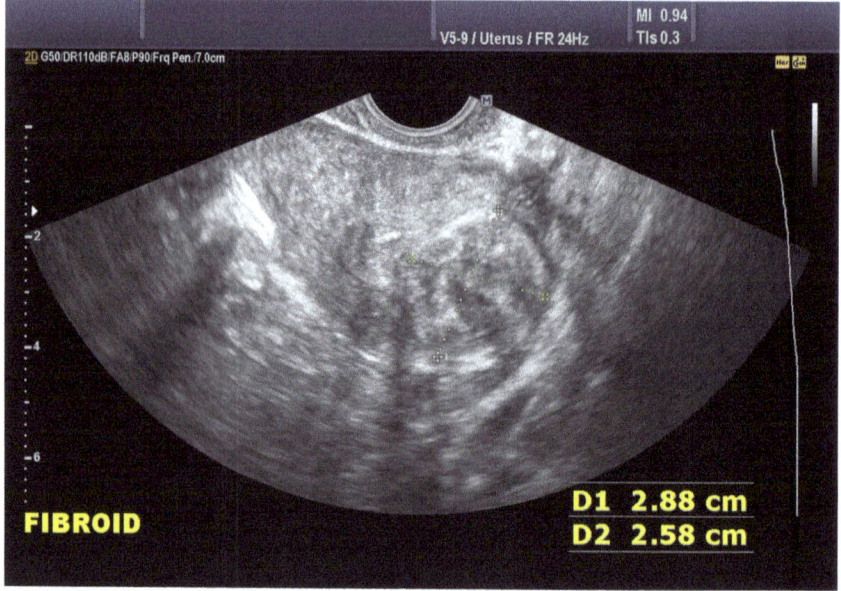

Fig. 6.2.22: Submucous fibroid impinging the cavity

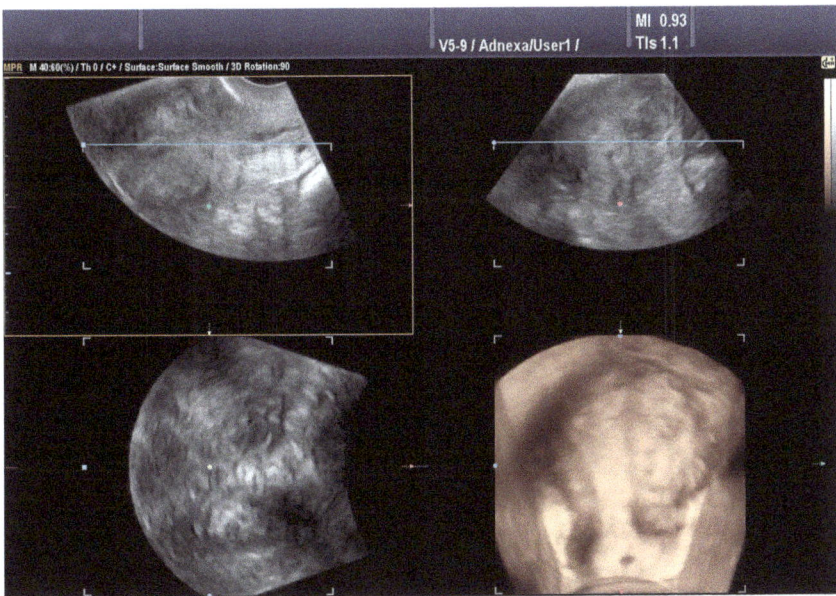

Fig. 6.2.23: Fundal fibroid and endometrium as seen on MPR

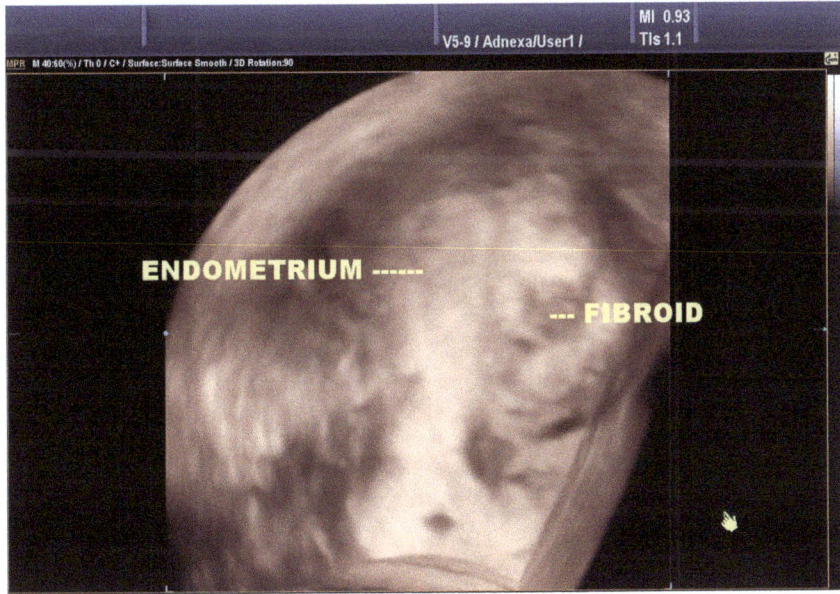

Fig. 6.2.24: The same as seen on 3D

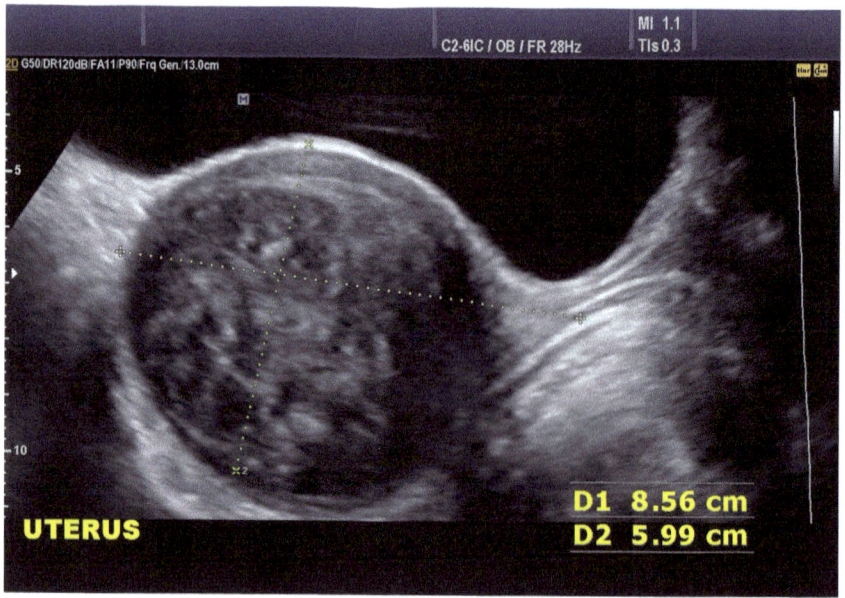

Fig. 6.2.25: Large posterior wall panmural fibroid

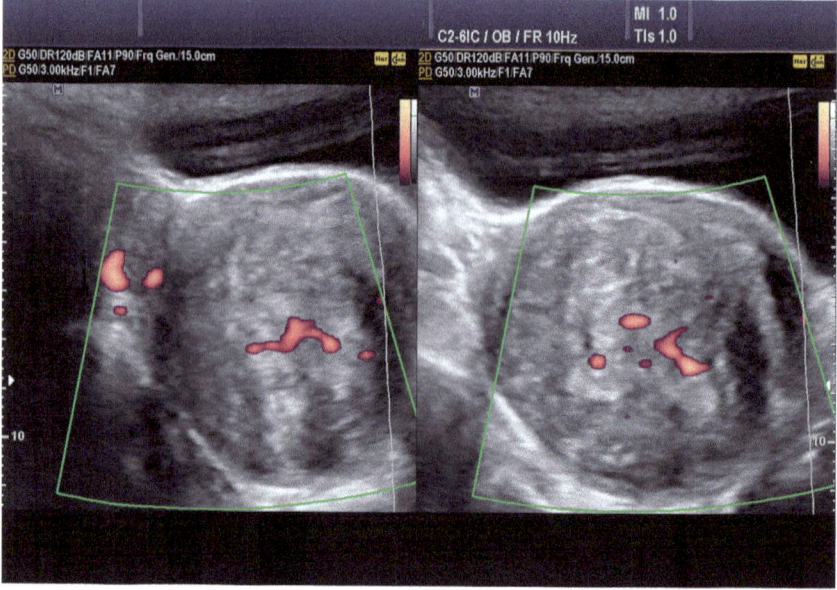

Fig. 6.2.26: Color flow mapping and power angio studies of the fibroid

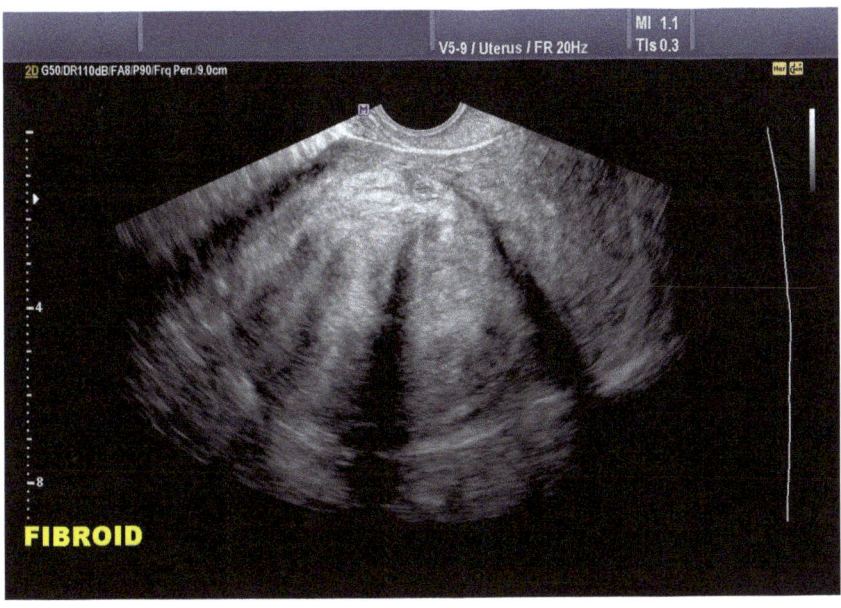

Fig. 6.2.27: Panmural fibroid with degeneration

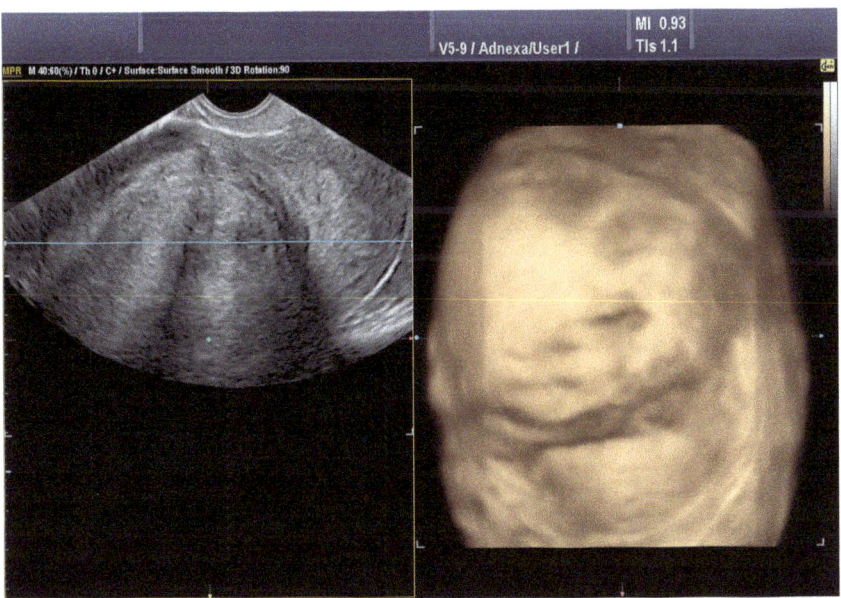

Fig. 6.2.28: Fibroid with rim calcification

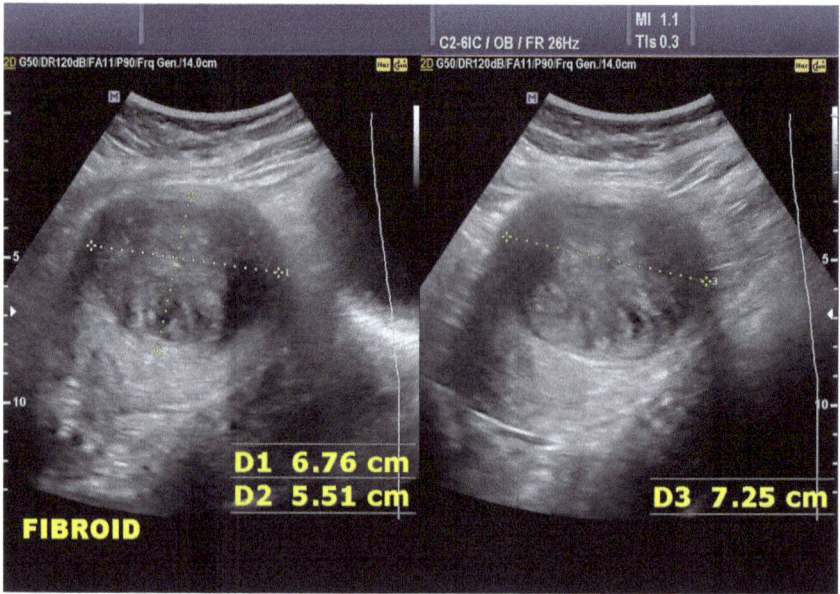

Fig. 6.2.29: Panmural fibroid seen from uterine surface till cavity

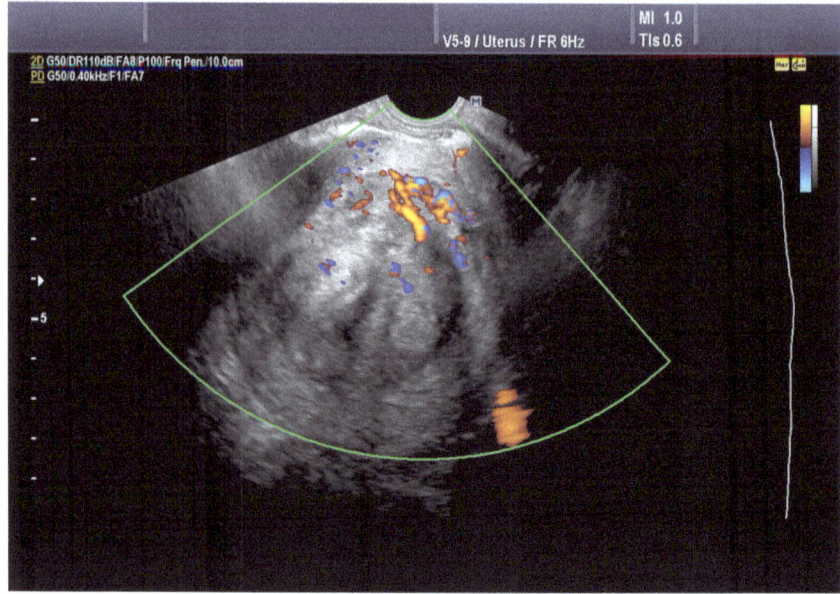

Fig. 6.2.30: Vascularity of the fibroid

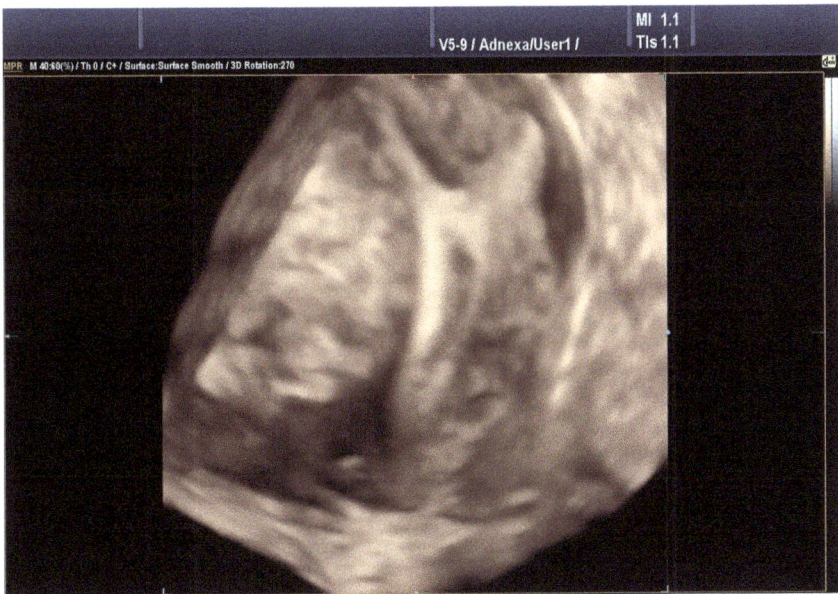

Fig. 6.2.31: 3D of panmural fibroid

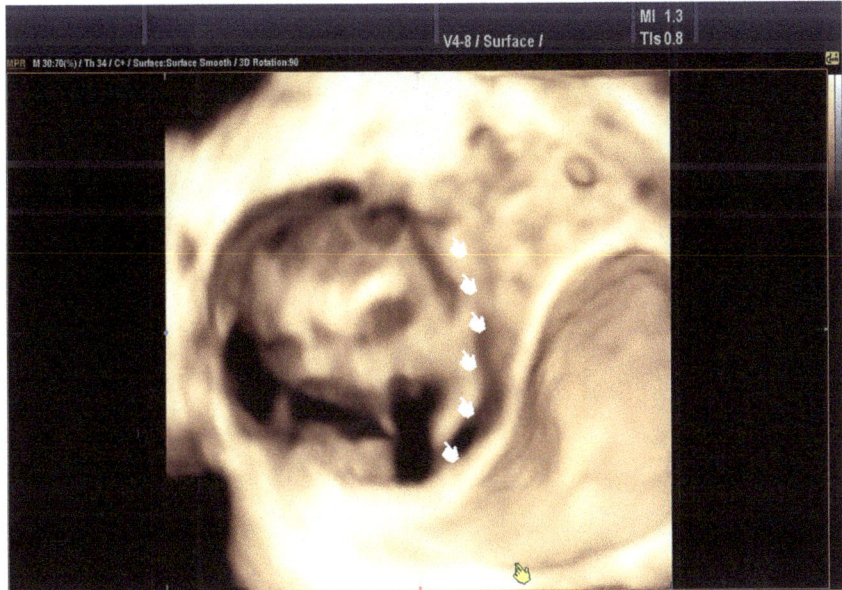

Fig. 6.2.32: 3D of panmural fibroid

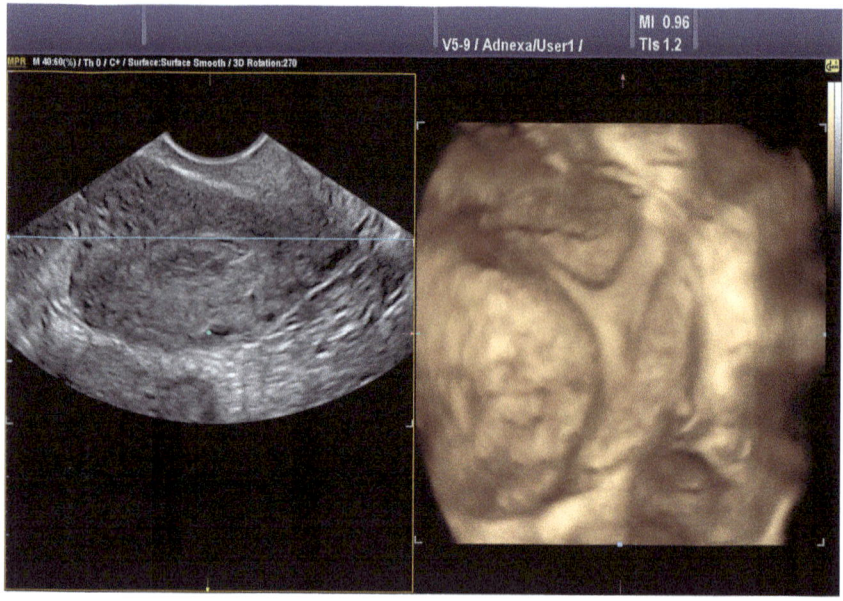

Fig. 6.2.33: 3D of panmural fibroid

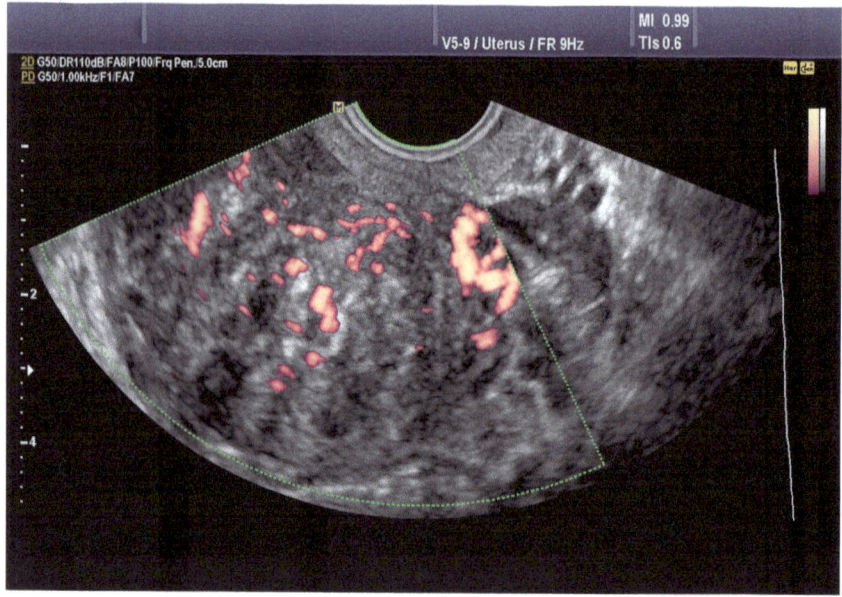

Fig. 6.2.34: Color flow mapping of panmural fibroid

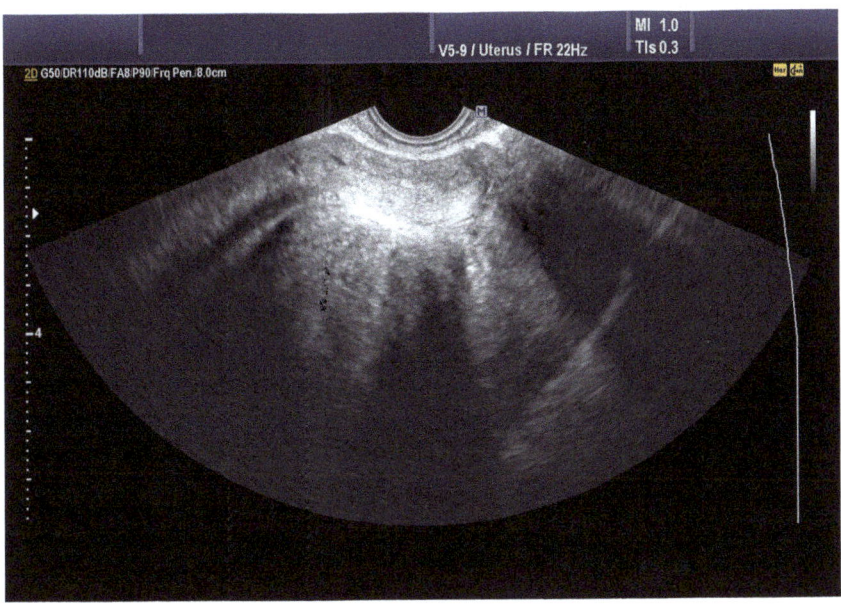

Fig. 6.2.35: Posterior wall panmural fibroid impinging the uterine cavity

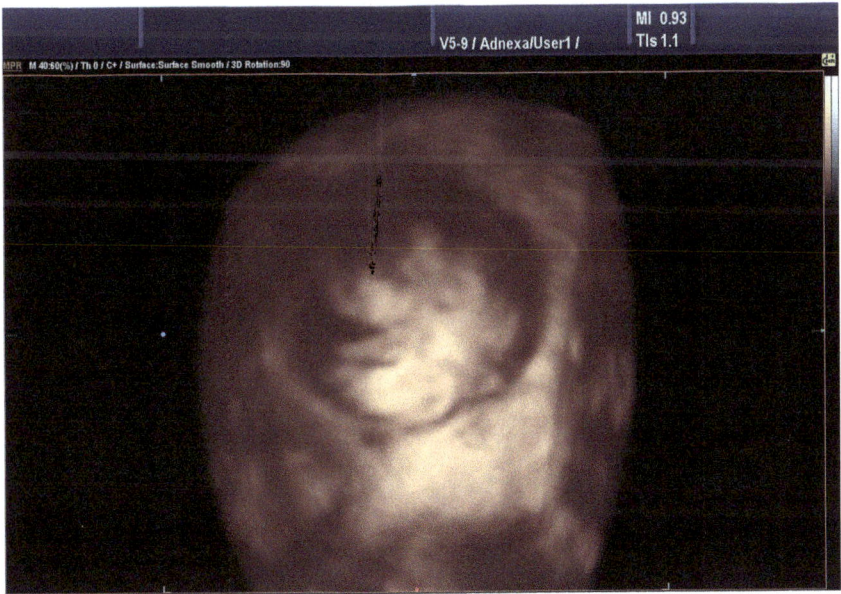

Fig. 6.2.36: Panmural fibroid as seen on 3D

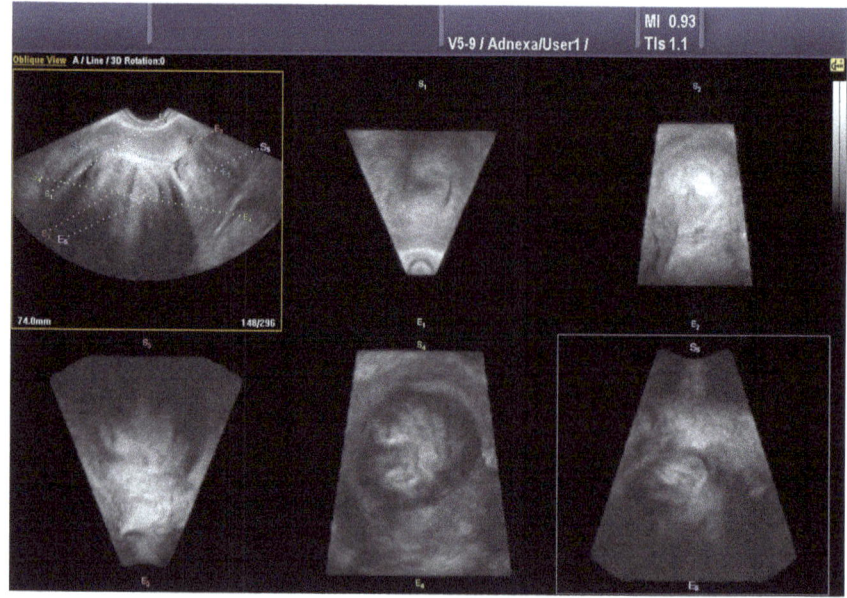

Fig. 6.2.37: Panmural fibroid as seen on MSV

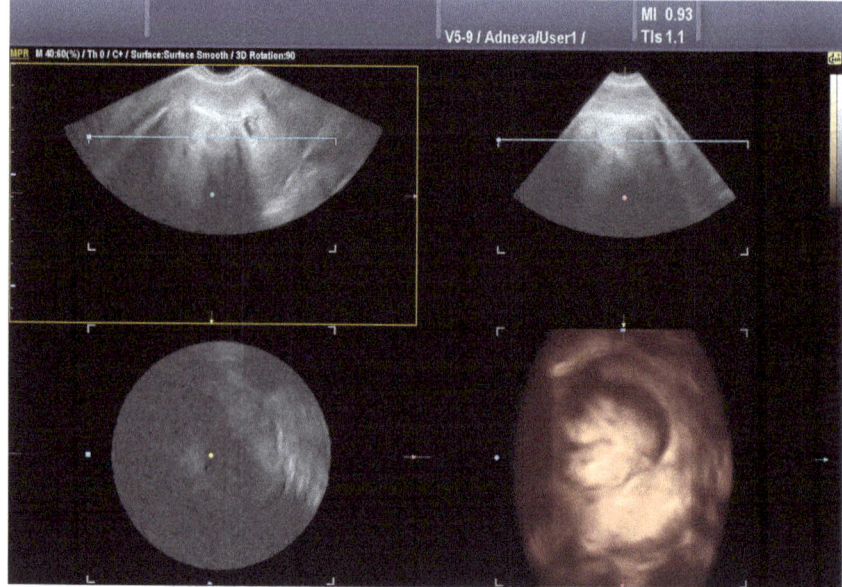

Fig. 6.2.38: Panmural fibroid as seen on MPR

6.2. Fibroids

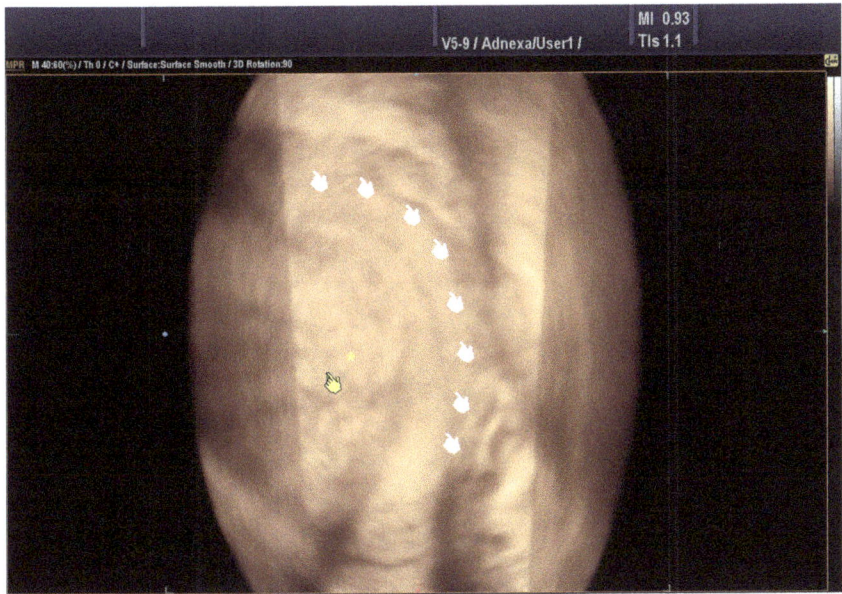

Fig. 6.2.39: Panmural fibroid displacing the uterine cavity

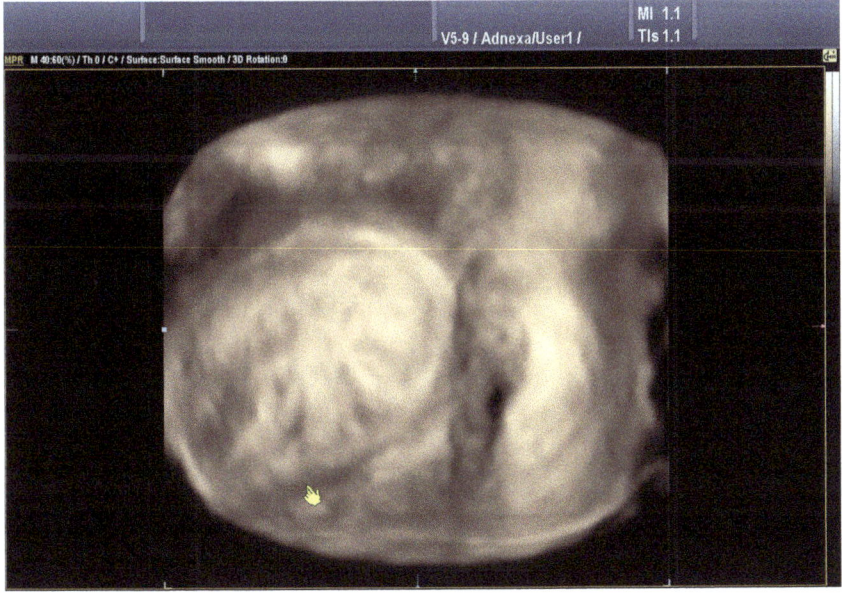

Fig. 6.2.40: Fibroid and endometrium as seen on 3D

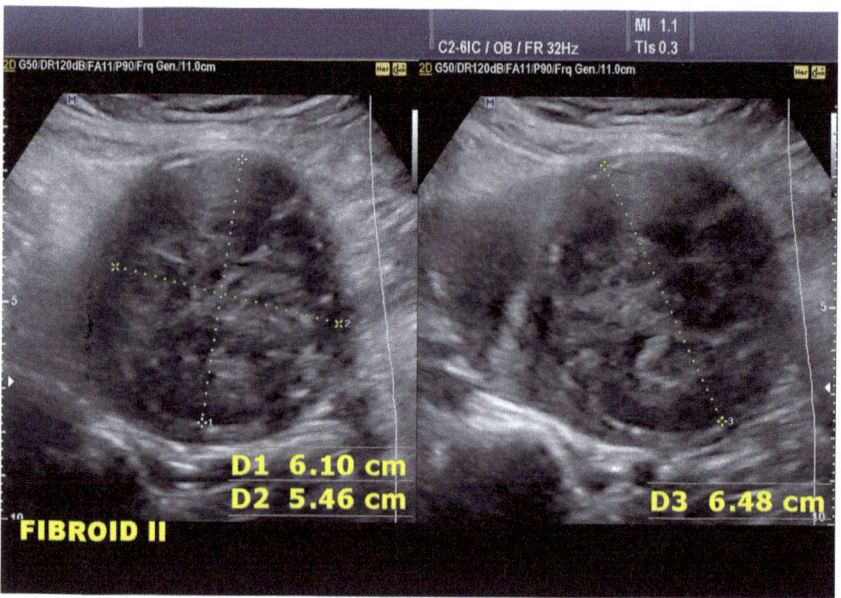

Fig. 6.2.41: Panmural fibroid

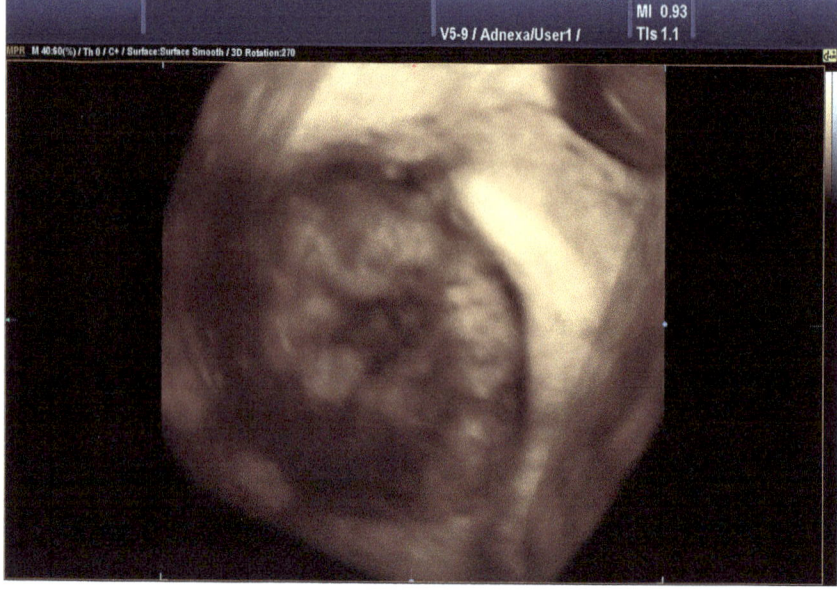

Fig. 6.2.42: Panmural fibroid on 3D

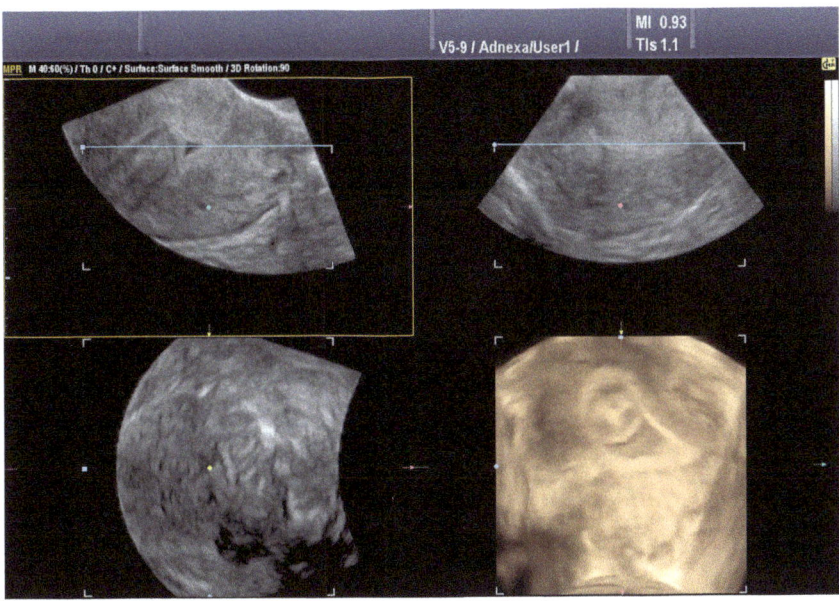

Fig. 6.2.43: Fibroid polyp as seen on 3D

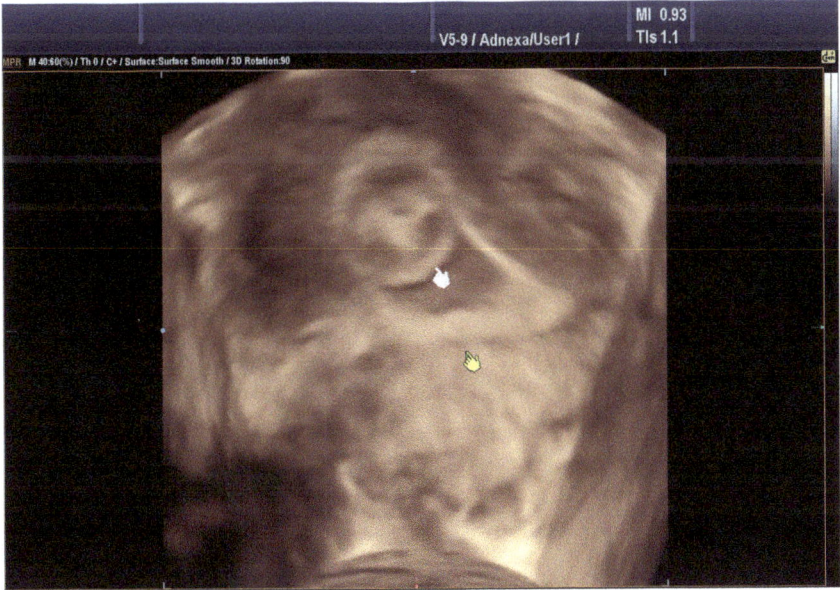

Fig. 6.2.44: Fibroid polyp as seen on 3D

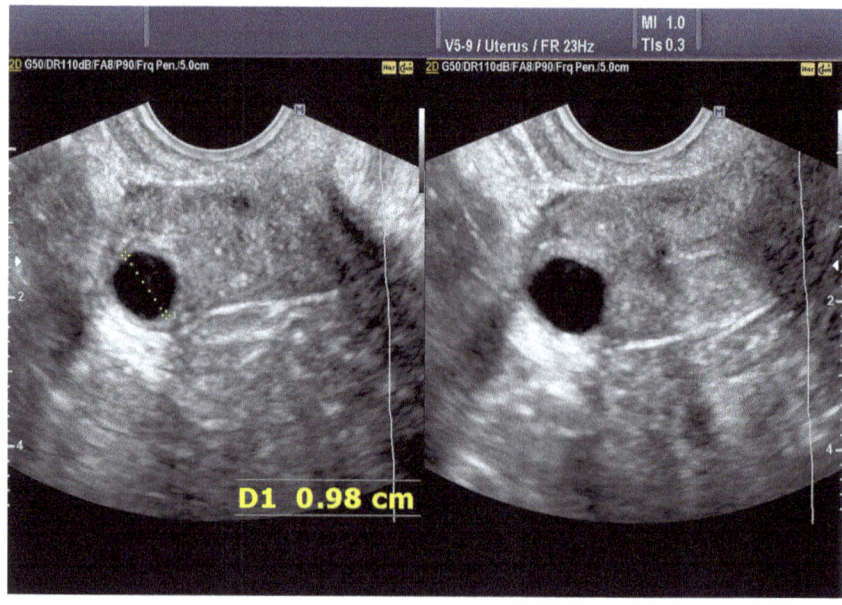

Fig. 6.2.45: Anechoic area in the myometrium, cystic degeneration of fibroid

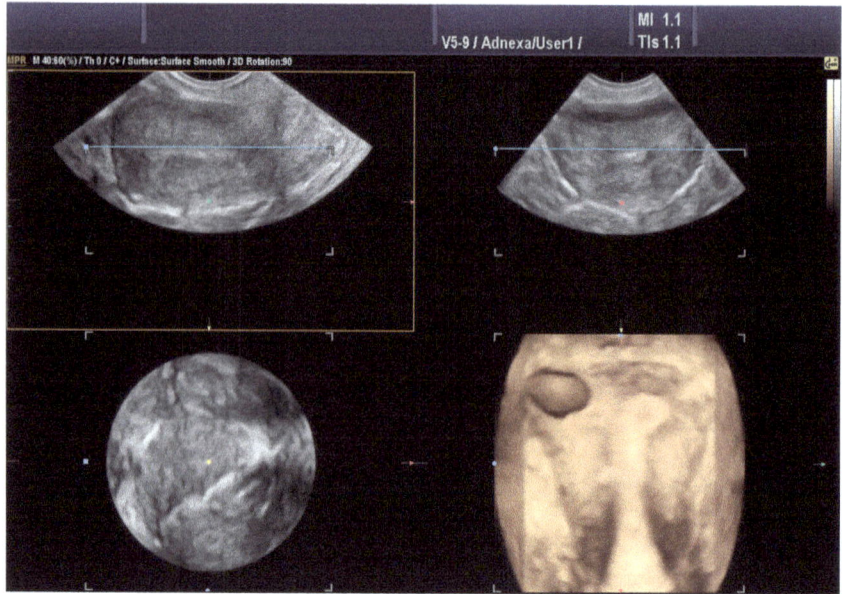

Fig. 6.2.46: Cystic fibroid seen on MPR

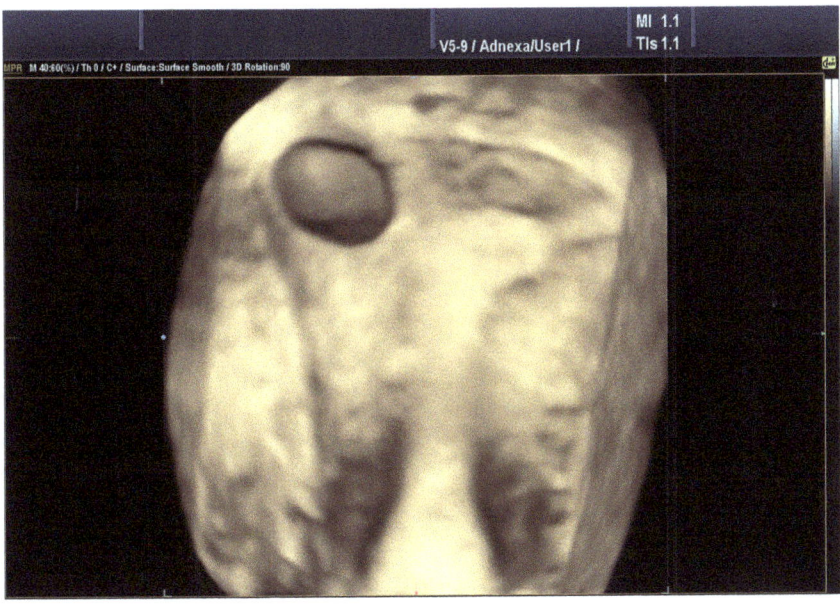

Fig. 6.2.47: Fibroid with cystic degeneration on 3D

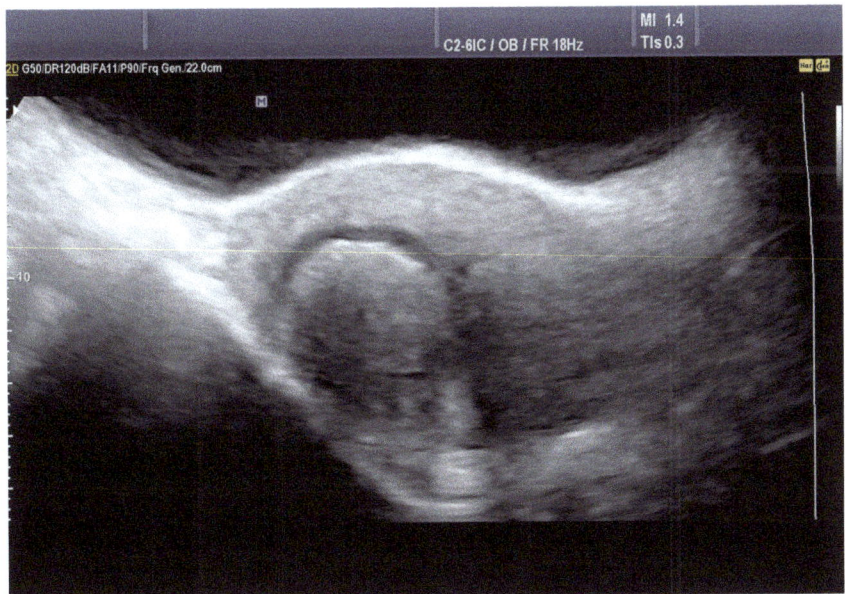

Fig. 6.2.48: Fibroid with rim calcification

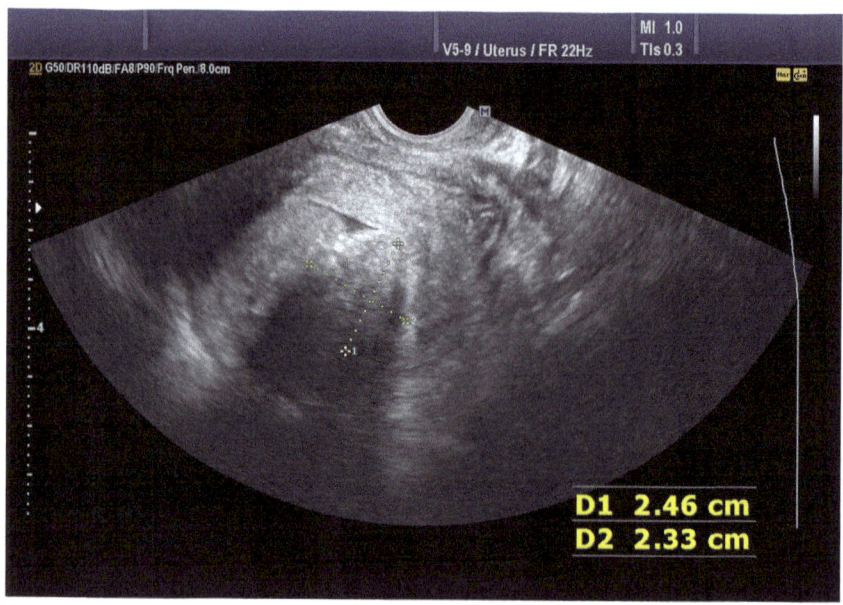

Fig. 6.2.49: Fibroid with calcification showing shadowing

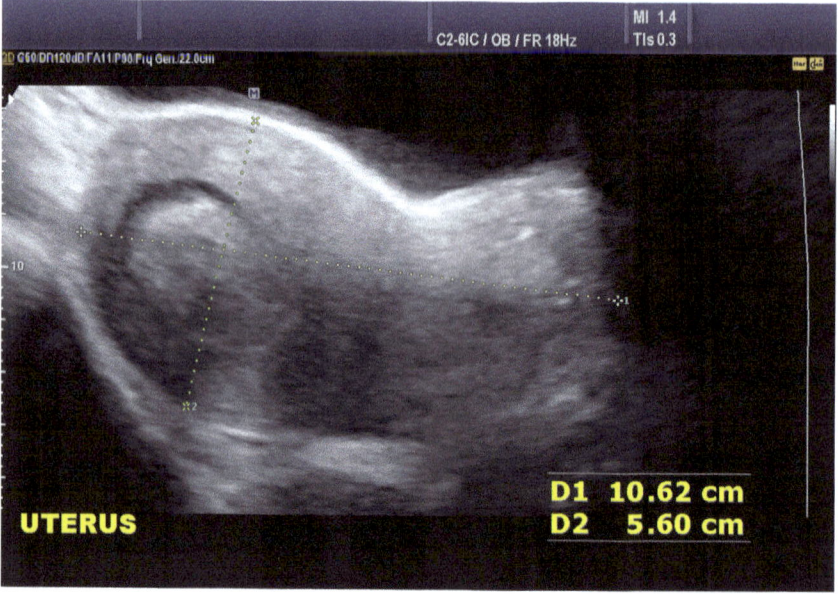

Fig. 6.2.50: Calcified fibroid

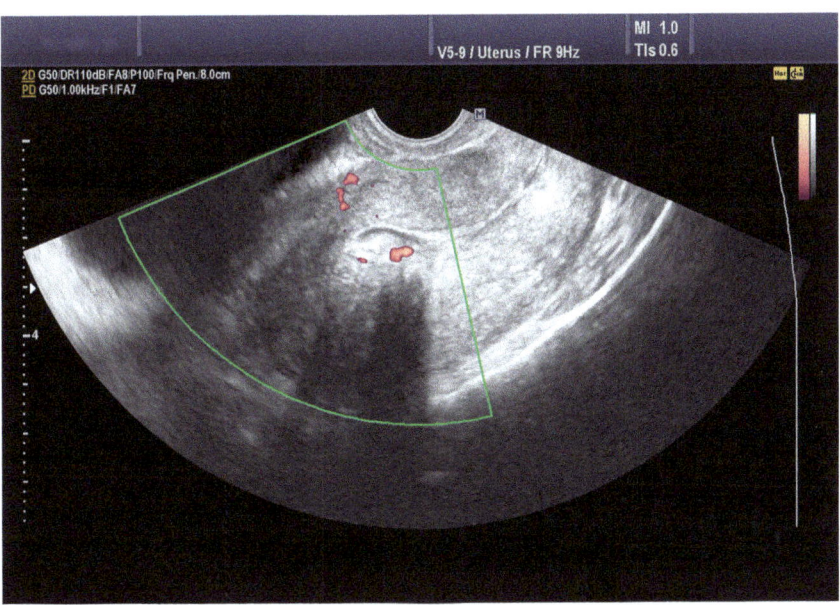

Fig. 6.2.51: Minimal vascularity seen in the fibroid

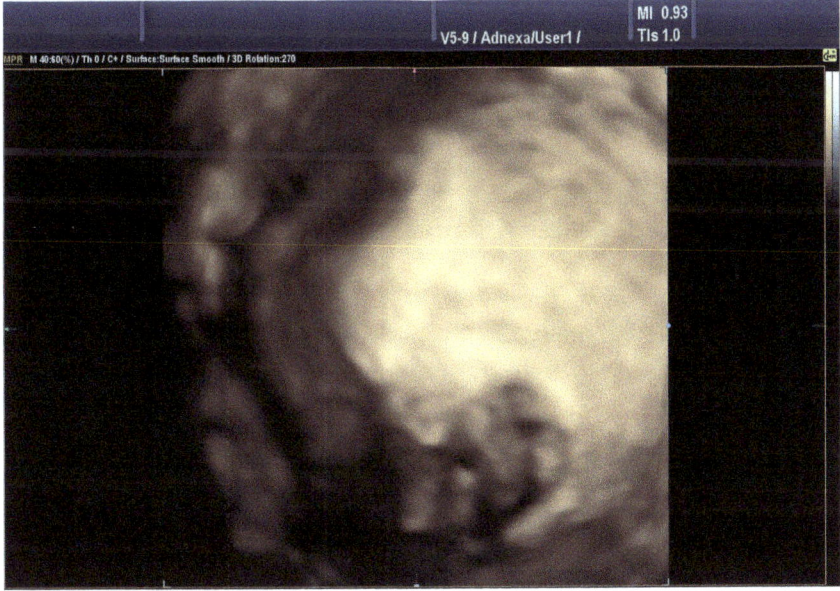

Fig. 6.2.52: Fibroid as seen on 3D

6.3. FIBROID POLYP

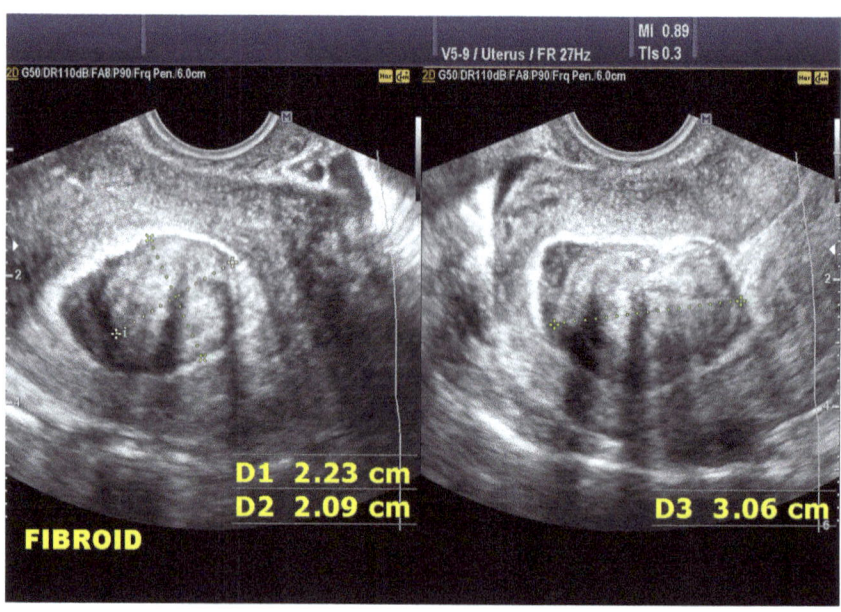

6.3. Fibroid Polyp

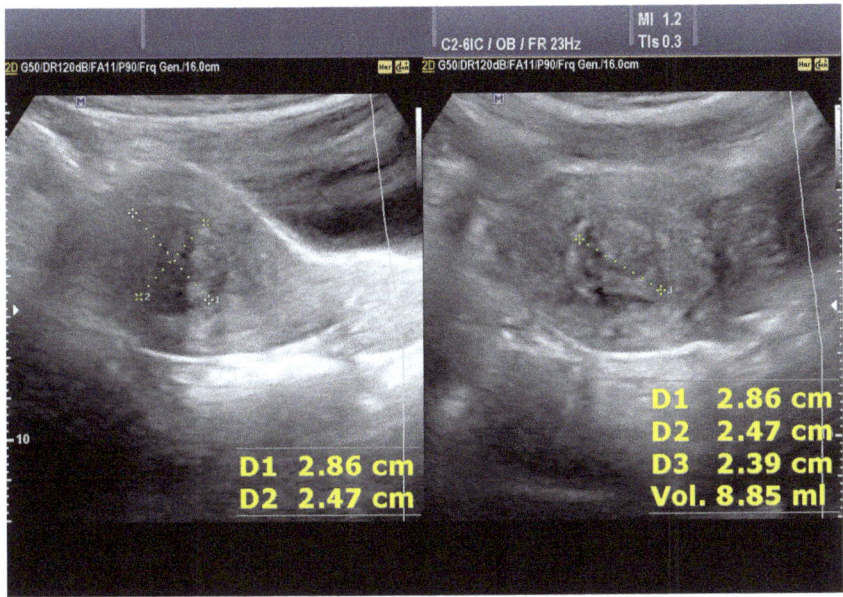

Fig. 6.3.1: Submucous fibroid polyp on TAS

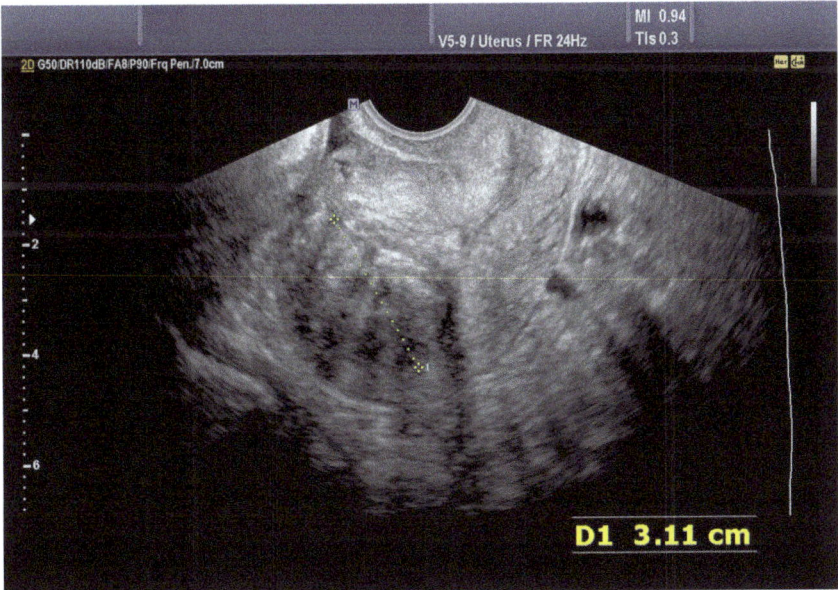

Fig. 6.3.2: Fibroid polyp on TVS

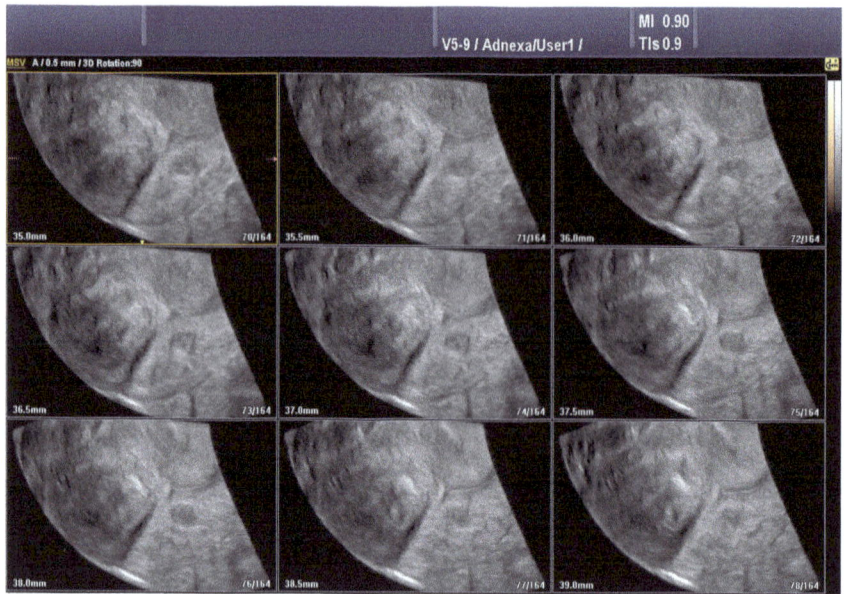

Fig. 6.3.3: Fibroid polyp as seen on MSV

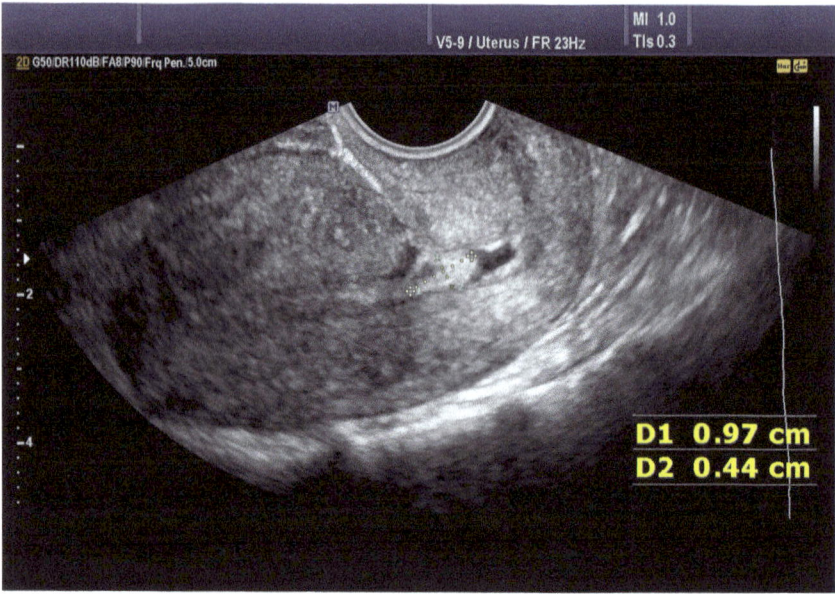

Fig. 6.3.4: Small polyp originating from the corpus extending into the cervical canal

6.3. Fibroid Polyp

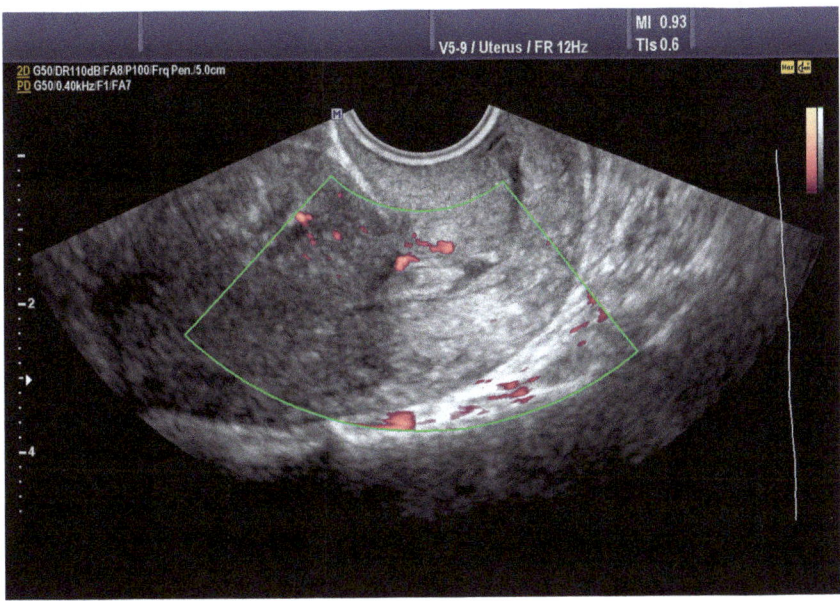

Fig. 6.3.5: Vascular pedicle of polyp on color flow mapping

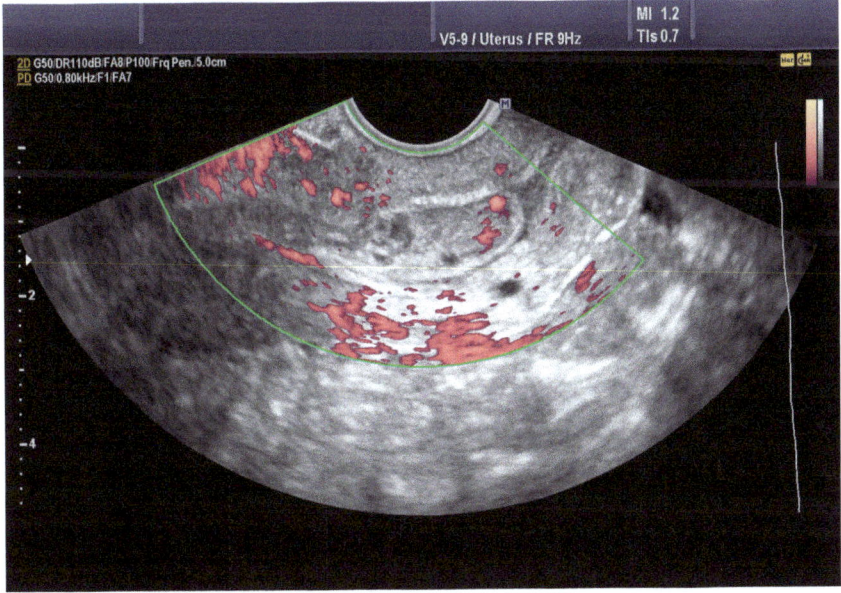

Fig. 6.3.6: Vascular polyp seen in the cervical canal

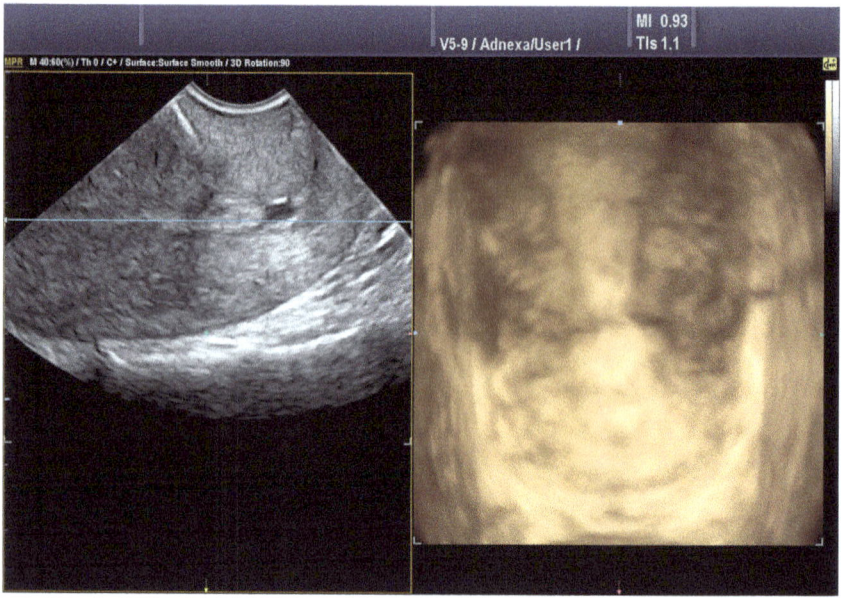

Fig. 6.3.7: Polyp as seen on 3D

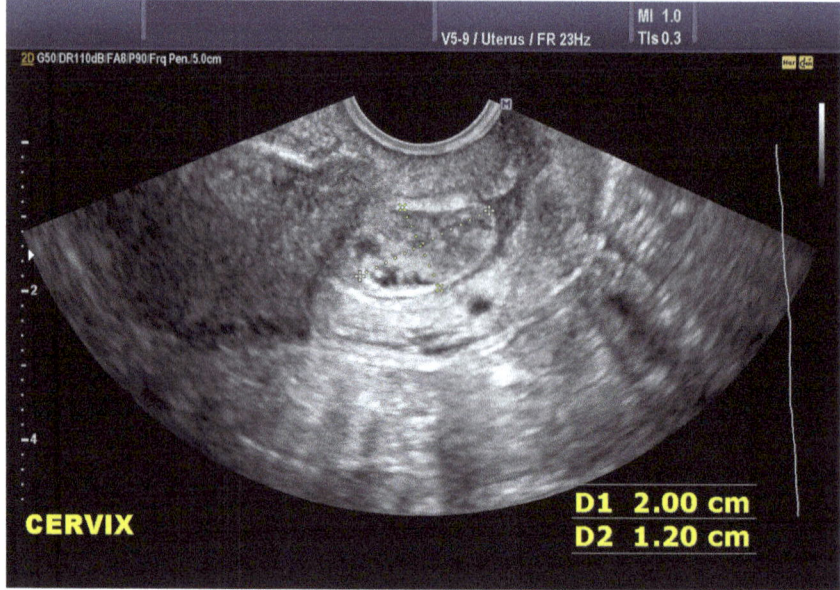

Fig. 6.3.8: Polyp seen in the cervix, inhomogeneous in echo pattern

6.3. Fibroid Polyp

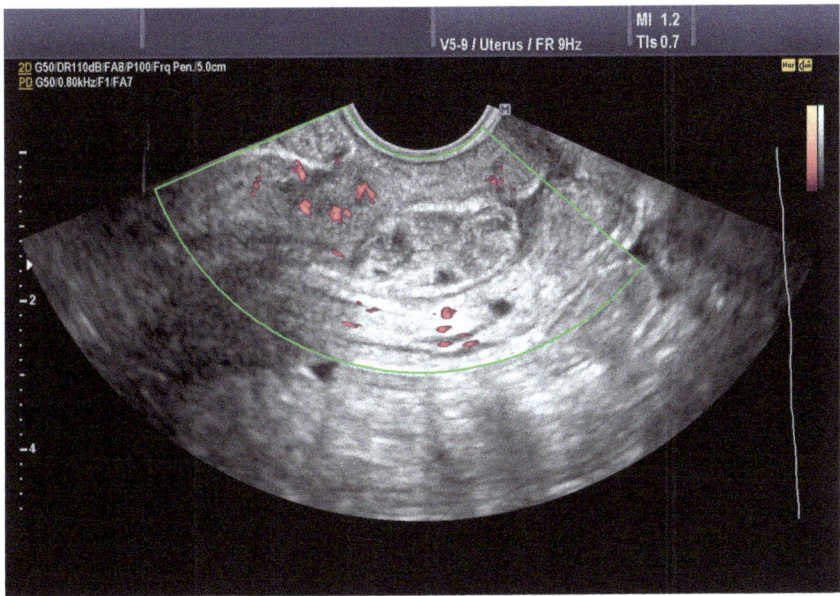

Fig. 6.3.9: On color flow mapping the vascular pedicle originating from the corpus anteriorly is delineated

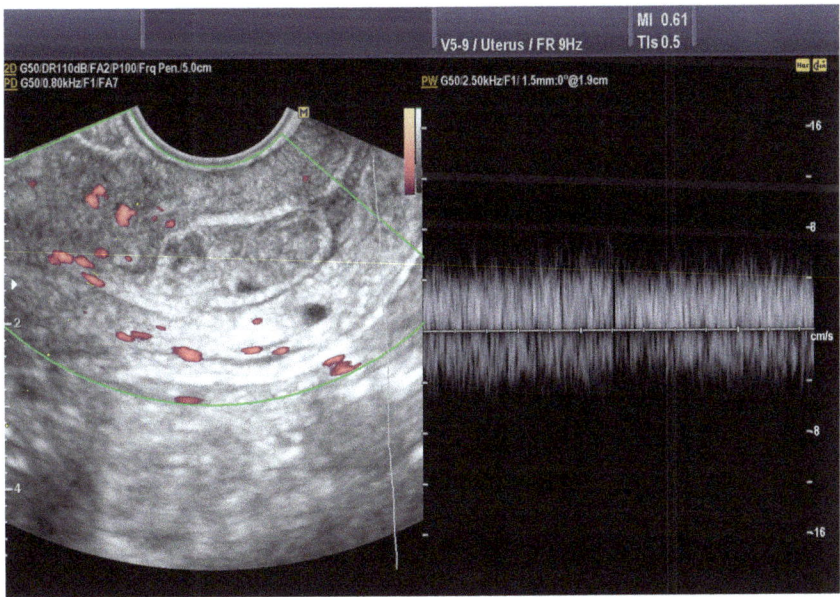

Fig. 6.3.10: Venous flow seen in the fibroid polyp

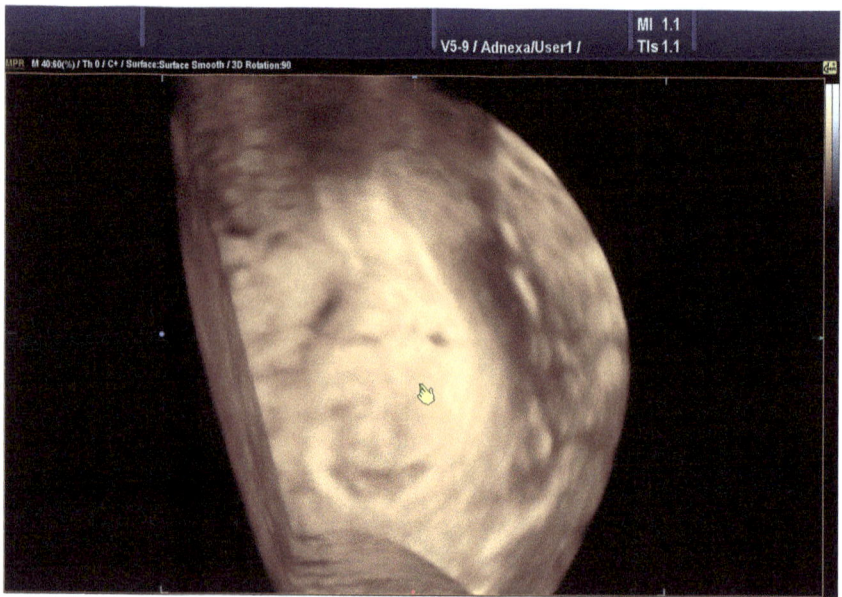

Fig. 6.3.11: Fibroid polyp as seen on 3D

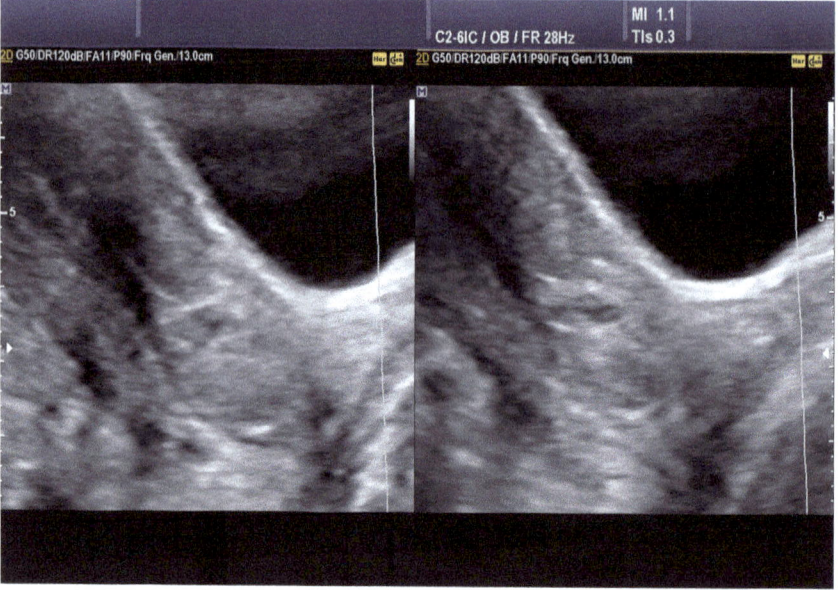

Fig. 6.3.12: Fibroid polyp seen on TAS

6.3. Fibroid Polyp

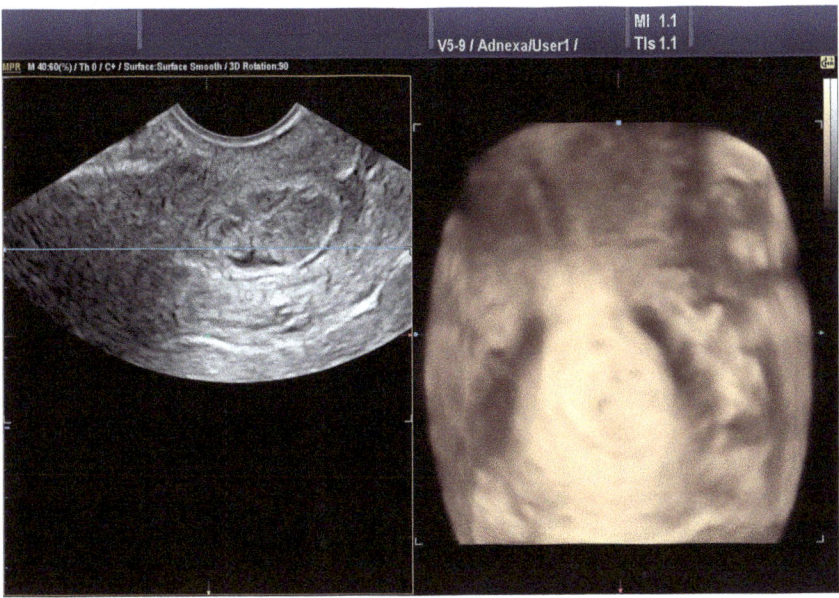

Fig. 6.3.13: Polyp seen on 3D

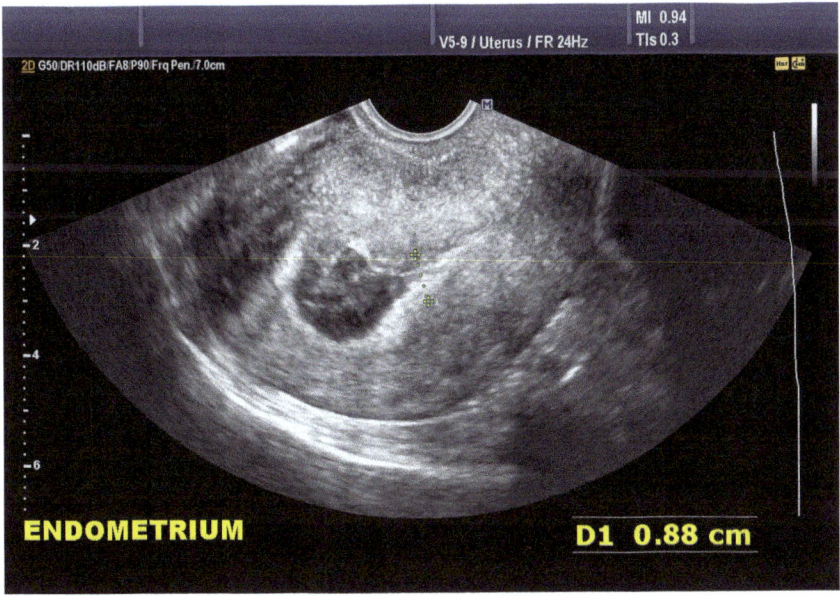

Fig. 6.3.14: Fibroid completely seen in the cavity

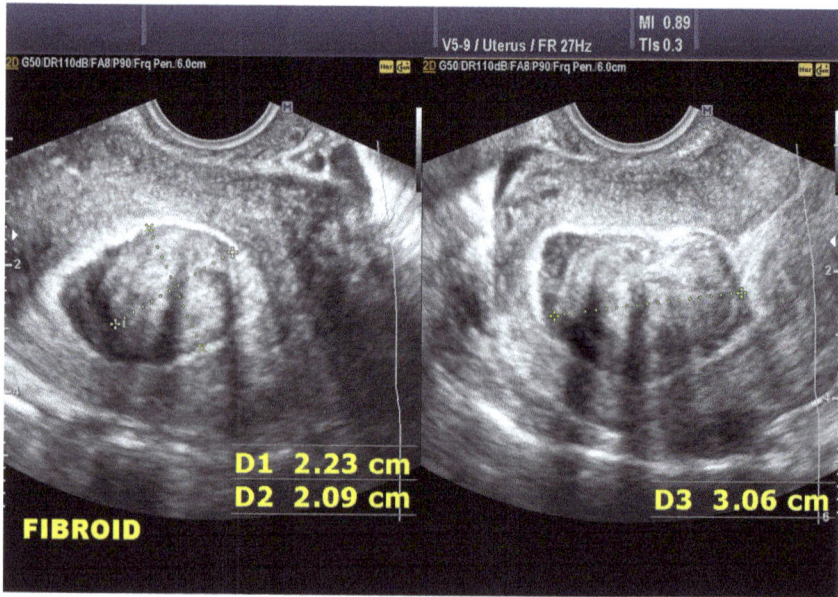

Fig. 6.3.15: Mixed echo pattern of the fibroid is seen

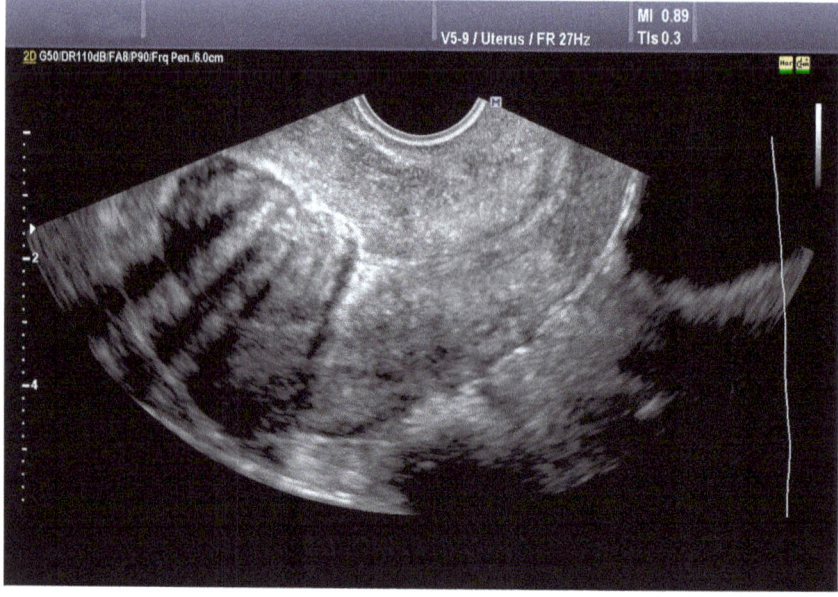

Fig. 6.3.16: Fibroid polyp seen in the fundus

6.3. Fibroid Polyp

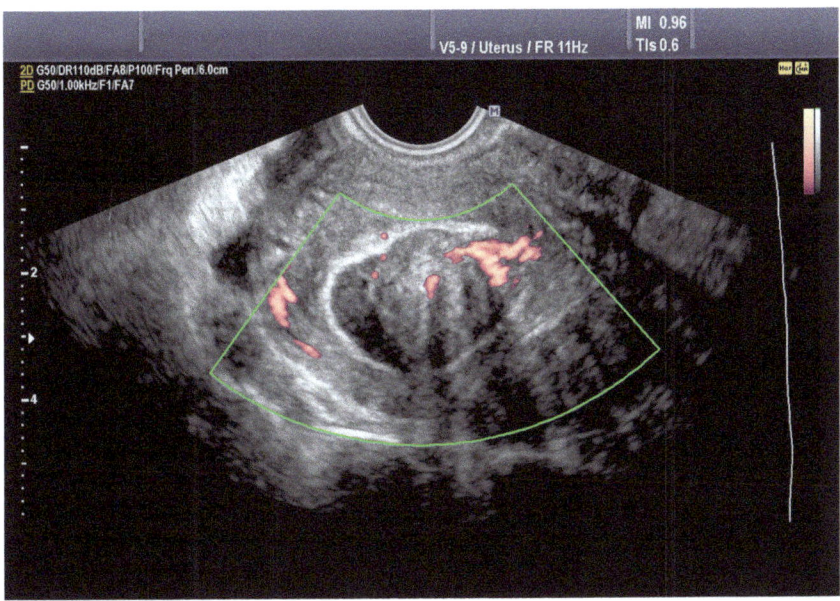

Fig. 6.3.17: Fibroid as seen on color flow mapping

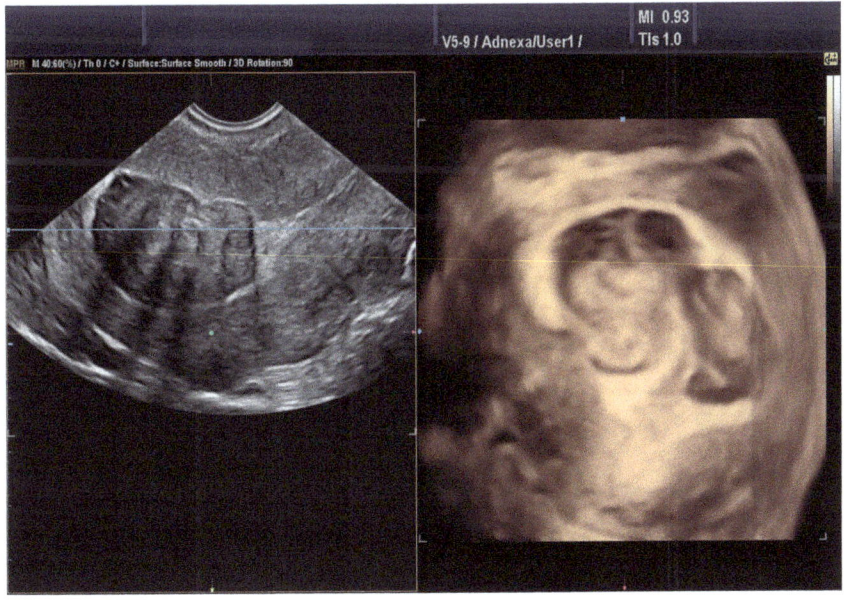

Fig. 6.3.18: As seen on 3D

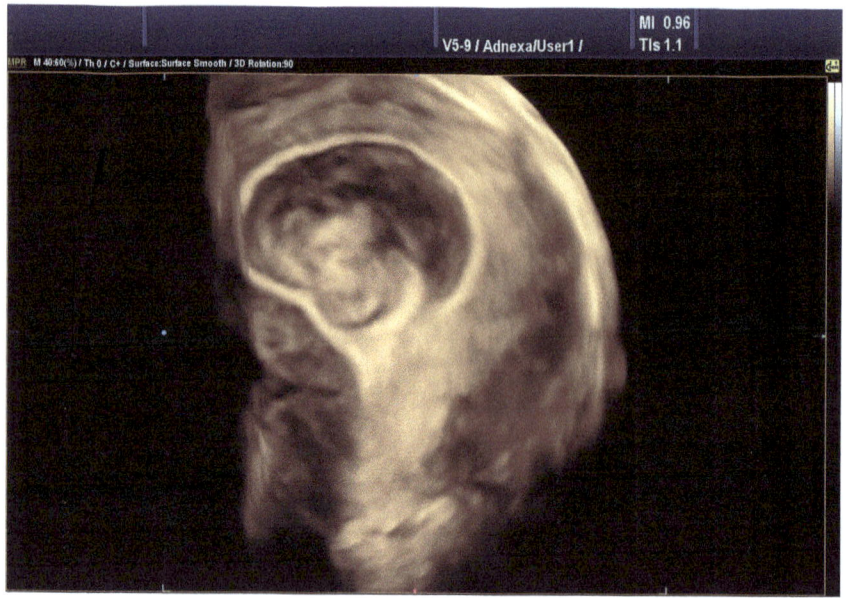

Fig. 6.3.19: As seen on 3D

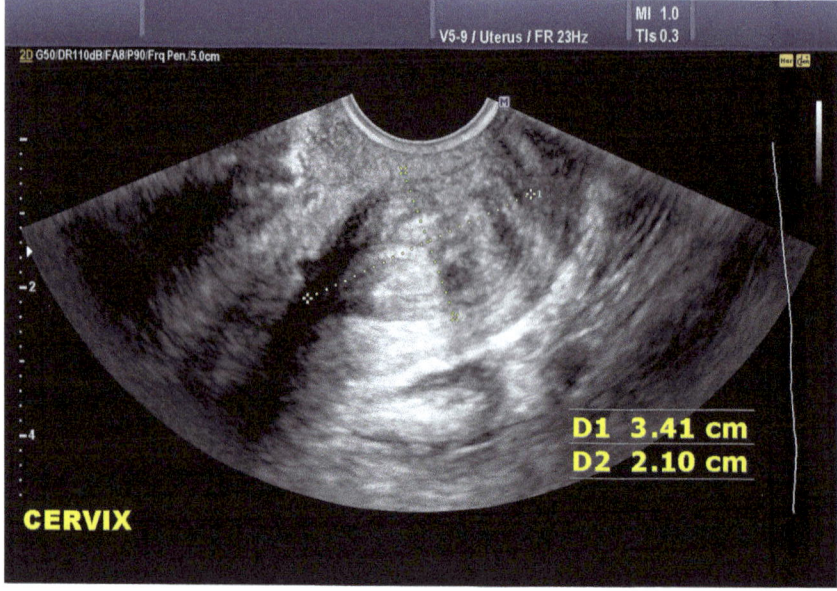

Fig. 6.3.20: Hypoechoic fibroid polyp seen in the cervix

6.3. Fibroid Polyp

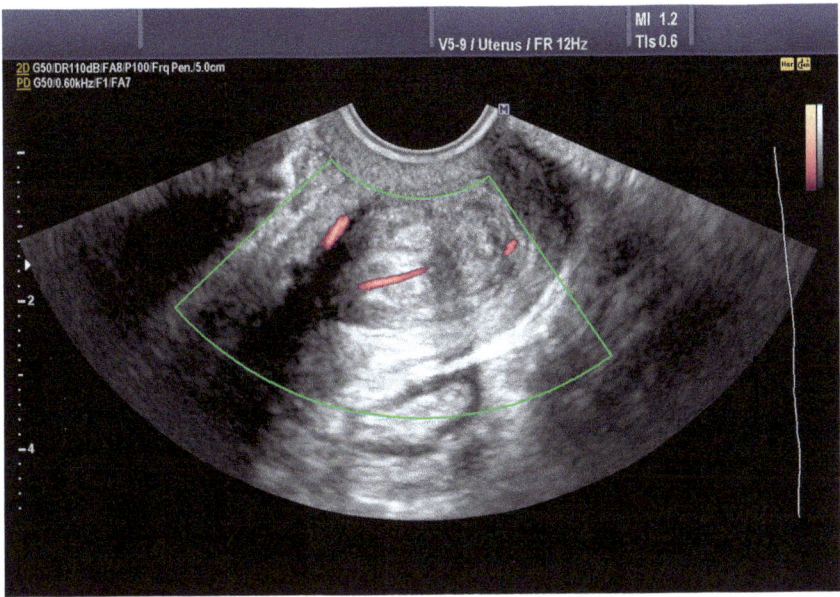

Fig. 6.3.21: Vascularity of the fibroid polyp

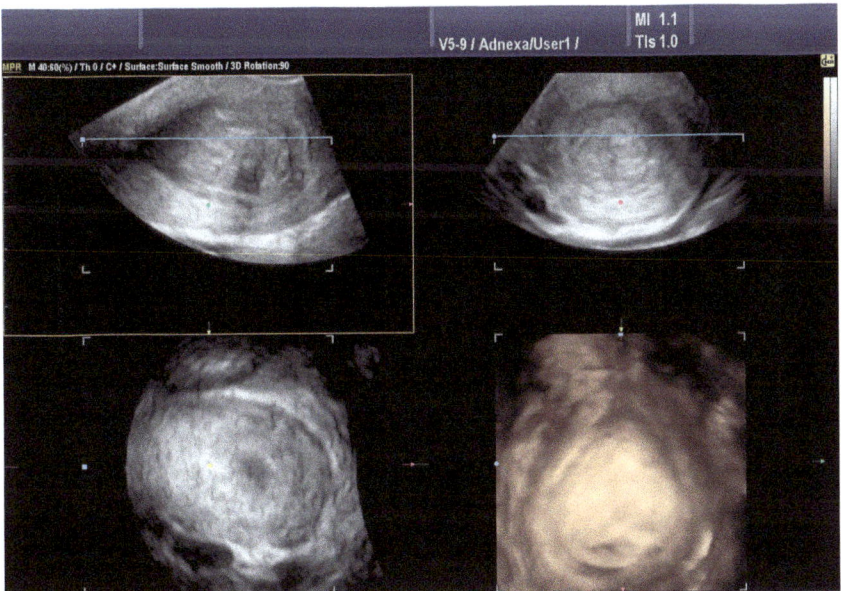

Fig. 6.3.22: As seen on MPR

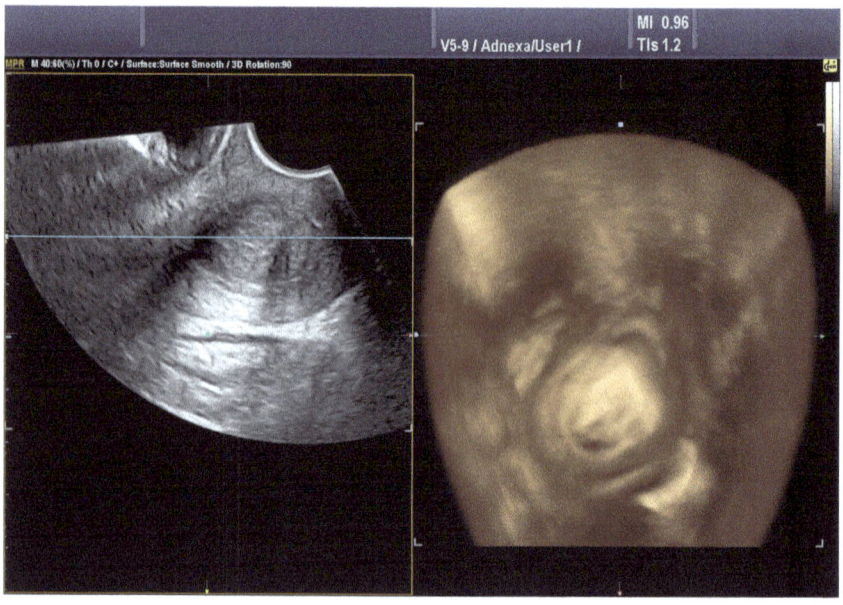

Fig. 6.3.23: As seen on 3D

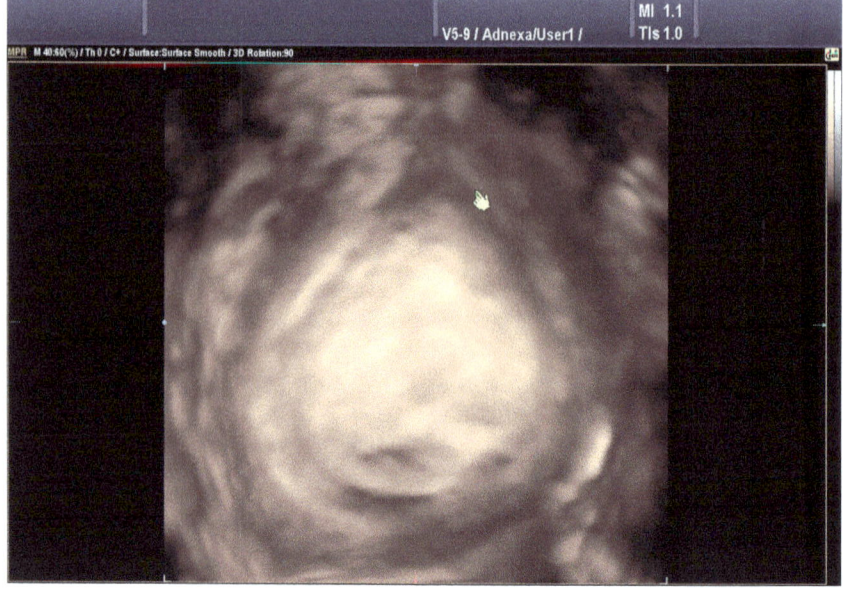

Fig. 6.3.24: As seen on 3D

6.4. ADENOMYOSIS

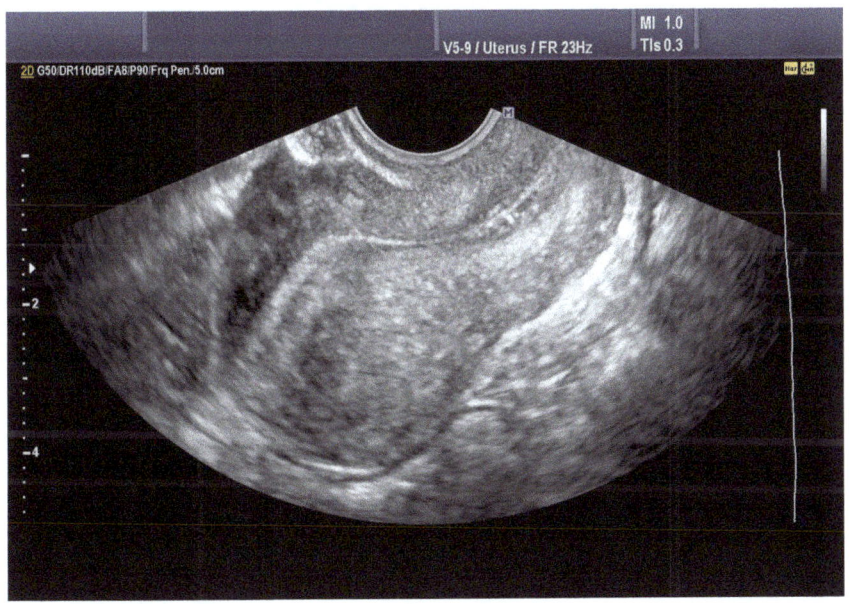

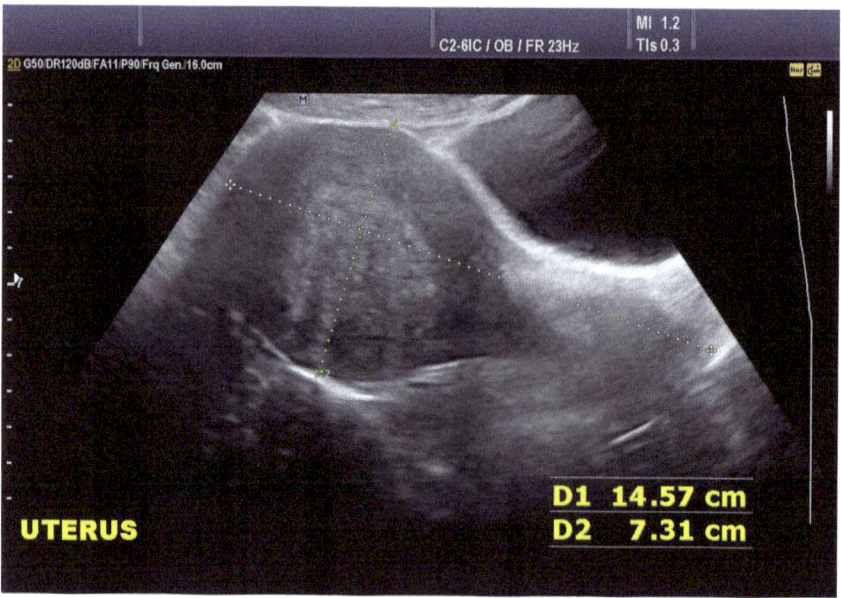

Fig. 6.4.1: Enlarged and globular uterus as seen on TAS

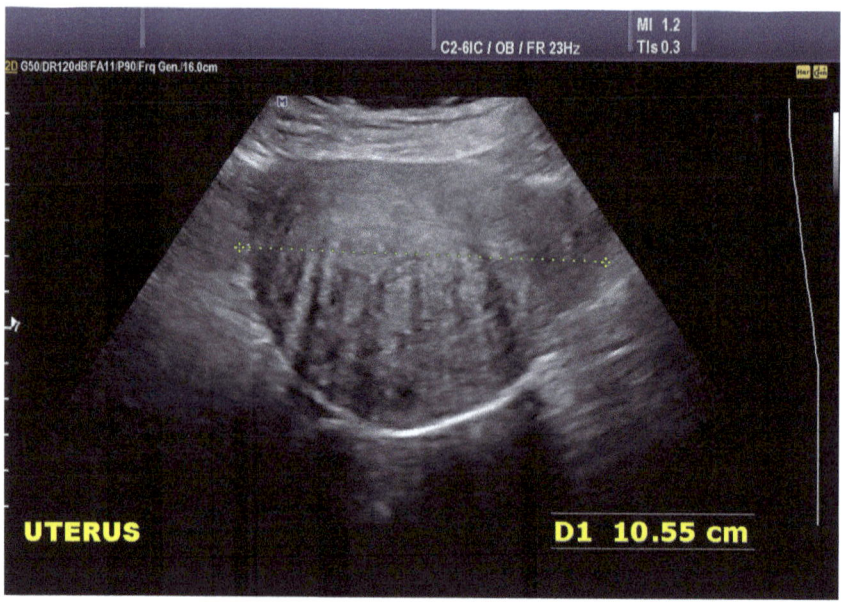

Fig. 6.4.2: Globular and bosselated uterus. Transverse section as seen on TAS

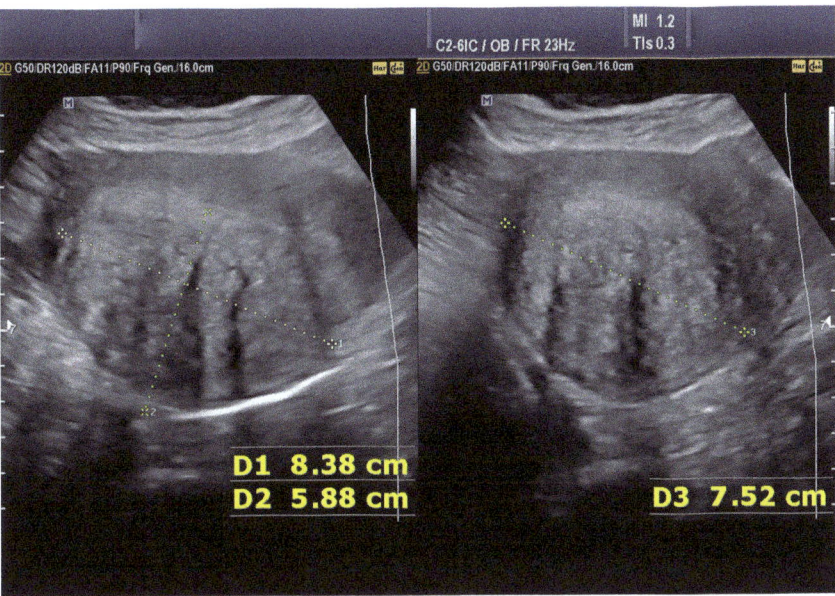

Fig. 6.4.3: Large panmural adenomyoma seen in the posterior wall

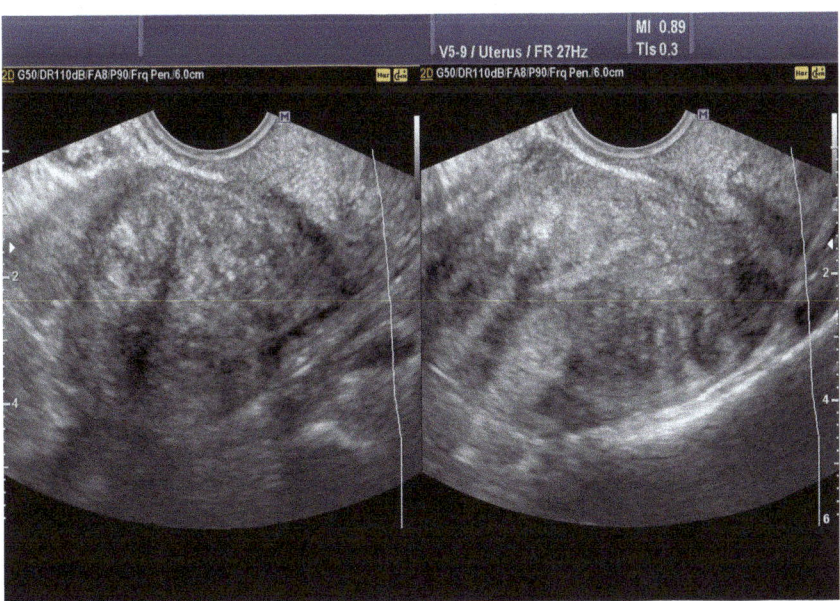

Fig. 6.4.4A: Adenomyosis presents with dysmenorrhea, menorrhagia and metrorrhagia

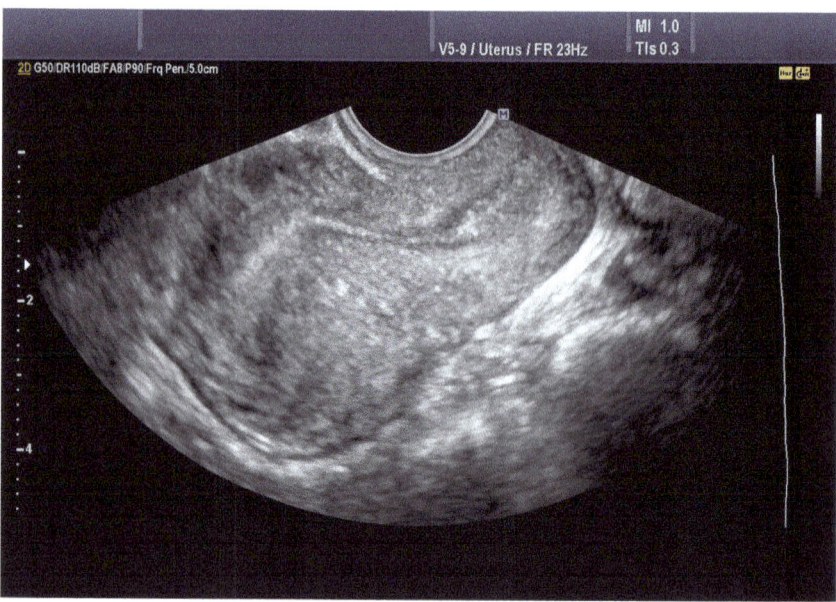

Fig. 6.4.4B: Thickening of the posterior myometrium is routinely seen in adenomyosis

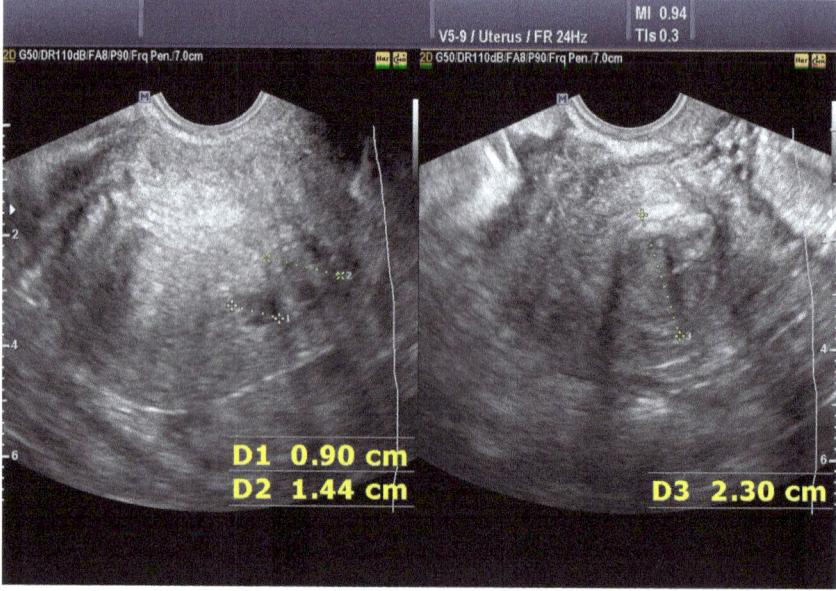

Fig. 6.4.5: Interstitial adenomyomas seen in the posterior myometrium

6.4. Adenomyosis

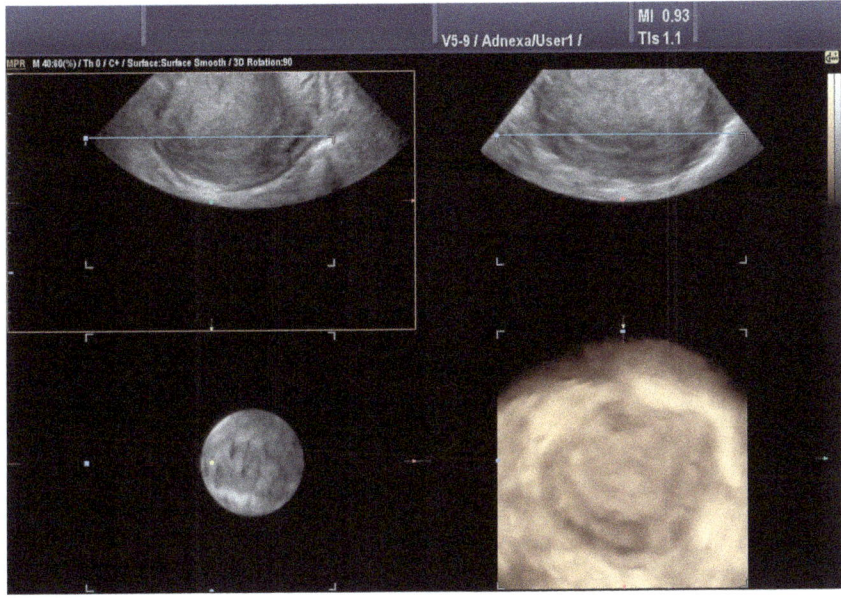

Fig. 6.4.6: Adenomyosis as seen on 3D

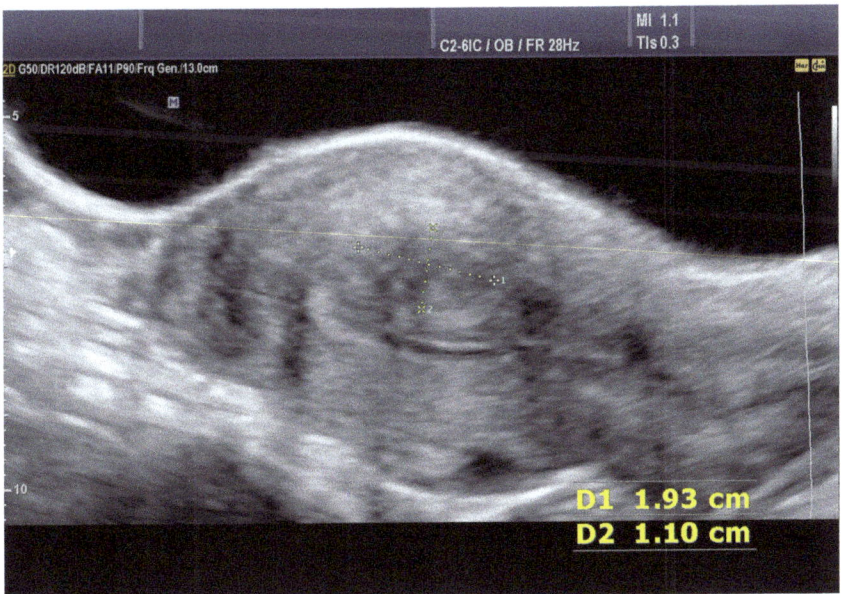

Fig. 6.4.7: Submucous adenomyoma seen in the anterior wall

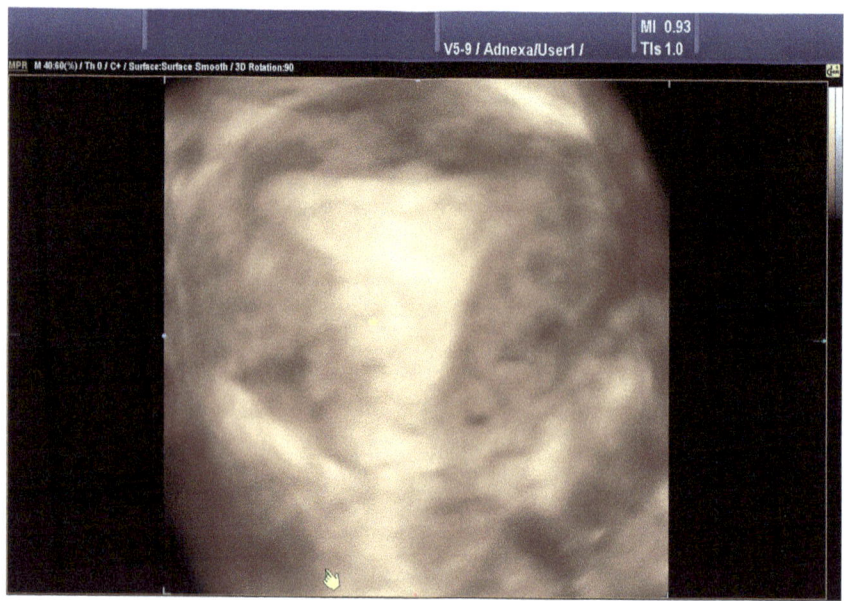

Fig. 6.4.8: Submucous adenomyoma seen impinging the uterine cavity on 3D

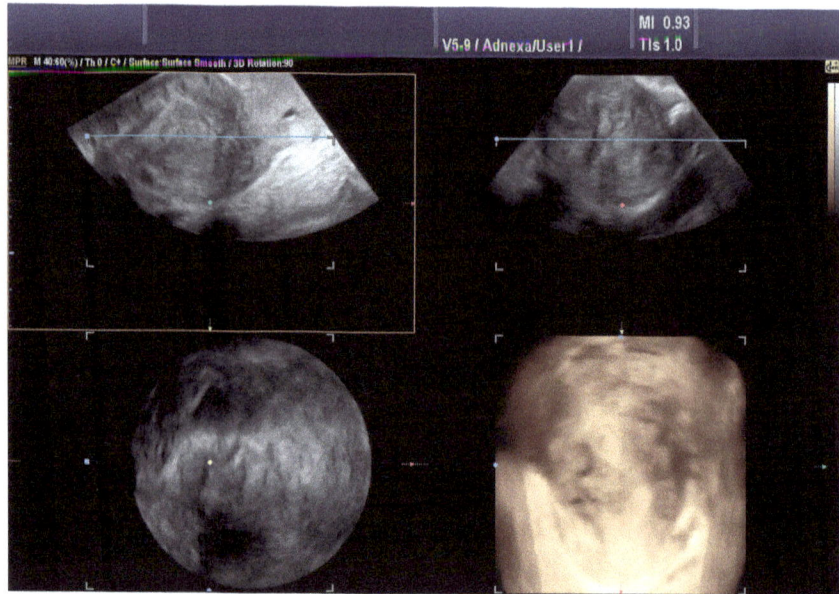

Fig. 6.4.9: Adenomyosis seen on 3D

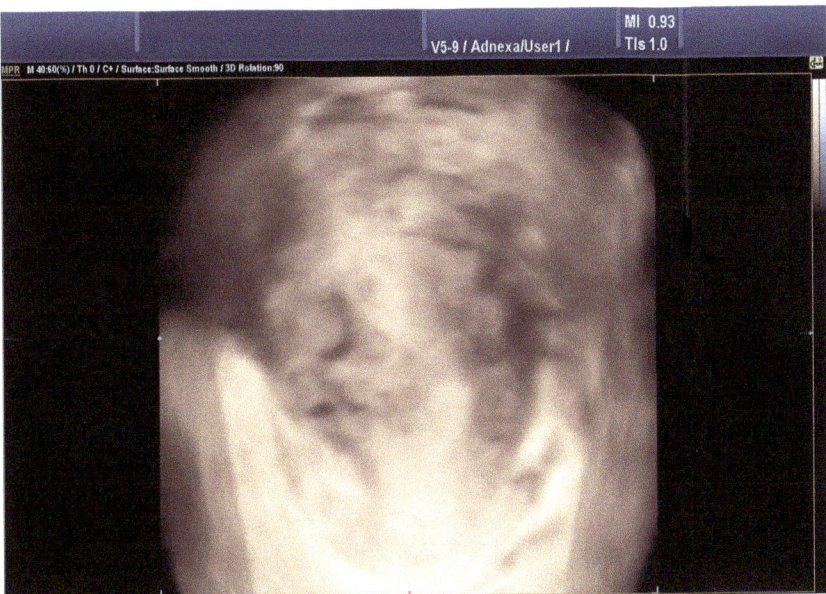

Fig. 6.4.10: 3D reconstruction of interstitial and submucous adenomyomas

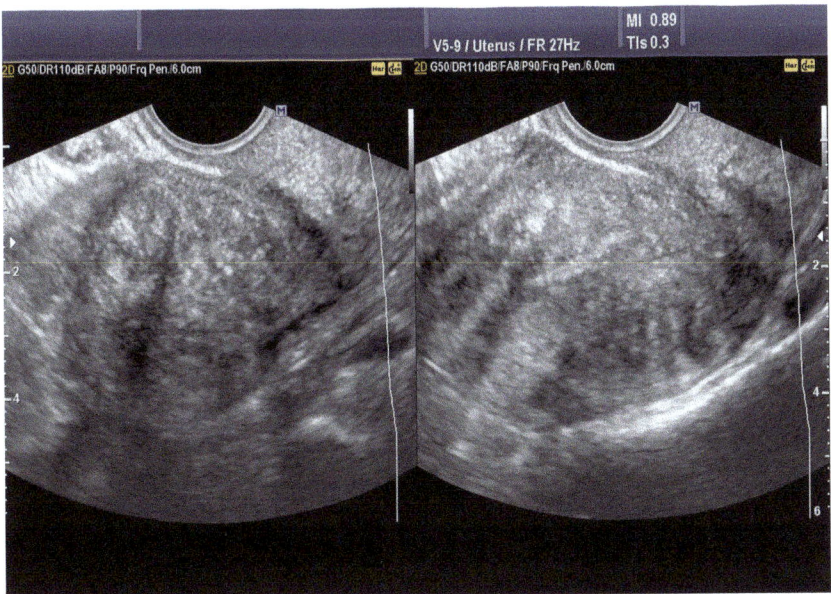

Fig. 6.4.11: Salt and pepper appearance of the myometrium

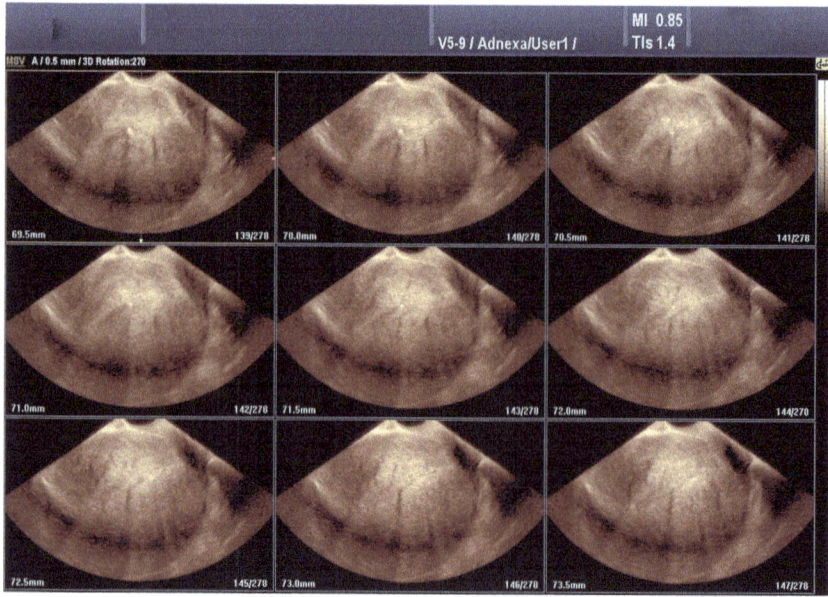

Fig. 6.4.12: Multislice view showing the swiss cheese appearance in adenomyosis

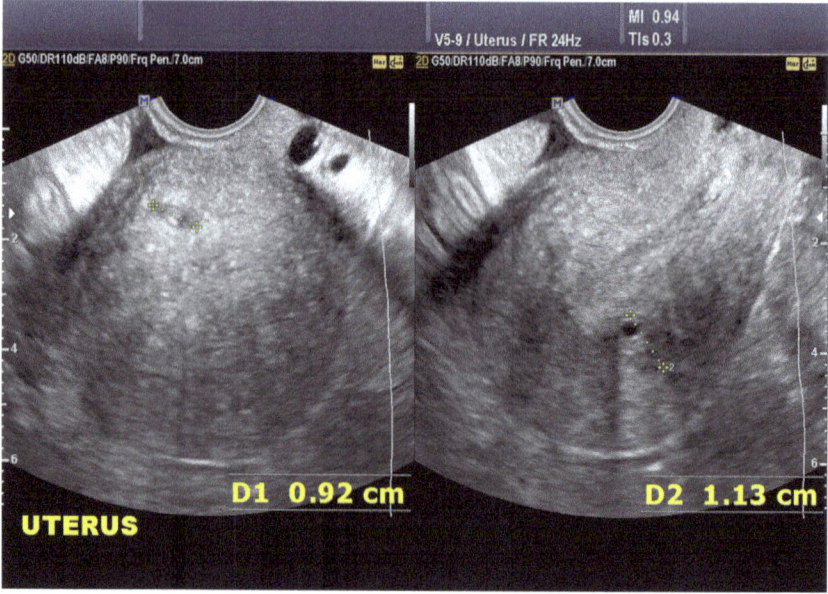

Fig. 6.4.13: Presence of multiple myometrial cysts also clinches the diagnosis of adenomyosis

6.4. Adenomyosis

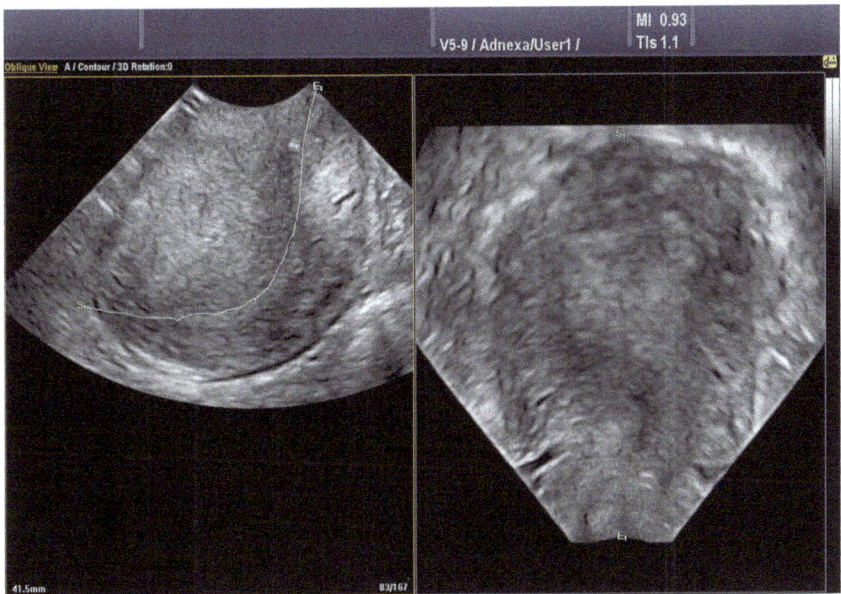

Fig. 6.4.14: Tracing the cavity rules out any submucous lesions on 3D

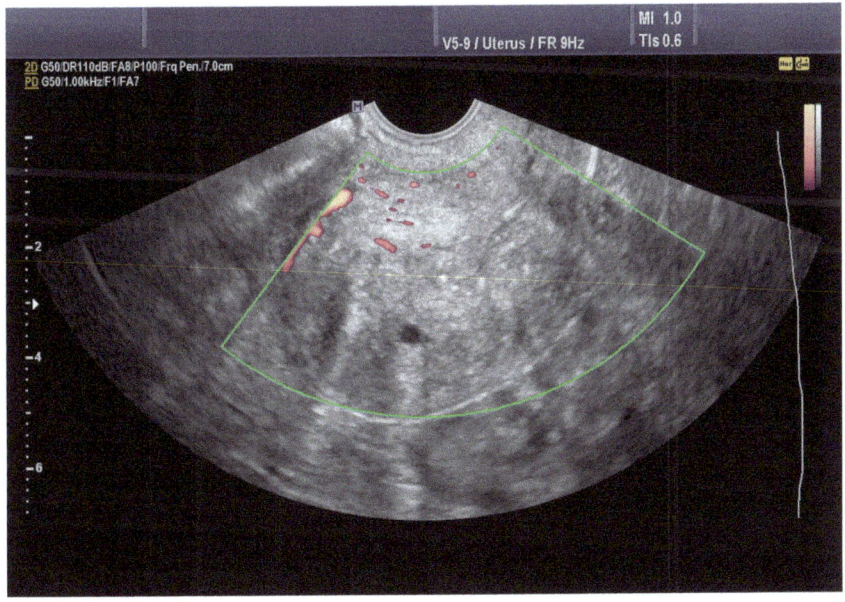

Fig. 6.4.15: Myometrial cysts and adenomyosis seen on TVS

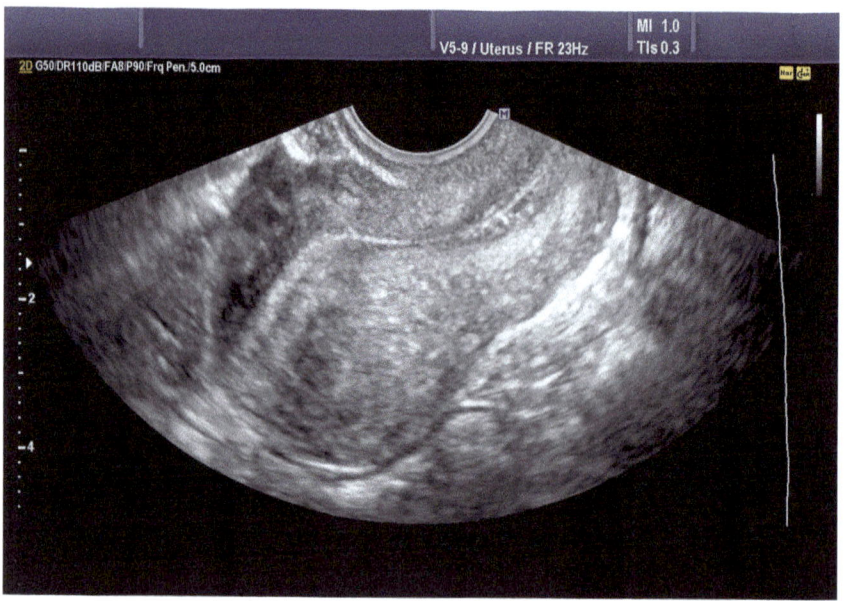

Fig. 6.4.16: Charecteristic myometrium as seen on adenomyosis

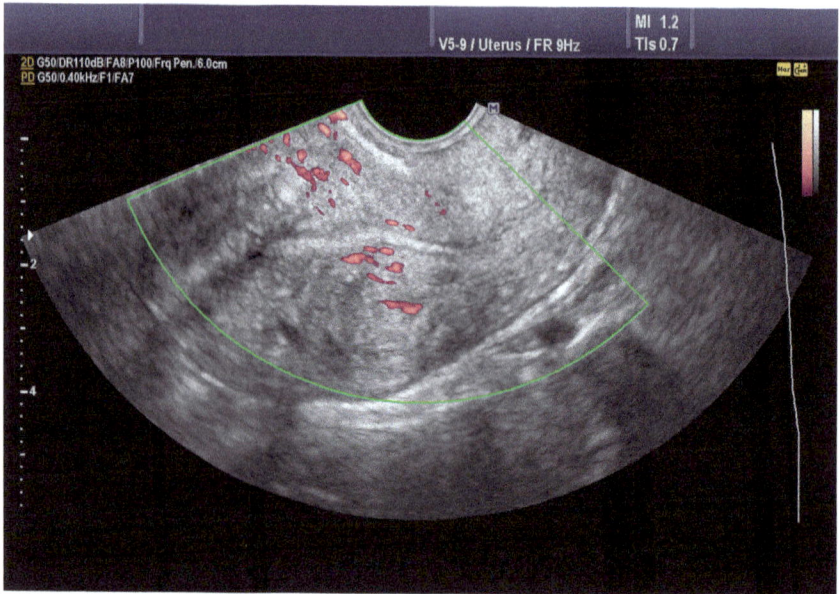

Fig. 6.4.17: Myometrial hyperemia as seen on color flow mapping and power angio studies

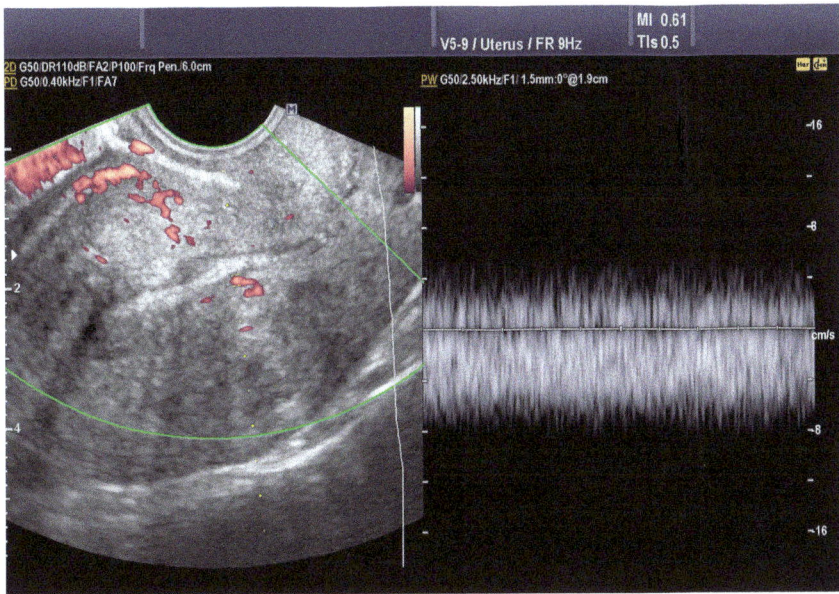

Fig. 6.4.18: Myometrial vascularity as seen on color flow in a patient with adenomyosis

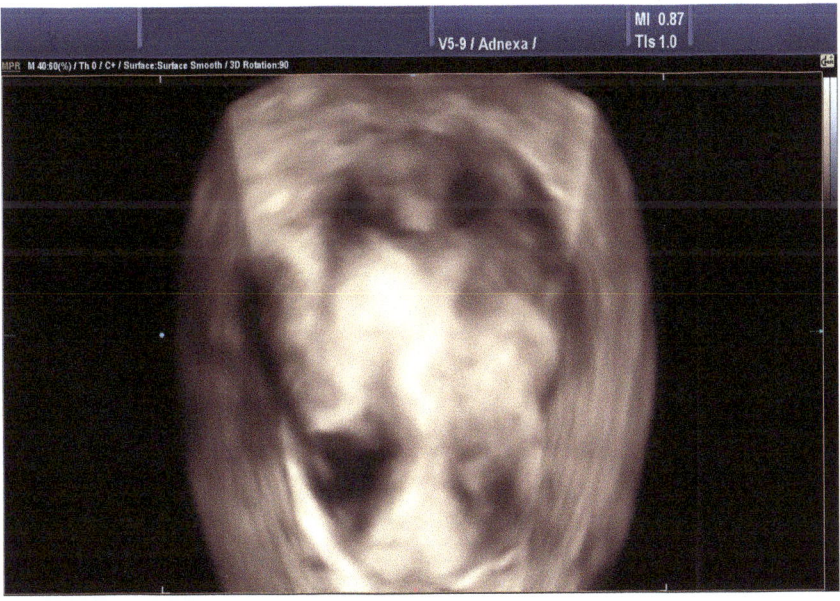

Fig. 6.4.19: 3D of an adenomyotic uterus

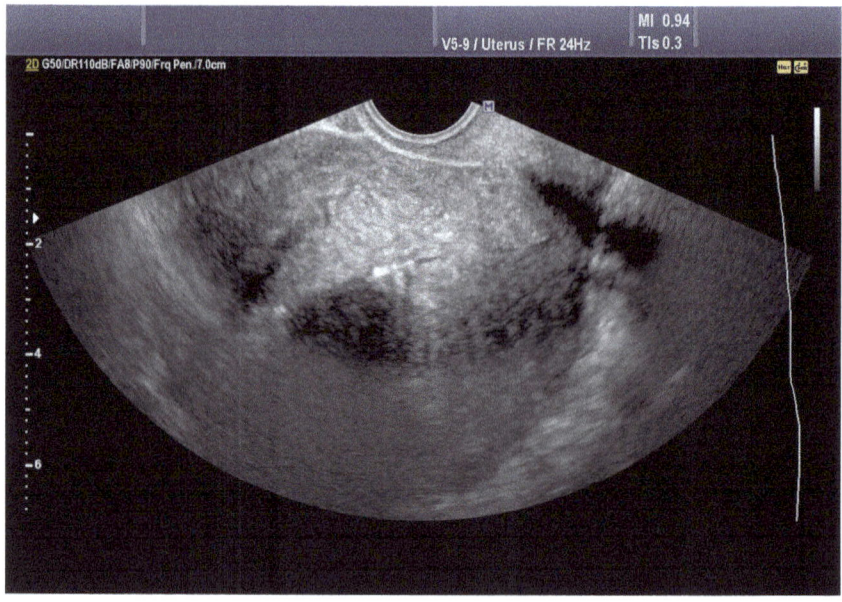

Fig. 6.4.20: IUCD in uterine cavity in an adenomyotic uterus

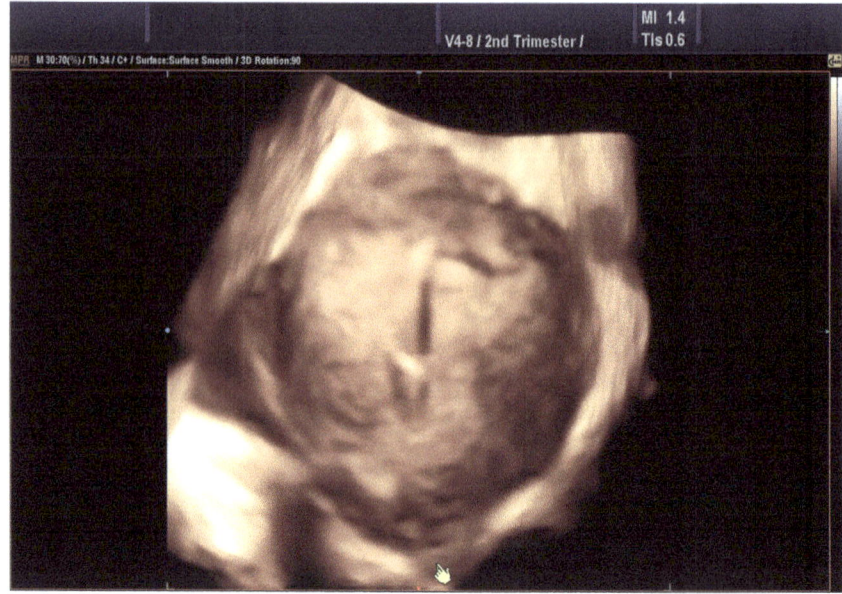

Fig. 6.4.21A: 3D of an IUCD and adenomyosis

6.4. Adenomyosis

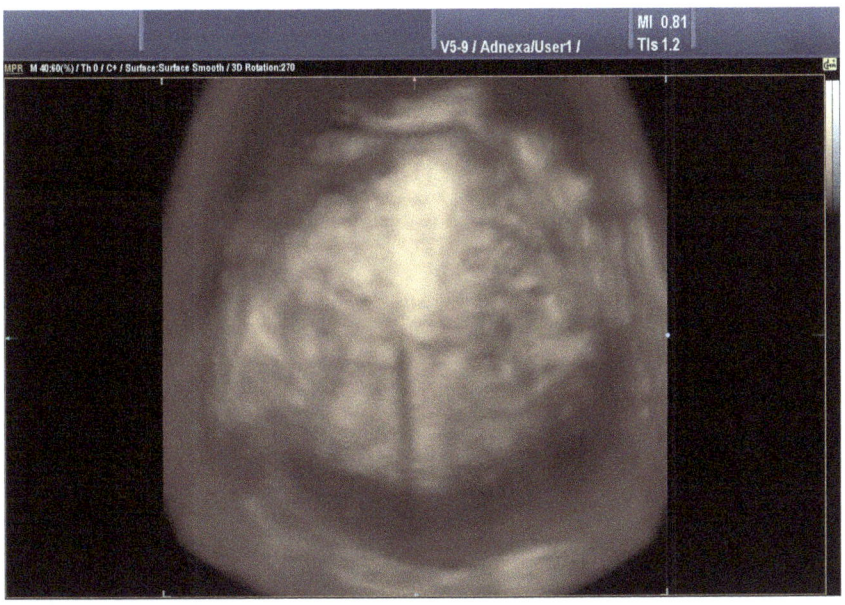

Fig. 6.4.21B: 3D reconstruction of the myometrium with an IUCD in the cavity

6.5. ASHERMAN'S SYNDROME

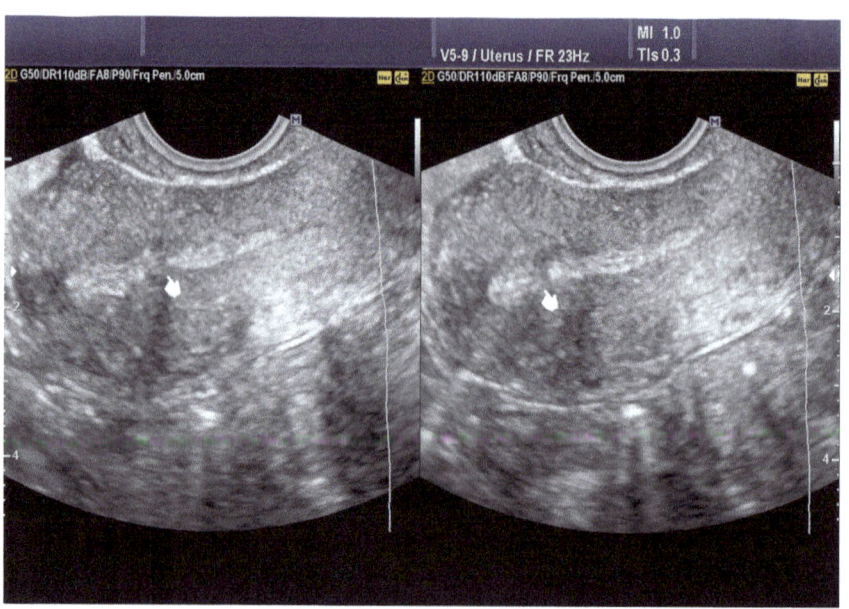

6.5. Asherman's Syndrome

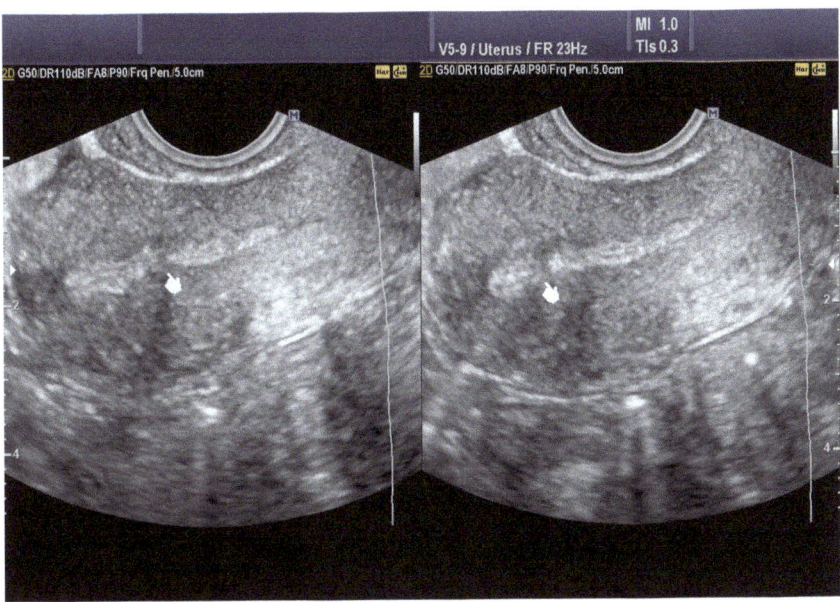

Fig. 6.5.1: Scarring in the endometrium with development of bands which are synechiae seen on TVS

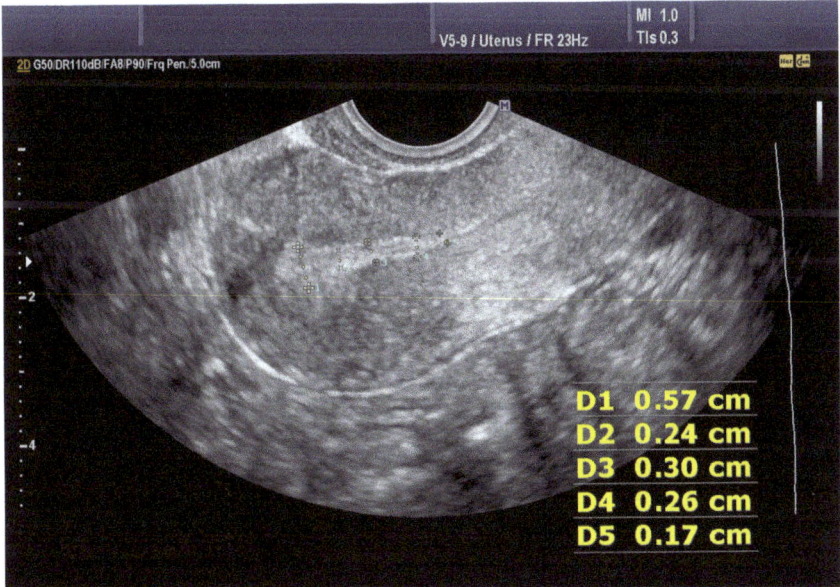

Fig. 6.5.2: Can result because of excessive curetting or tuberculosis. On TVS irregular thickening of endometrium with a careful history is important

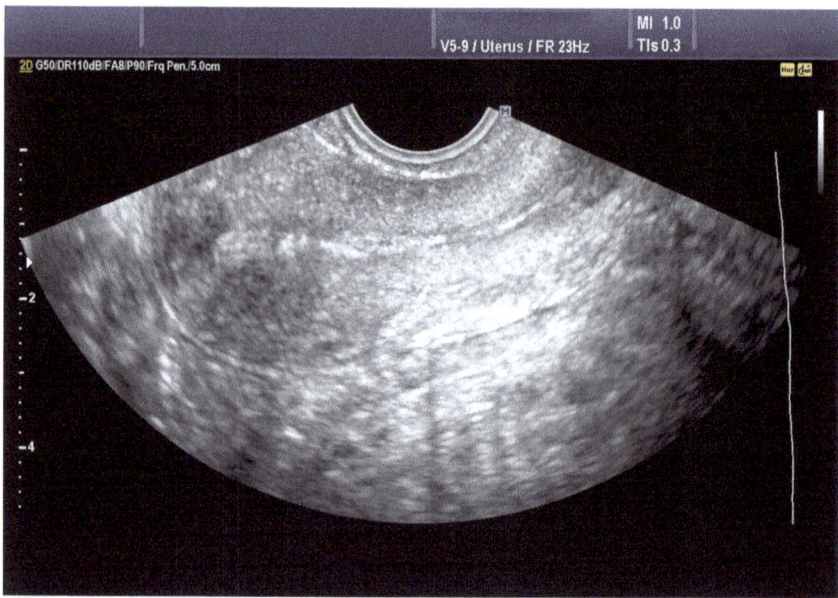

Fig. 6.5.3: Visualizing the cavity in the menstrual phase or sonohysterography (outline by fluid/blood) gives the best picture

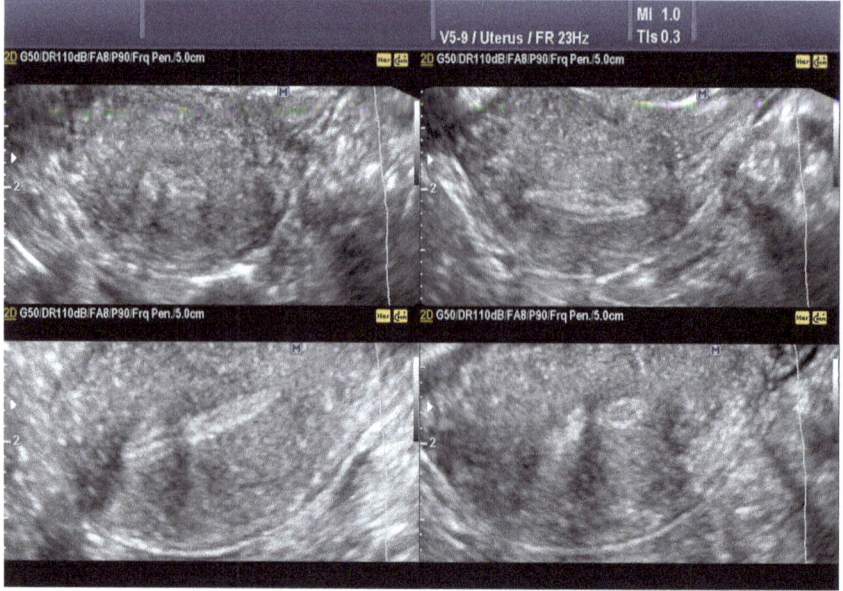

Fig. 6.5.4: Intrauterine adhesions can be accurately visualized in multiplaner imaging of the uterine cavity

6.5. Asherman's Syndrome

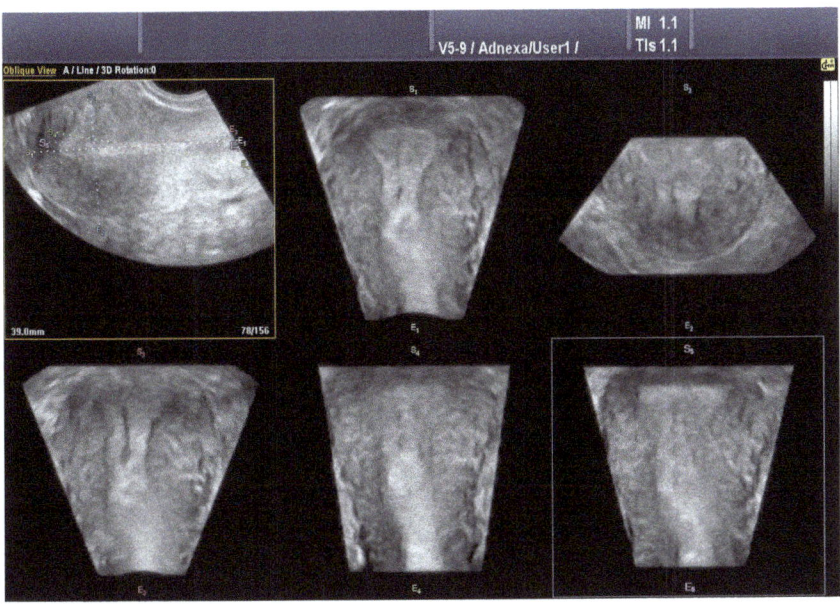

Fig. 6.5.5: 3D rendering gives location of the bands traversing the uterine cavity

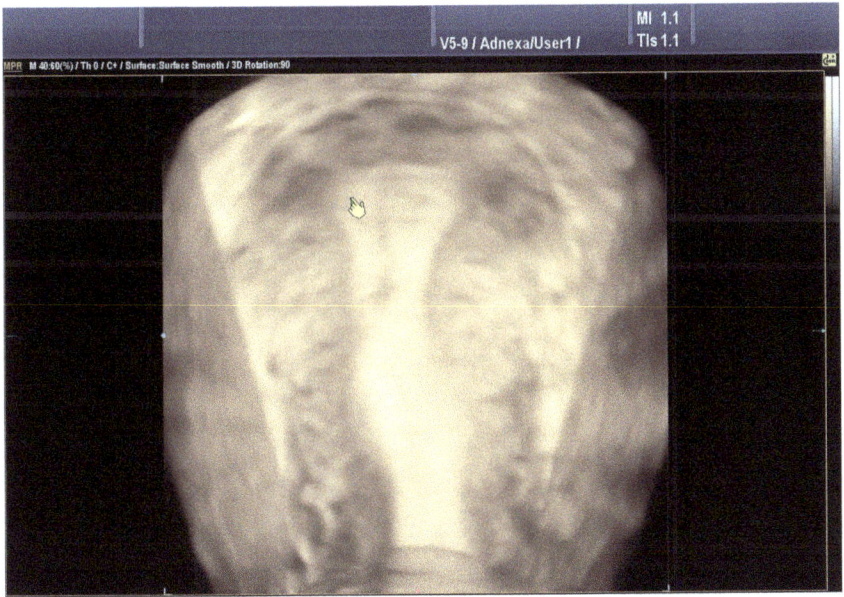

Fig. 6.5.6: 3D ultrasound helps in surgical planning

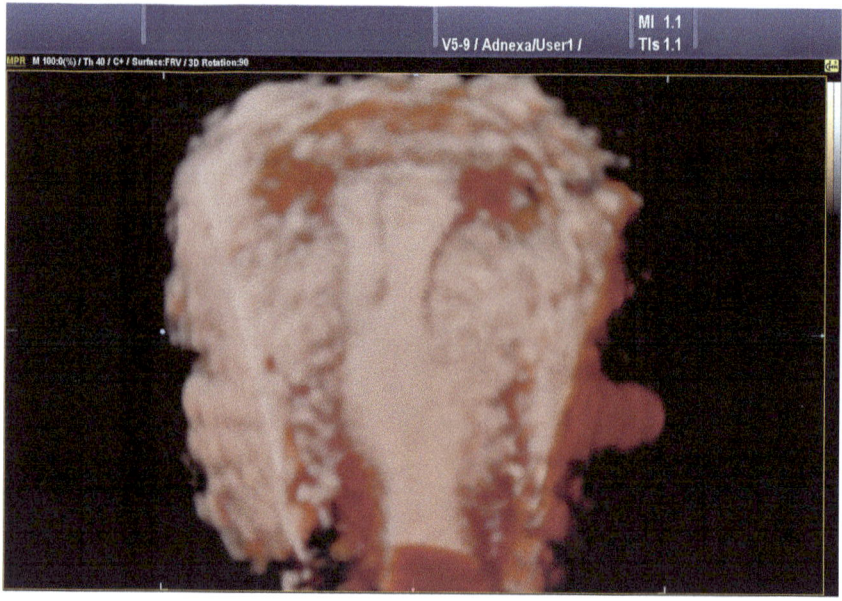

Fig. 6.5.7: The degree of obliteration can be assessed on 3D US

6.6. ENDOMETRIAL POLYP

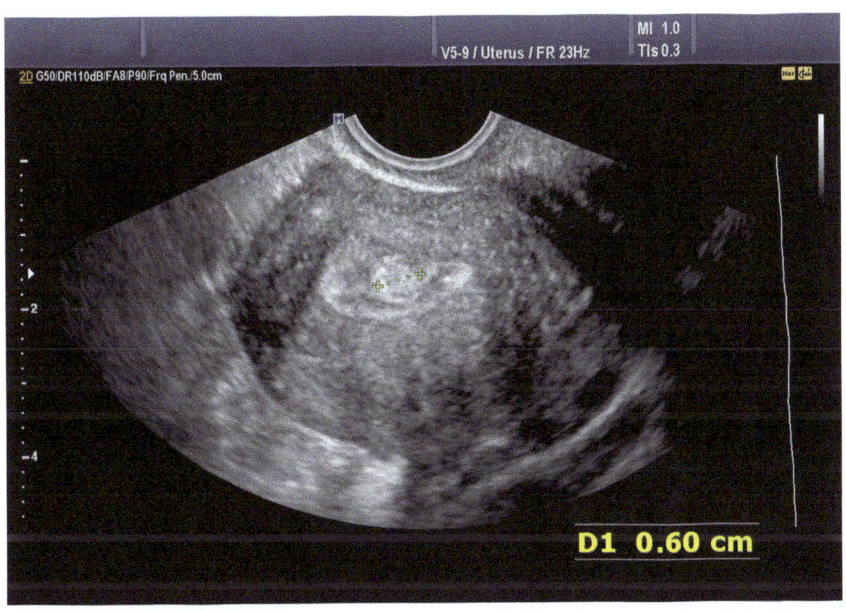

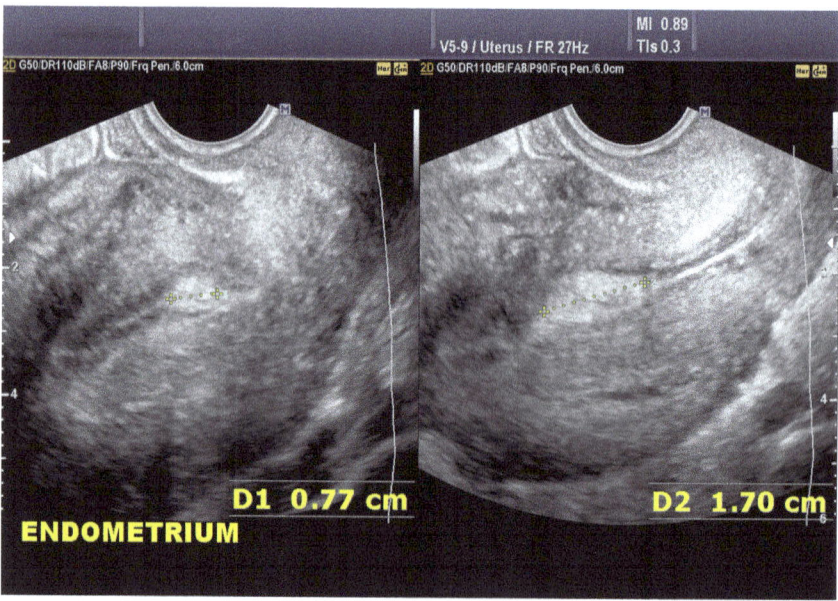

Fig. 6.6.1: Polyps can manifest as symptoms of infertility or menstrual problem

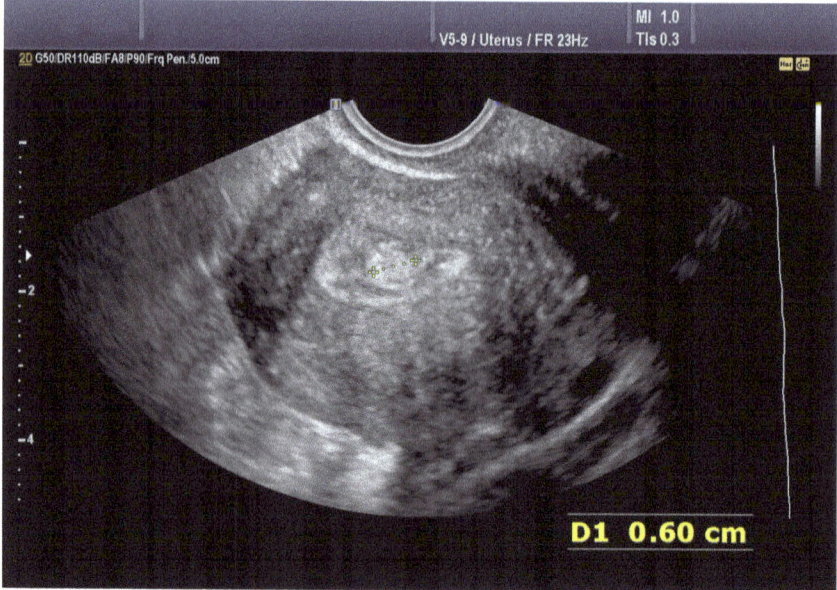

Fig. 6.6.2: Patient with irregular menstrual bleeding, bleeding between periods and menometrorrhagia should be evaluated for polyps

6.6. Endometrial Polyp

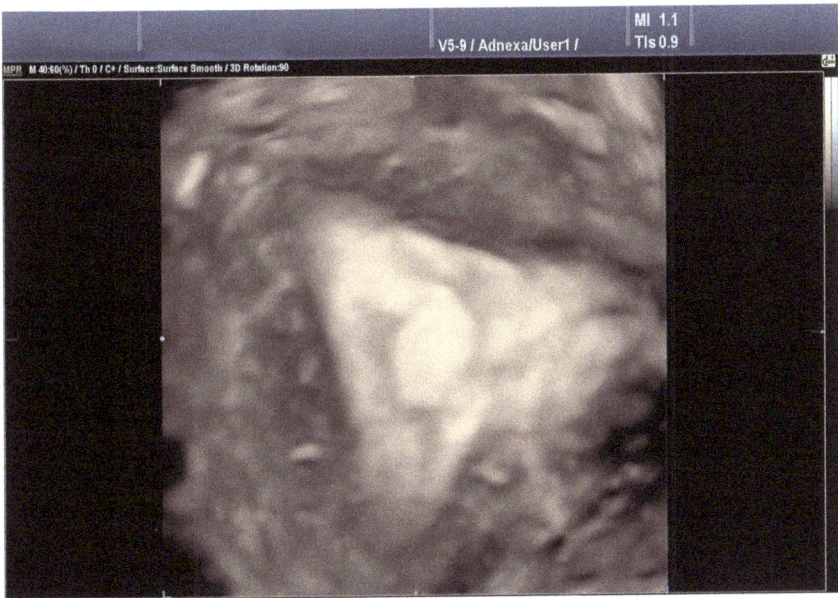

Fig. 6.6.3: Polyp on a 3D scan

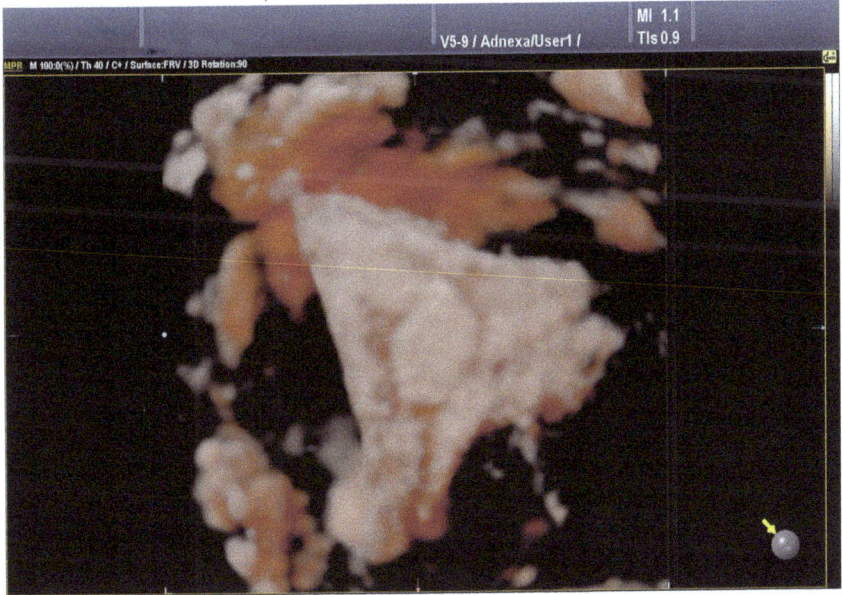

Fig. 6.6.4: Polyp on a 3D scan

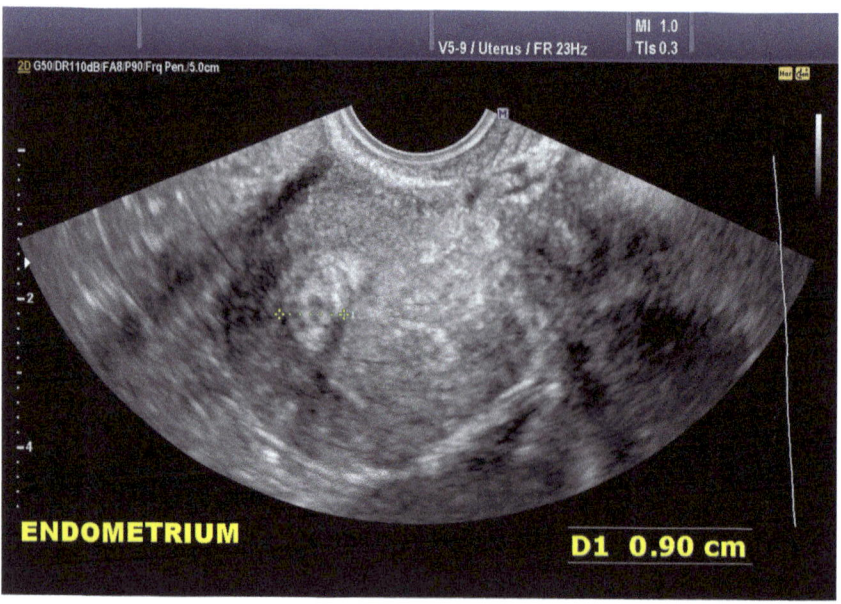

Fig. 6.6.5: Polyps should carefully be seen on a thickened hyperplastic endometrium

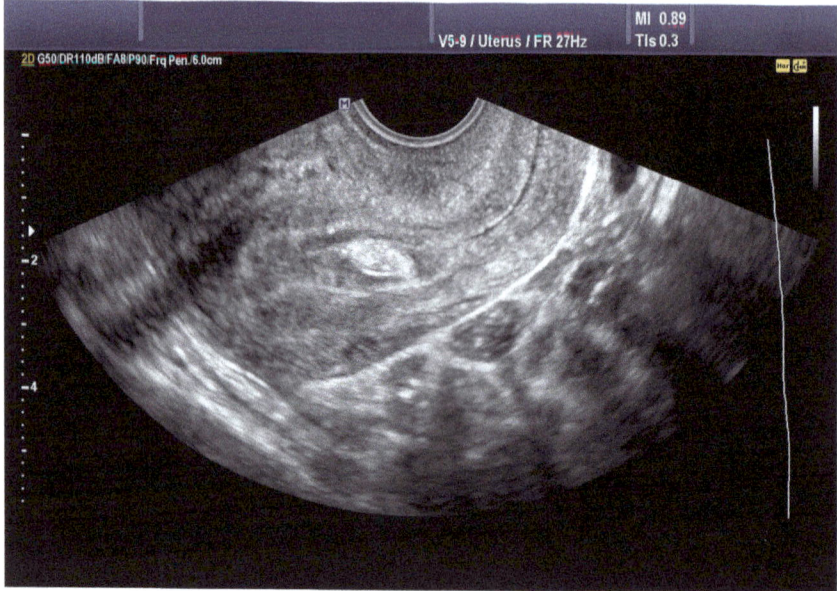

Fig. 6.6.6: Polyps can be seen in the corpus

6.6. Endometrial Polyp

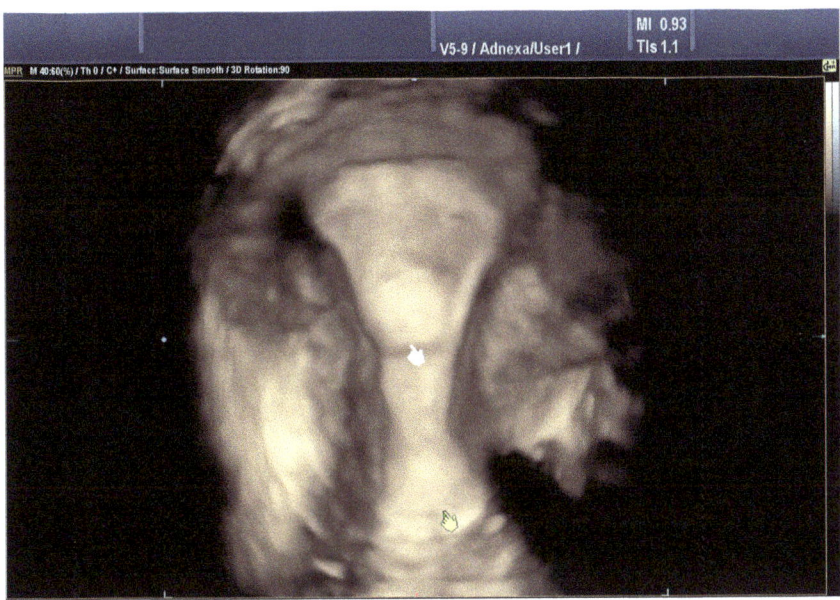

Fig. 6.6.7: Seen on 3D scan in the corpus

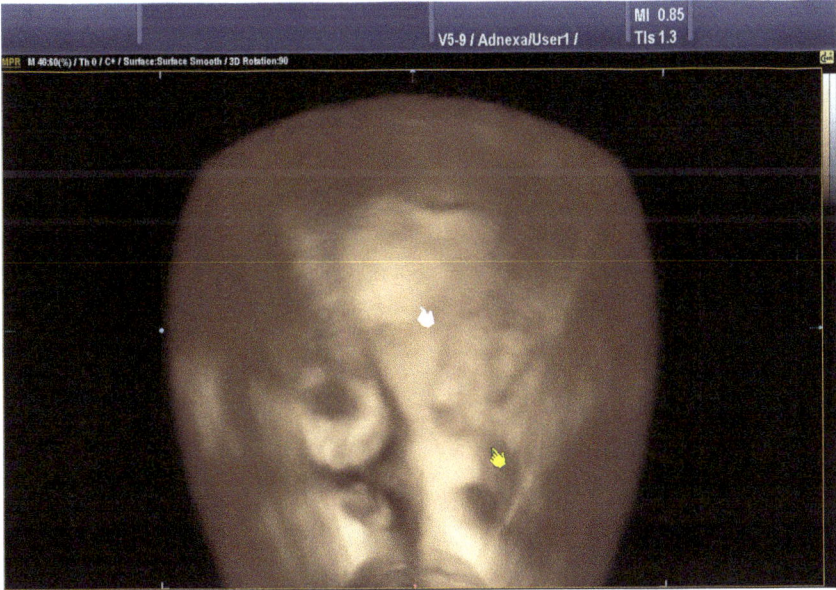

Fig. 6.6.8: Can be seen in the subfundal area

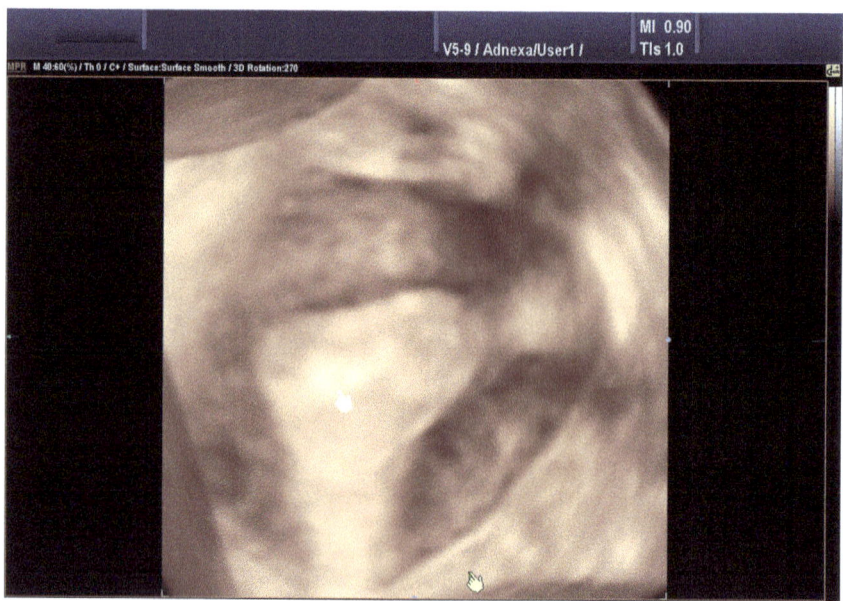

Fig. 6.6.9: Polyp seen in the right subfundal area

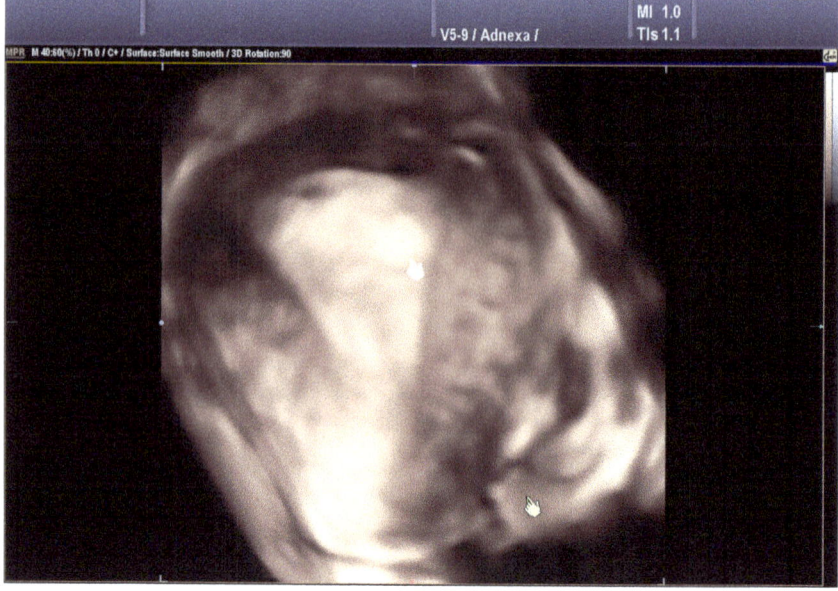

Fig. 6.6.10: Polyp seen in the left subfundal area

6.6. Endometrial Polyp

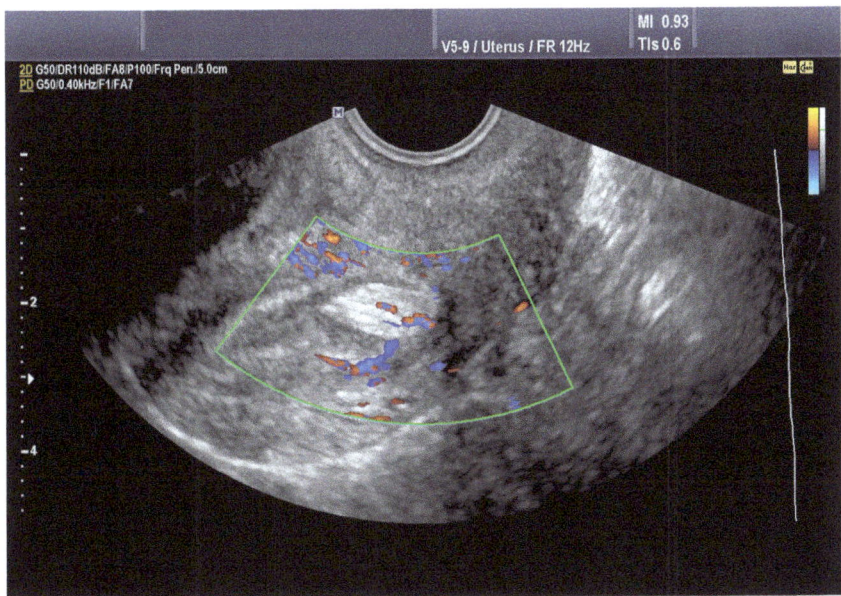

Fig. 6.6.11: Vascularity of the polyps as seen on color flow mapping

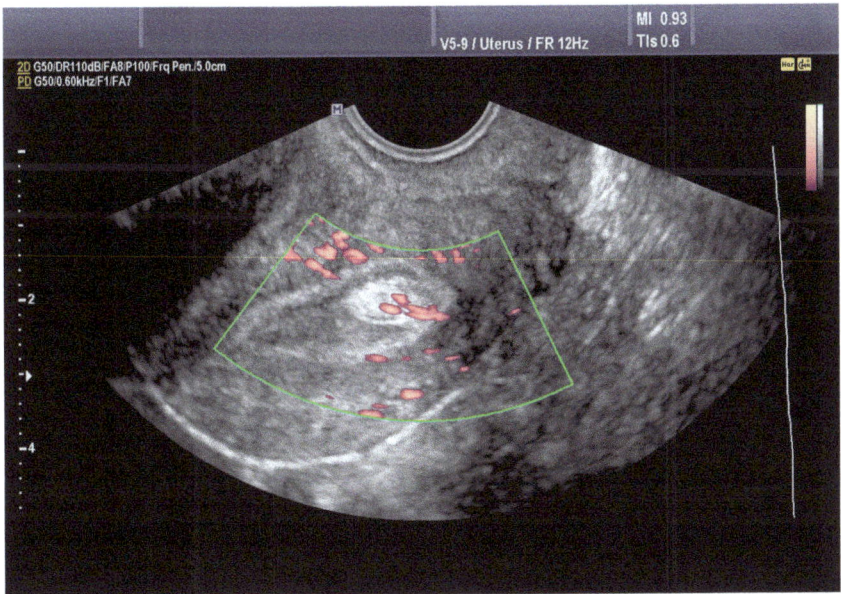

Fig. 6.6.12: Vascularity as seen on power angio studies

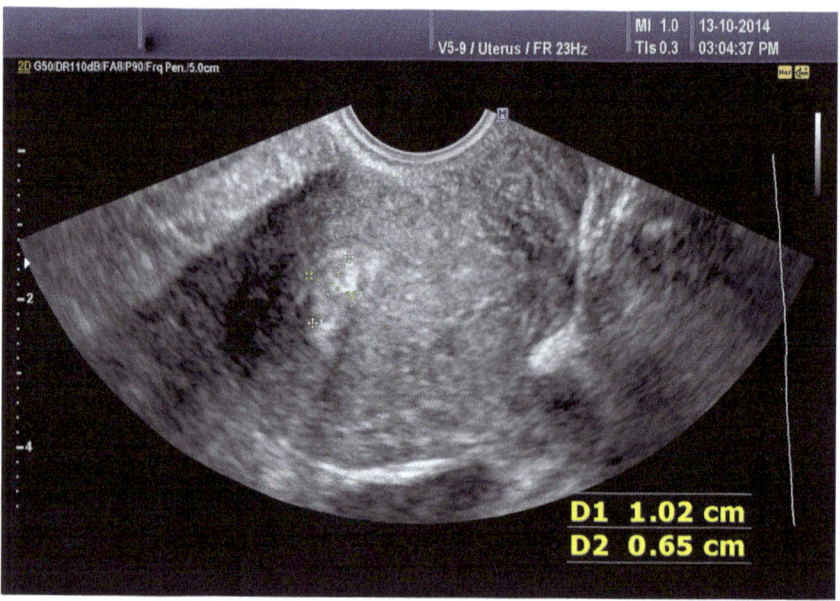

Fig. 6.6.13: Thick inhomogeneous endometrium with an endometrial polyp

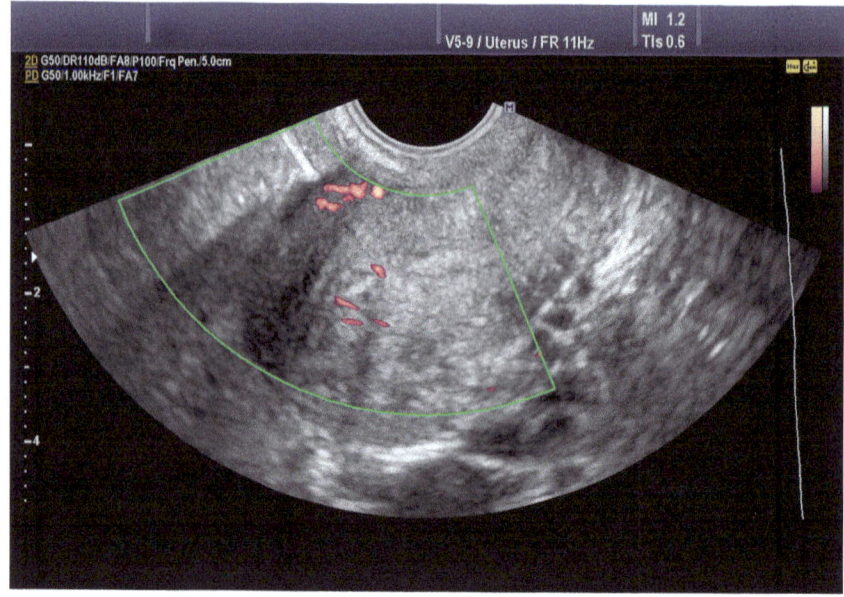

Fig. 6.6.14: Vascularity in the endometrial polyp

6.6. Endometrial Polyp

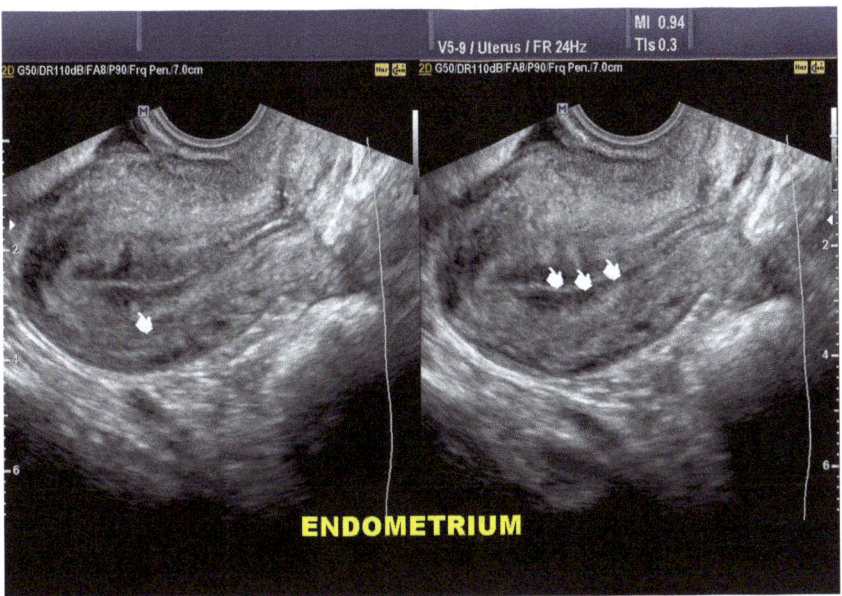

Fig. 6.6.15: Polyps can be solitary or multiple

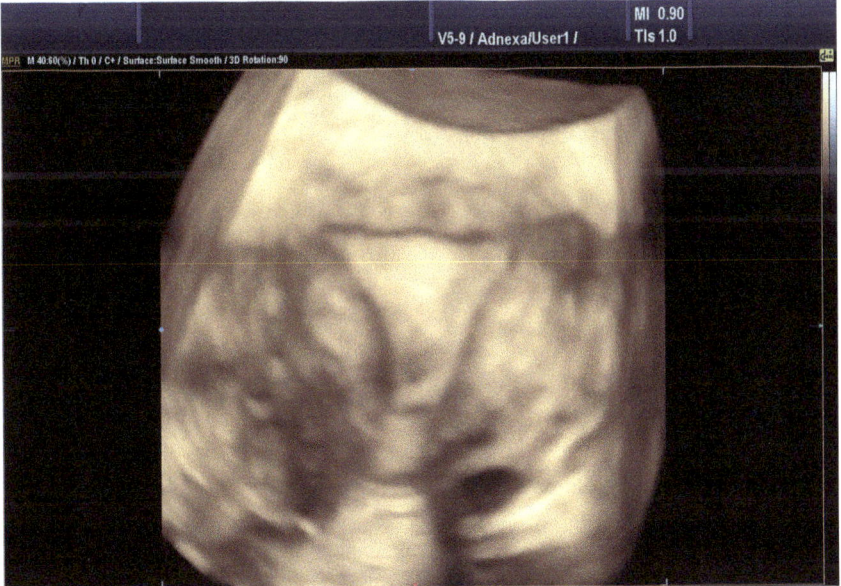

Fig. 6.6.16: Single polyp seen in the endometrium

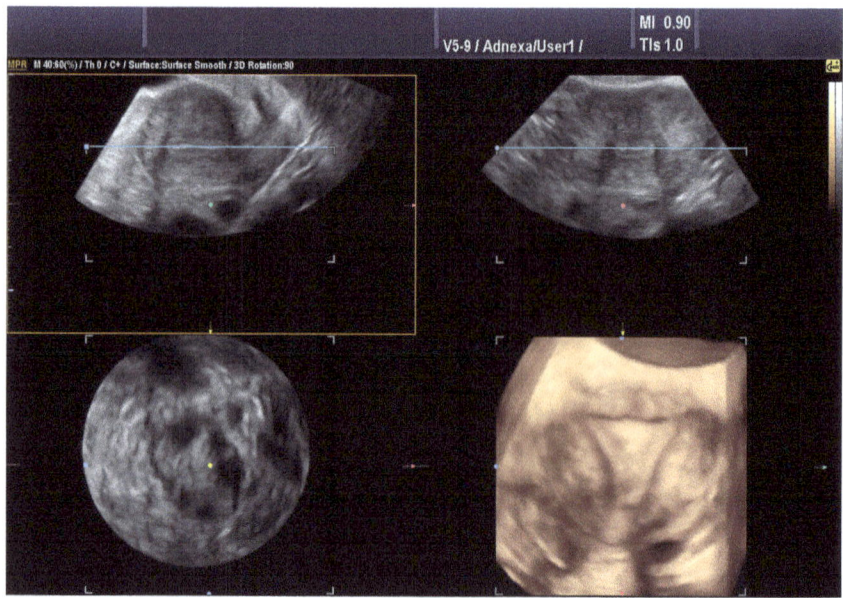

Fig. 6.6.17: As seen on 3D

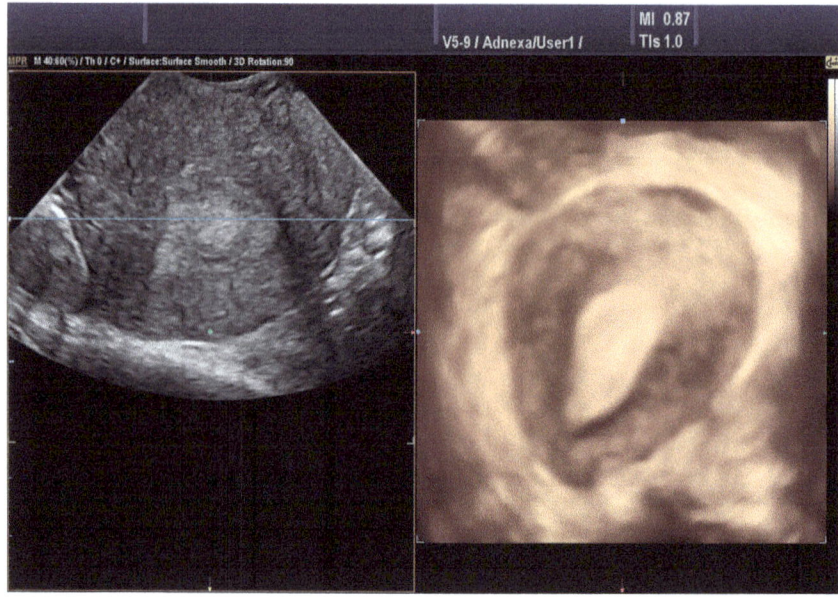

Fig. 6.6.18: Polyp on 3D

6.6. Endometrial Polyp

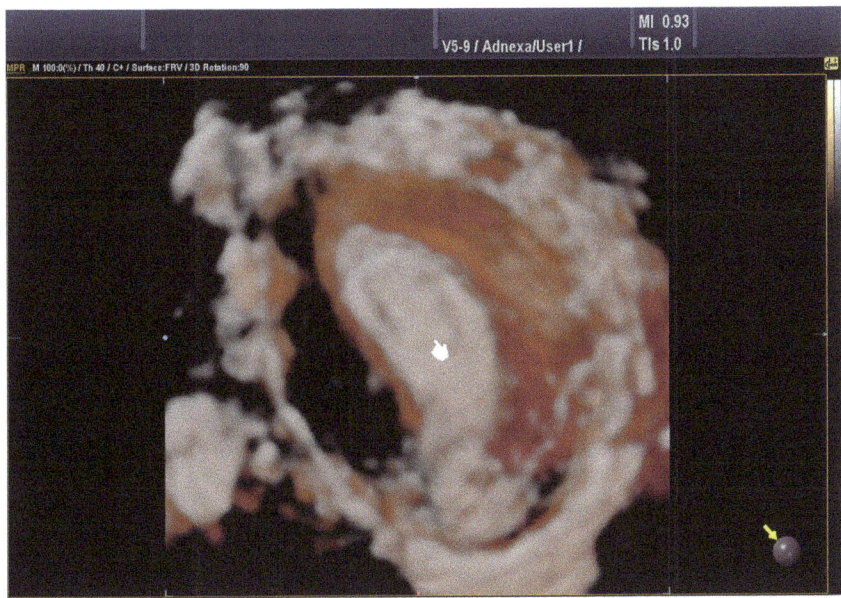

Fig. 6.6.19: Endometrial polyp on 3D

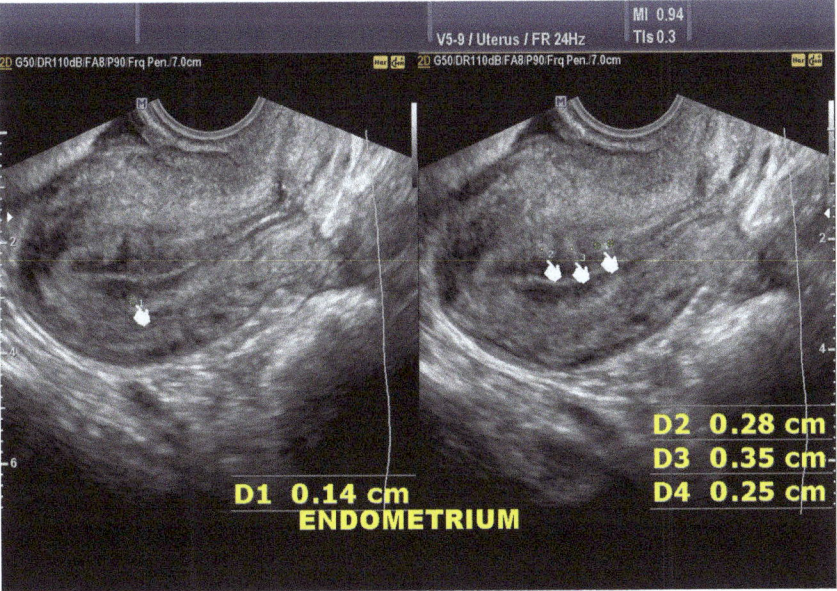

Fig. 6.6.20: Polyps can be small or large

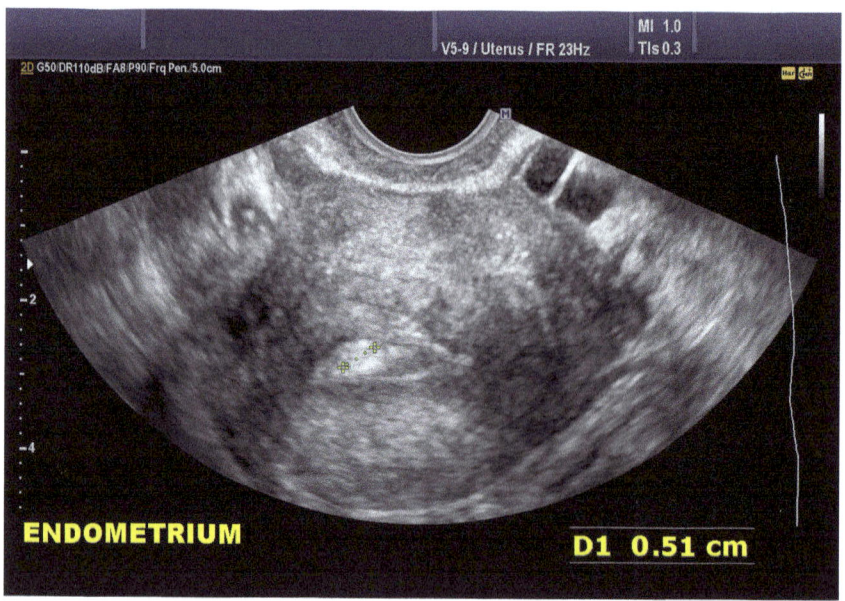

Fig. 6.6.21: 5.1 mm endometrial polyp

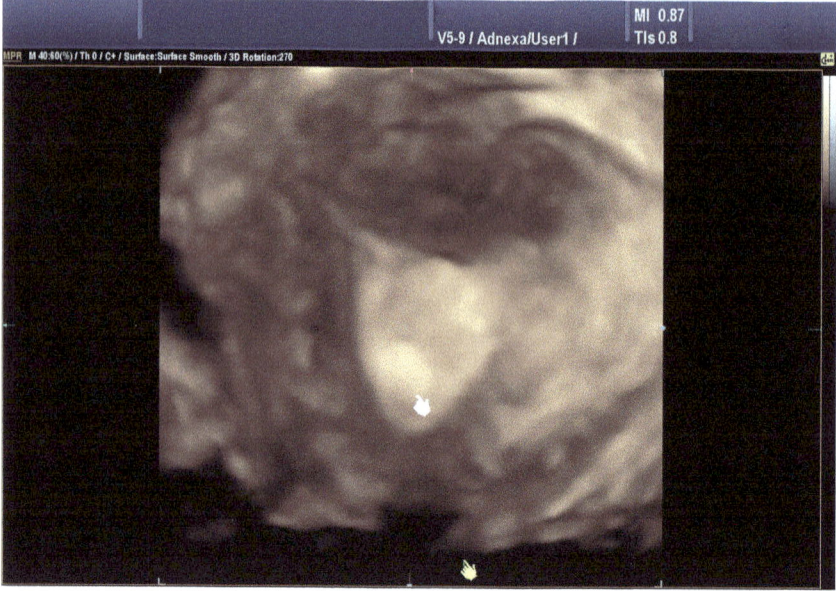

Fig. 6.6.22: As seen on 3D

6.6. Endometrial Polyp

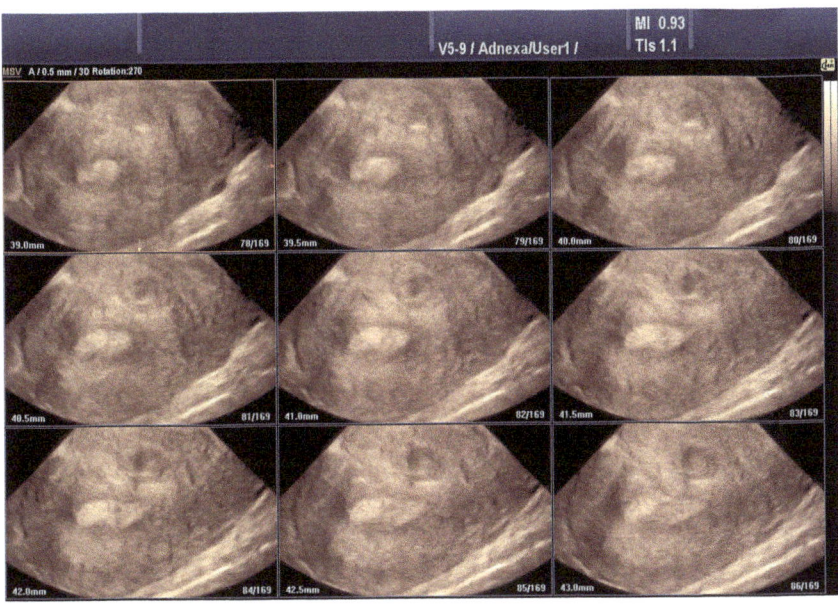

Fig. 6.6.23: As seen on multislice views

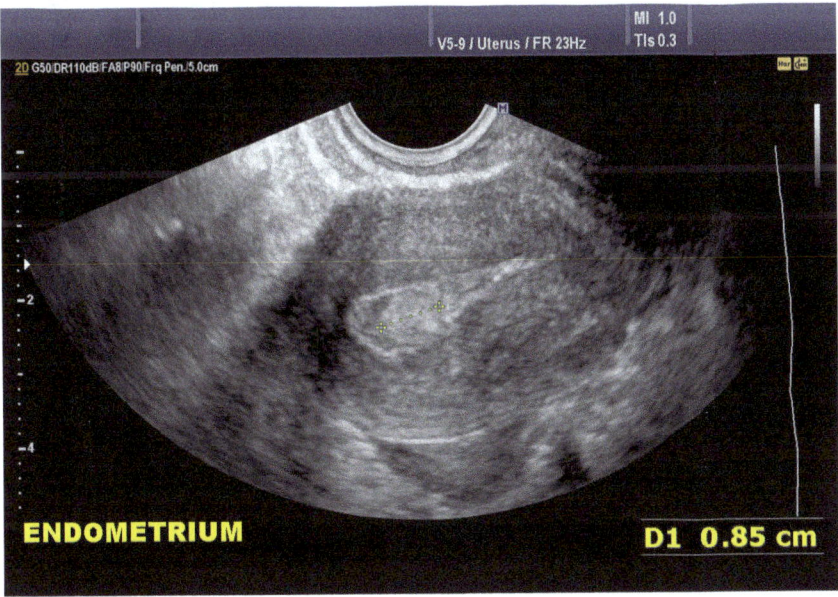

Fig. 6.6.24: An 8.5 mm polyp in the subfundal area

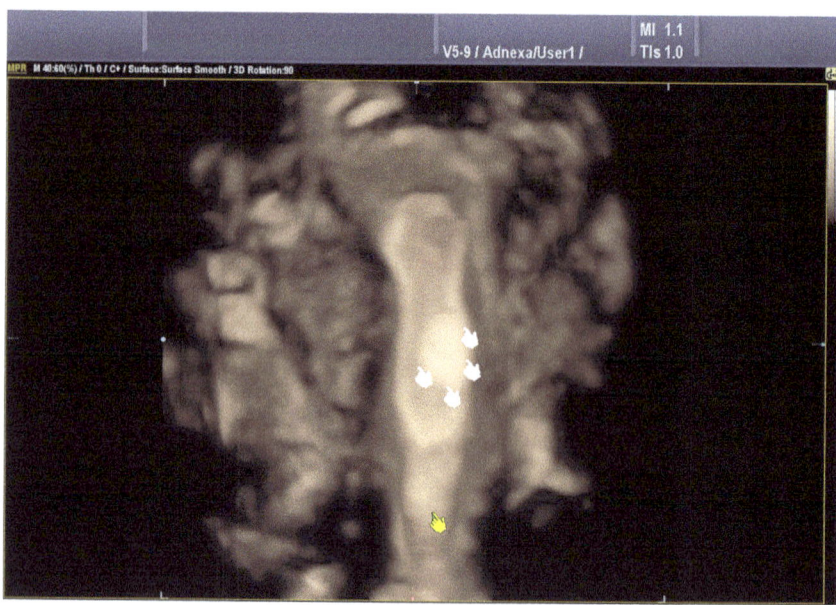

Fig. 6.6.25: Polyp in the uterine corpus left side

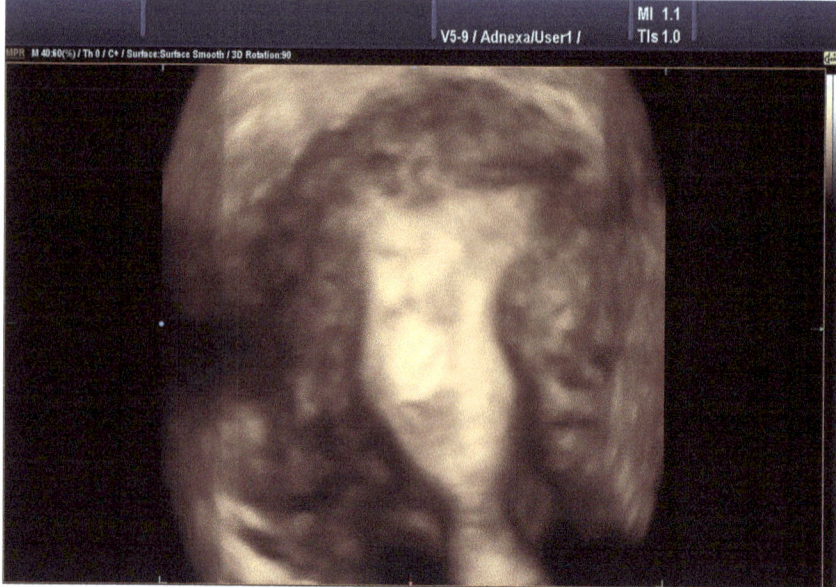

Fig. 6.6.26: Polyp in the uterine corpus right side

6.6. Endometrial Polyp

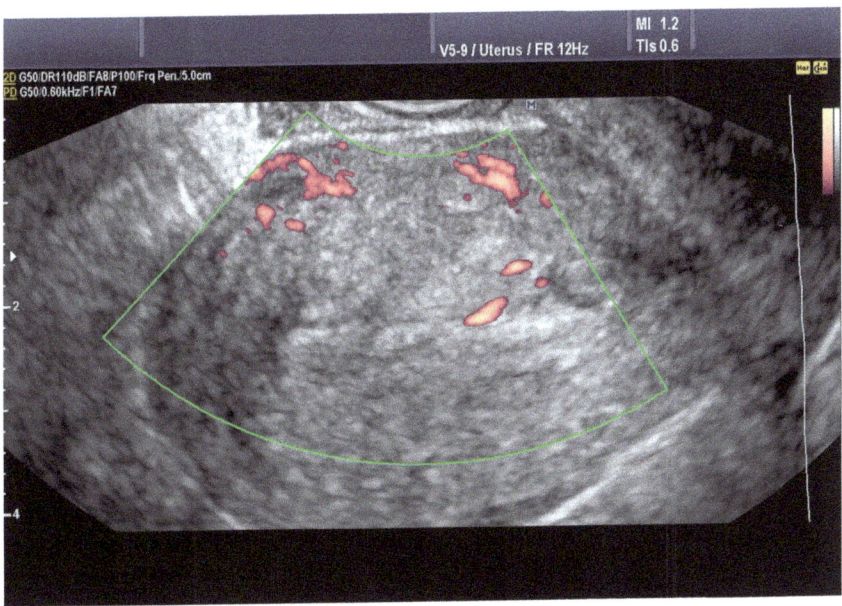

Fig. 6.6.27: In cases of infection associated with a polyp increased vascularity is delineated

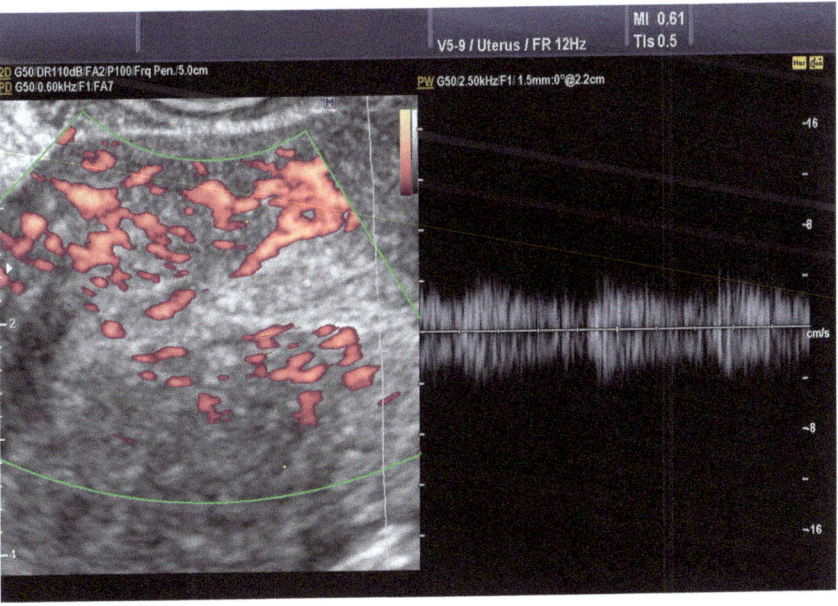

Fig. 6.6.28: Low impedance flow should not give a false risk of endometrial malignancy. Careful search for polyps should be done

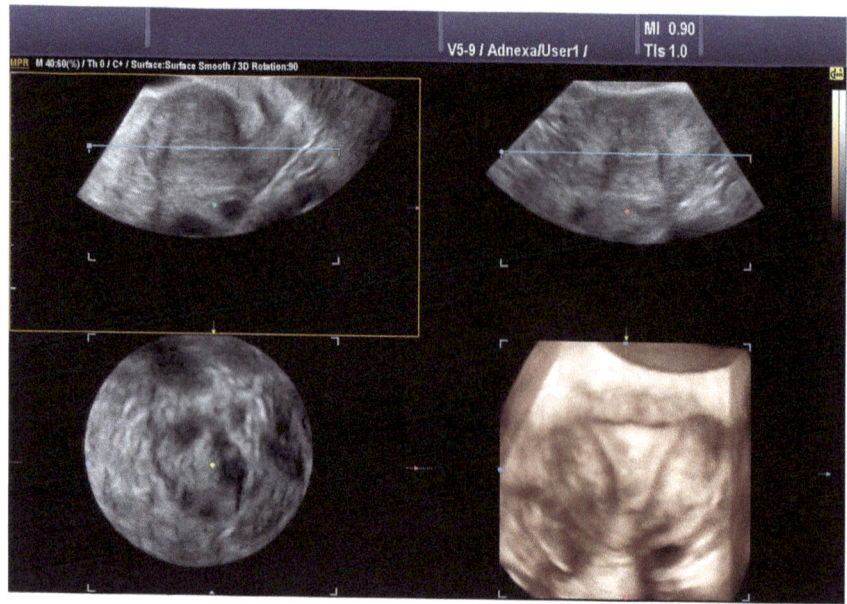

Fig. 6.6.29: Endometrial polyp on MPR

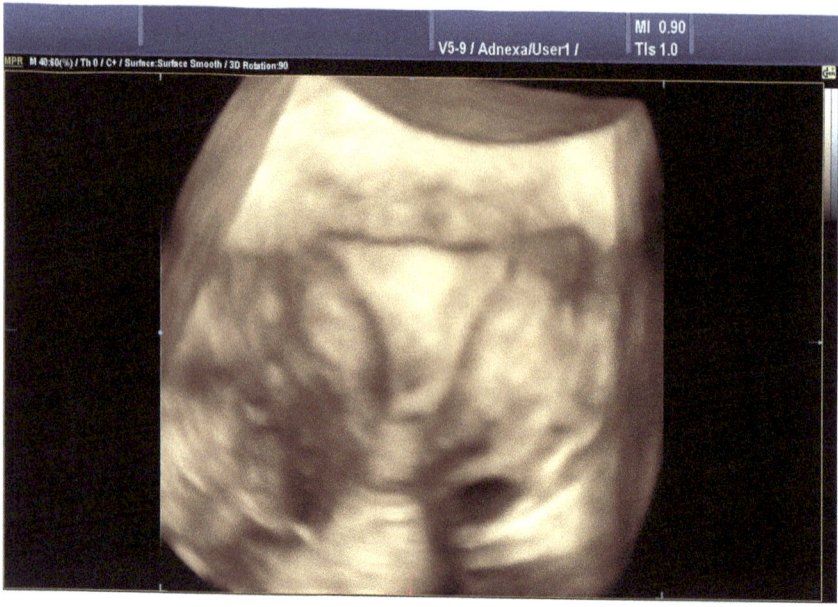

Fig. 6.6.30: 3D scan of endometrial polyp seen at the fundus

6.7. ENDOMETRIUM: ABNORMAL THICKNESS AND ECHO PATTERN

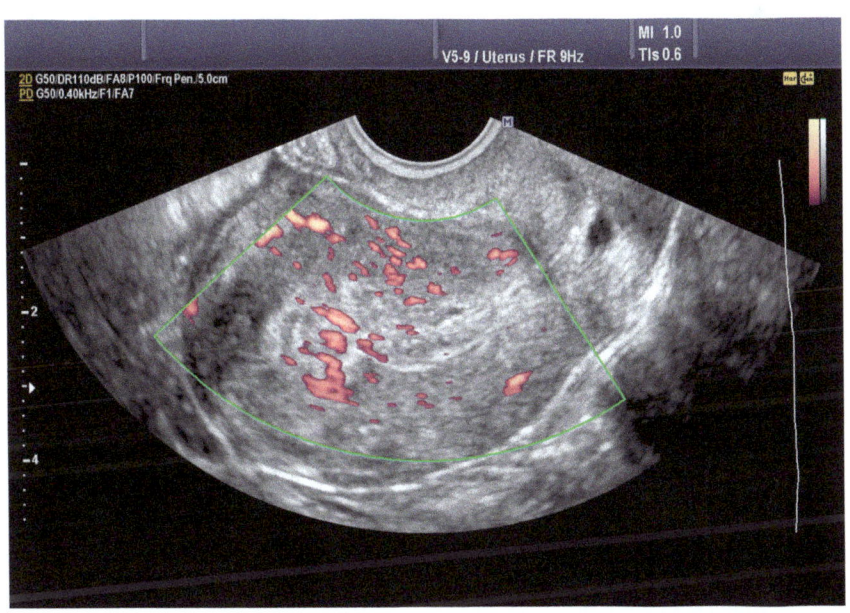

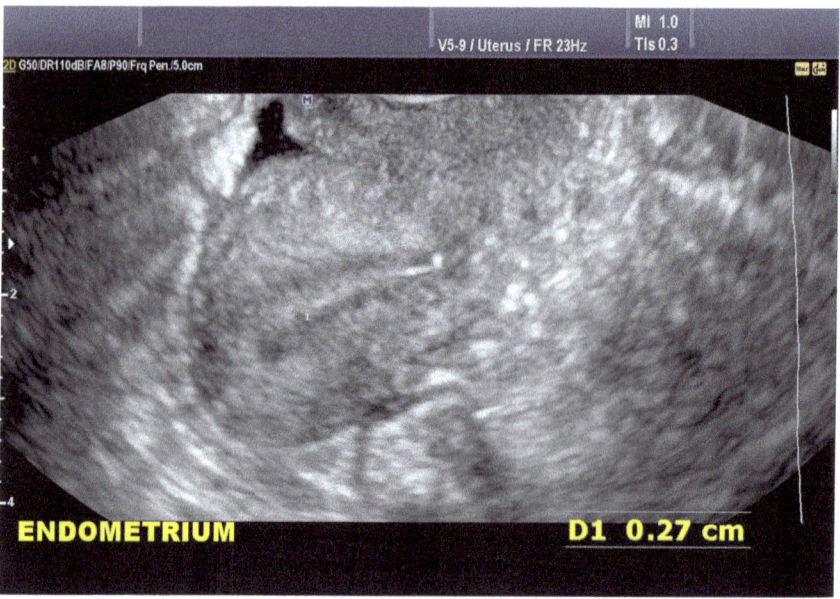

Fig. 6.7.1: Thin endometrium (homogeneous) in a postmenopausal woman

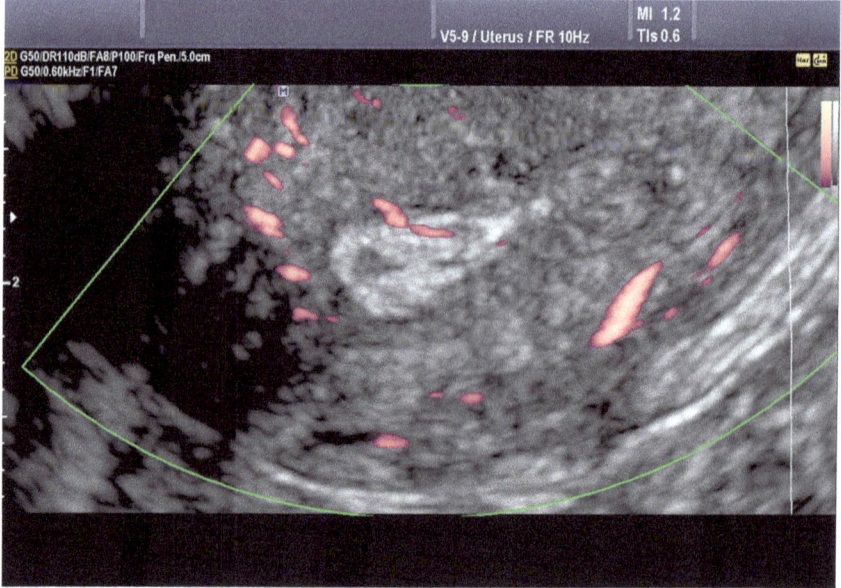

Fig. 6.7.2: Increased vascularity on the anterior aspect needs to be sampled

6.7. Endometrium: Abnormal Thickness and Echo Pattern

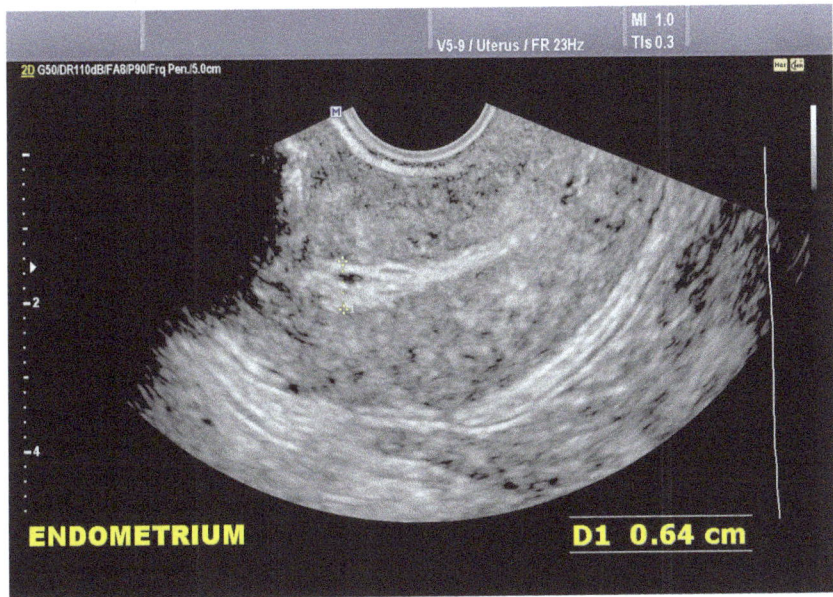

Fig. 6.7.3: Thick irregular endometrium in a postmenopausal woman

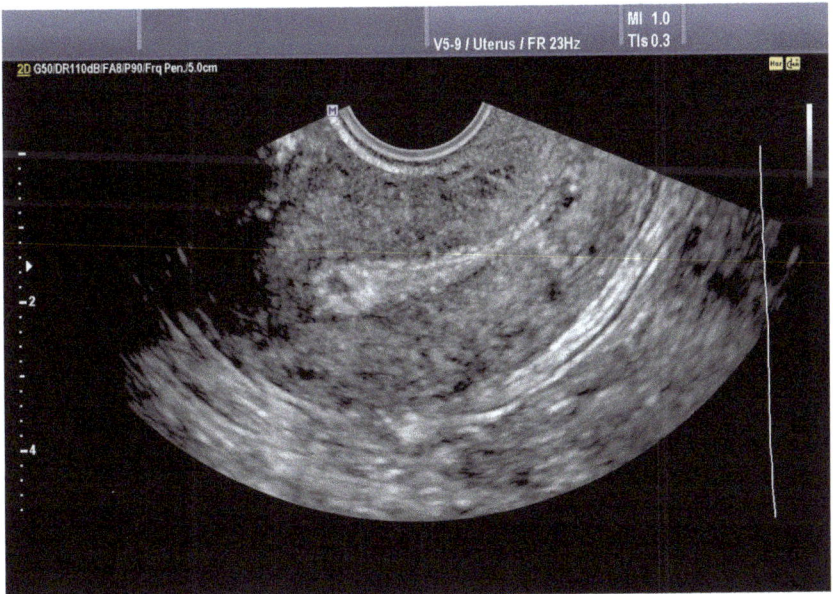

Fig. 6.7.4: Endometrium in a postmenopausal woman with bleeding

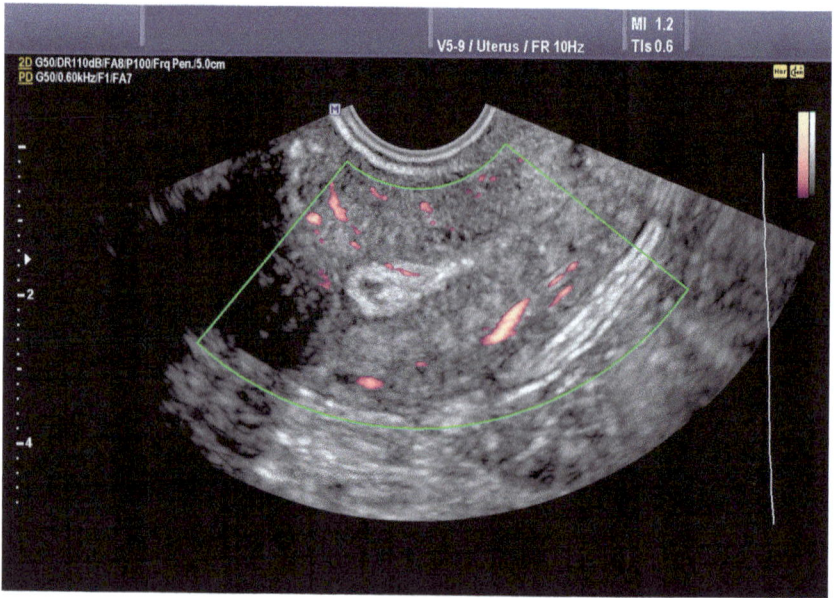

Fig. 6.7.5: Same as seen on color flow mapping

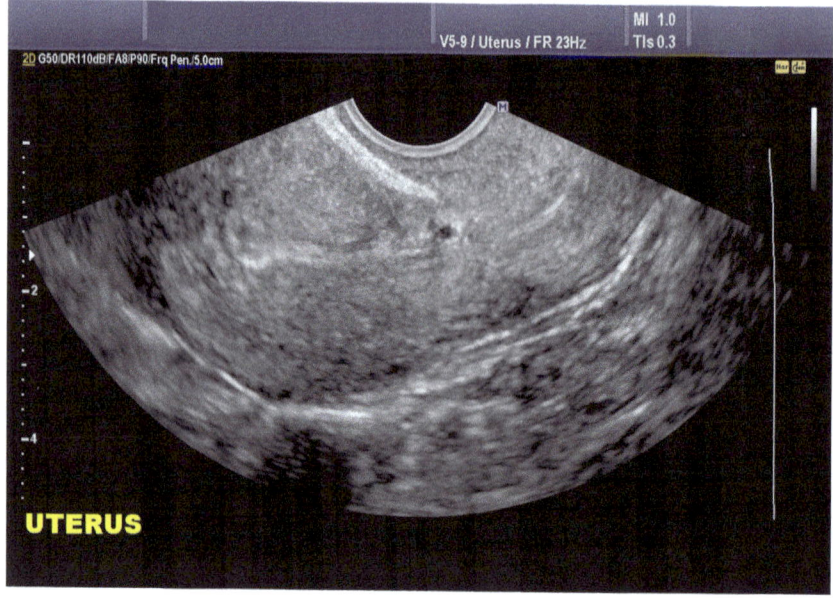

Fig. 6.7.6: Irregularly thickened endometrium

6.7. Endometrium: Abnormal Thickness and Echo Pattern

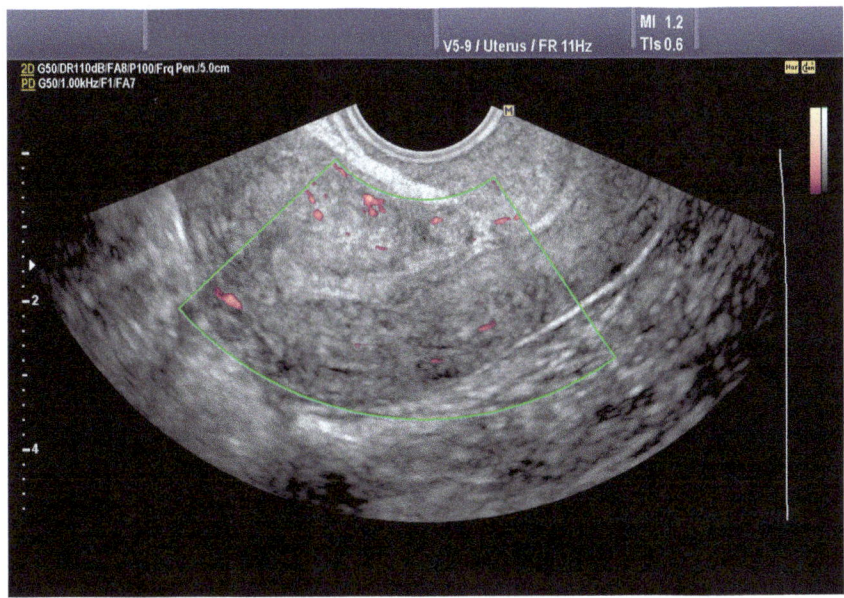

Fig. 6.7.7: Irregularly thickened endometrium as seen on color flow mapping

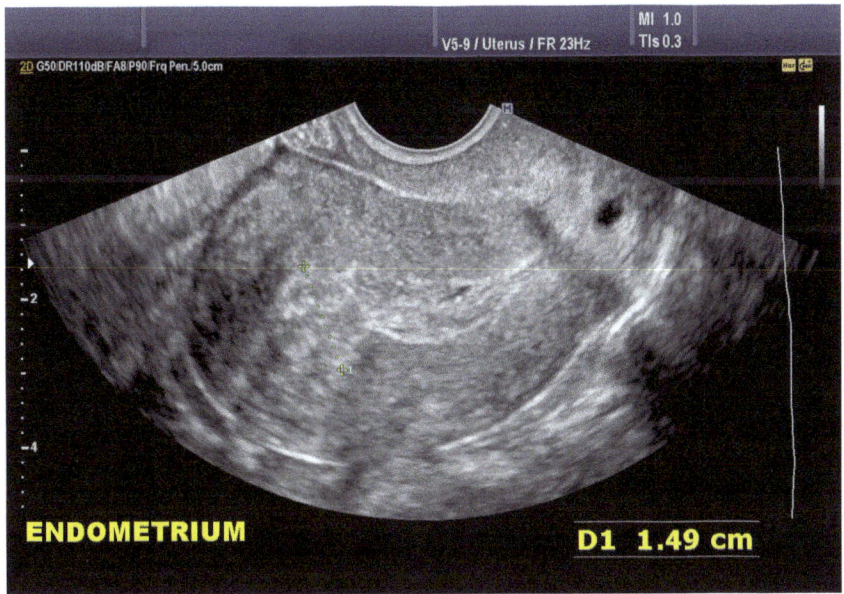

Fig. 6.7.8: Thick endometrium

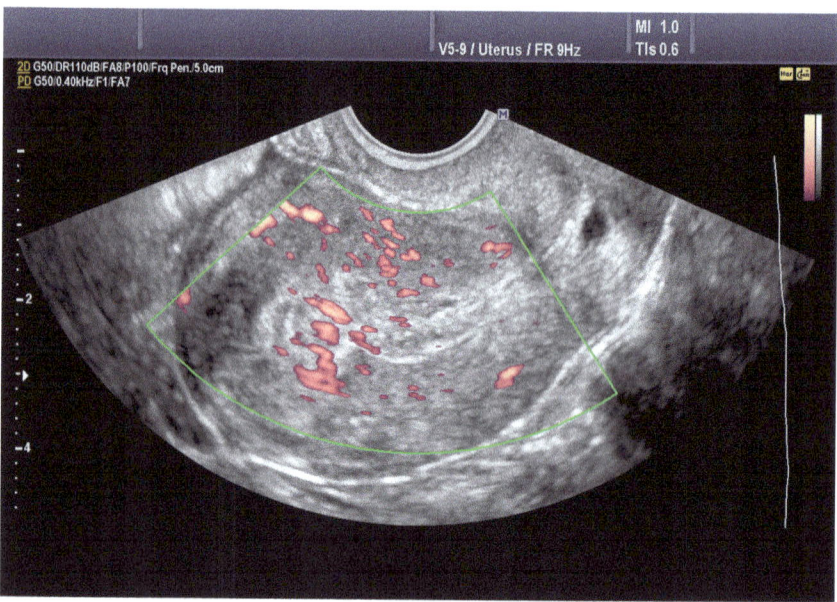

Fig. 6.7.9: Thick endometrium with increased vascularity in the posterior subfundal area

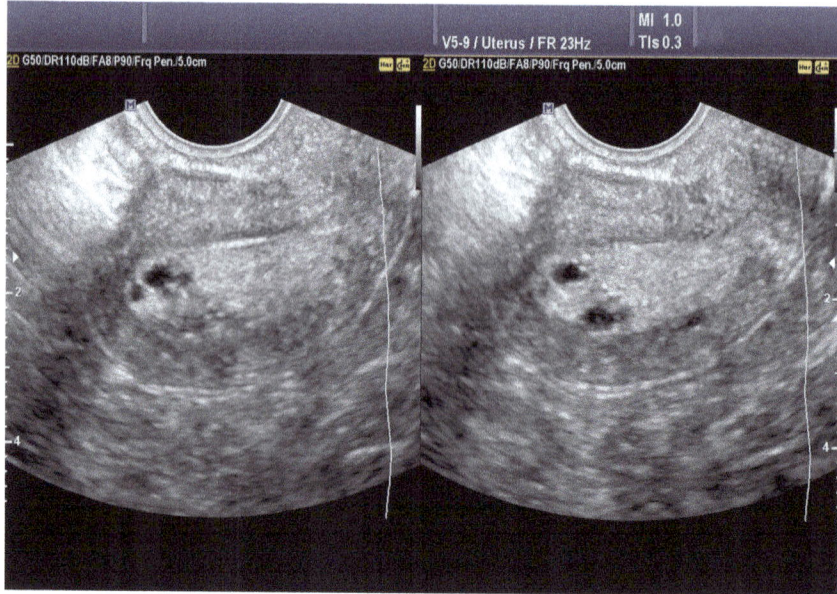

Fig. 6.7.10: Endometrium with multiple cystic spaces

6.7. Endometrium: Abnormal Thickness and Echo Pattern

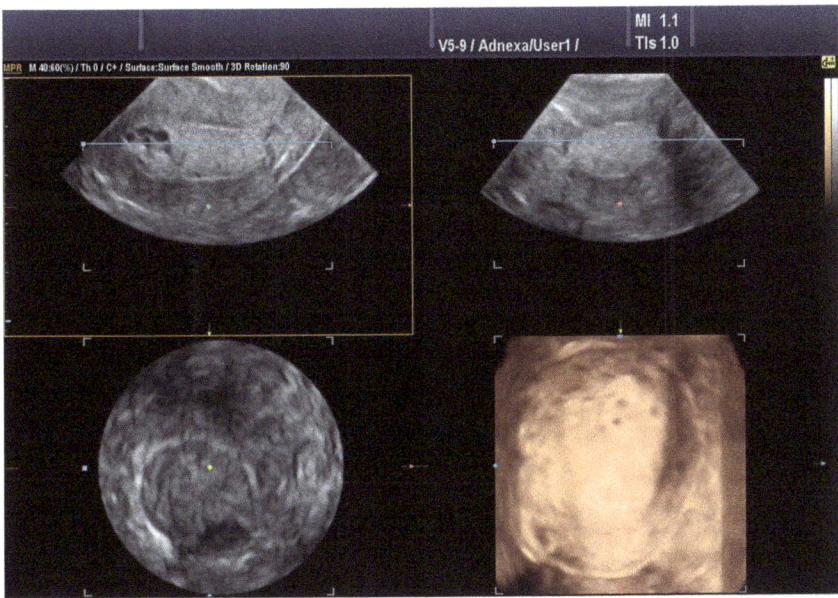

Fig. 6.7.11: As seen on MPR

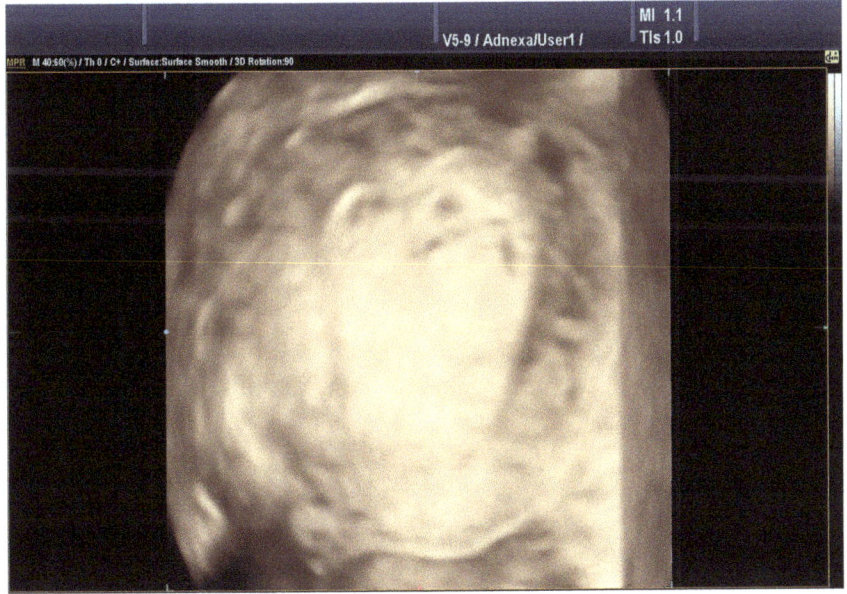

Fig. 6.7.12: As seen on 3D

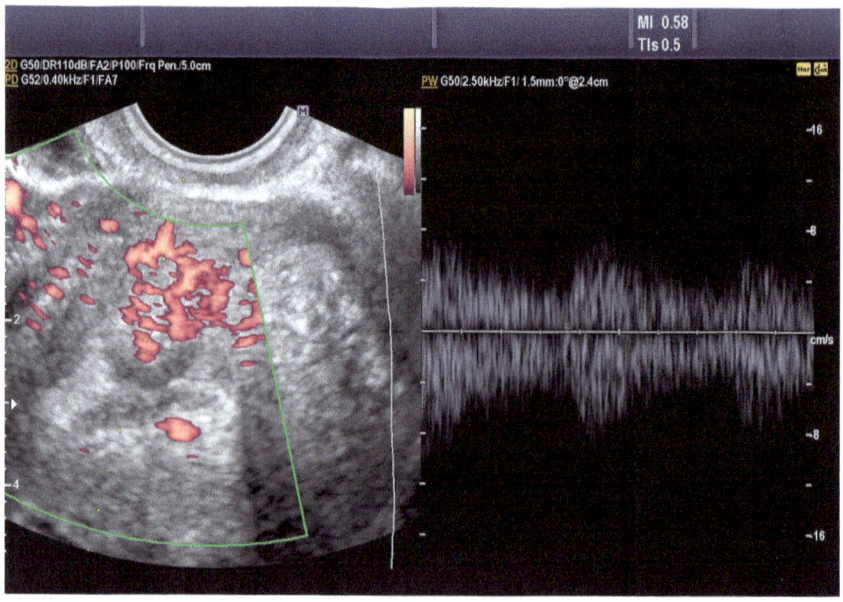

Fig. 6.7.13: Moderate low impedance vascularity seen on color flow mapping and duplex Doppler

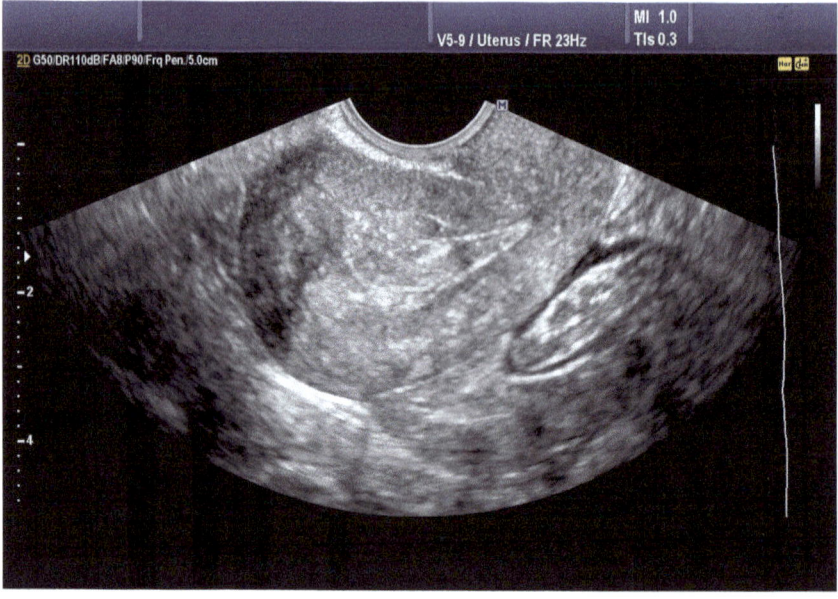

Fig. 6.7.14: Inhomogeneous endometrium

6.7. Endometrium: Abnormal Thickness and Echo Pattern

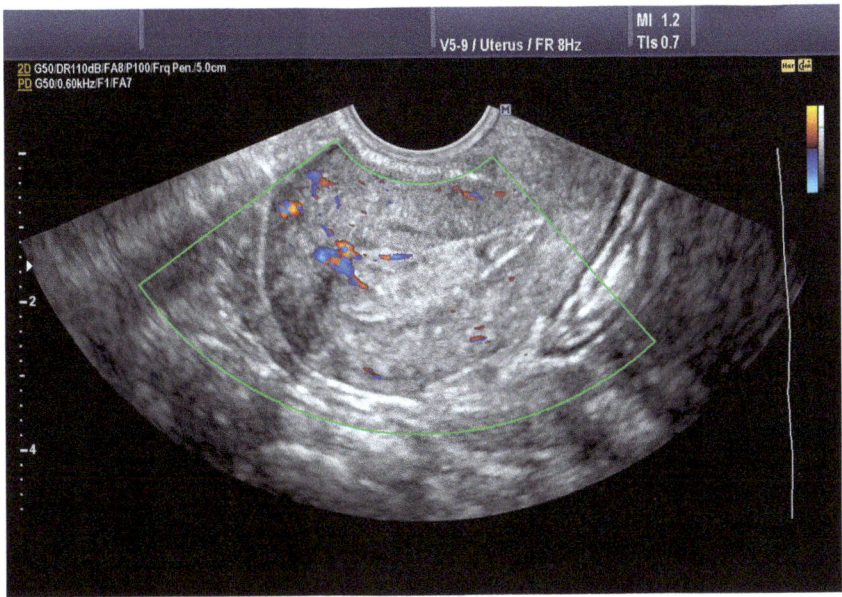

Fig. 6.7.15: Inhomogeneous endometrium

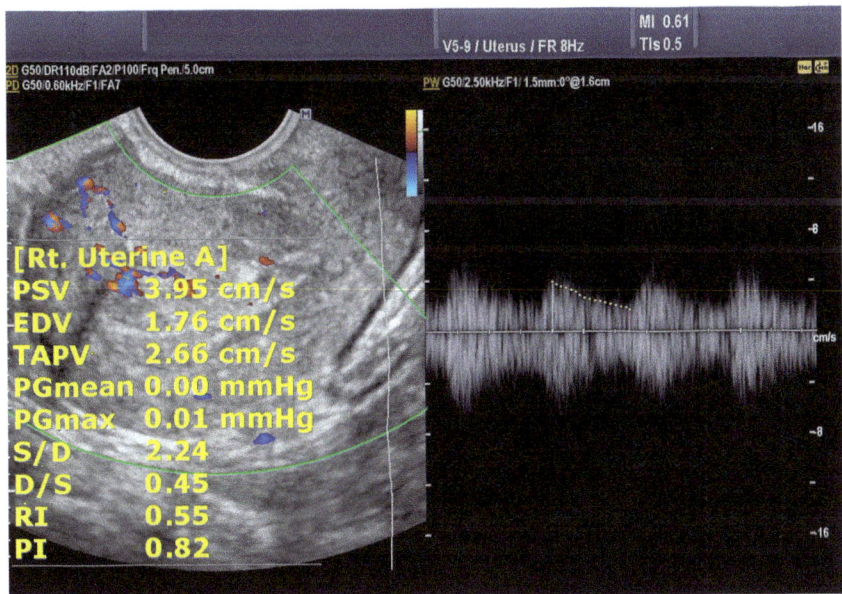

Fig. 6.7.16: Inhomogeneous endometrium showing low impedance vascularity

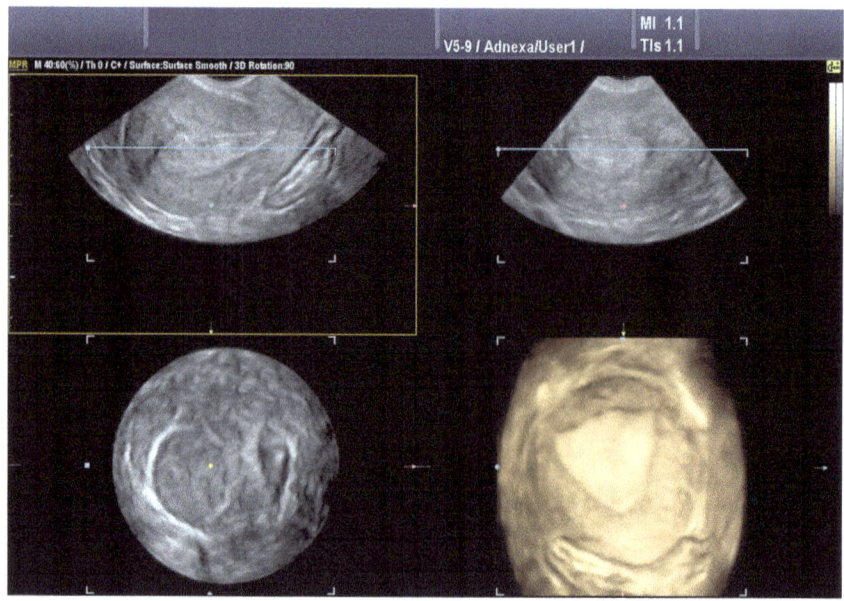

Fig. 6.7.17: Thickened endometrium on MPR

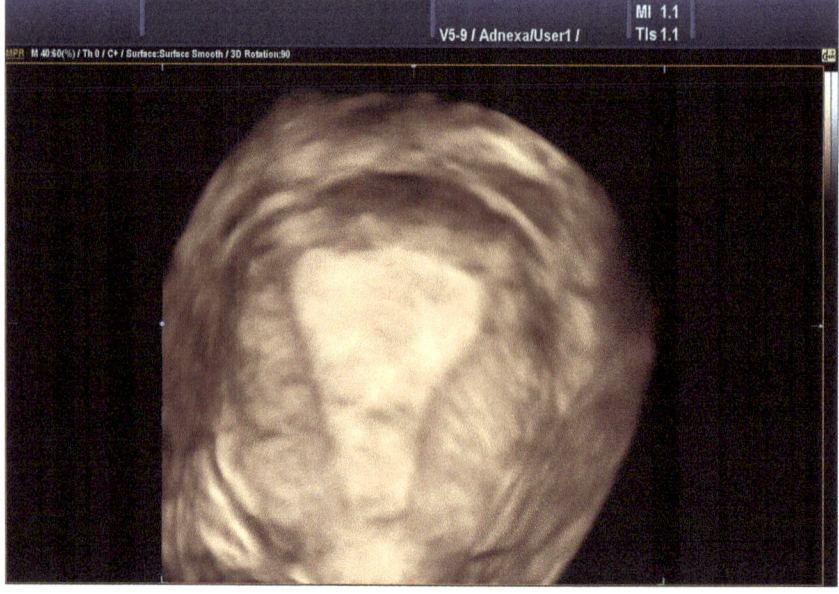

Fig. 6.7.18: Endometrium on 3D

6.7. Endometrium: Abnormal Thickness and Echo Pattern

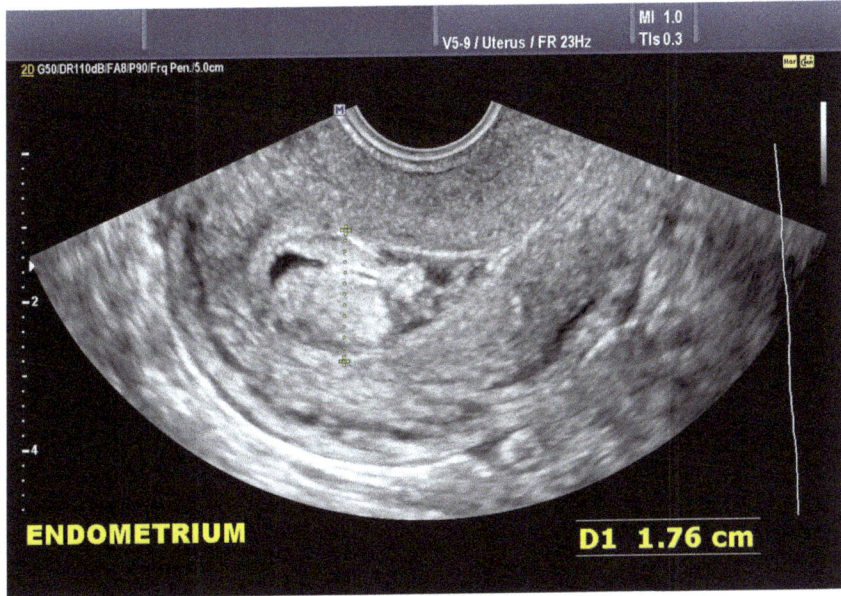

Fig. 6.7.19: Thickened endometrium (17.6 mm)

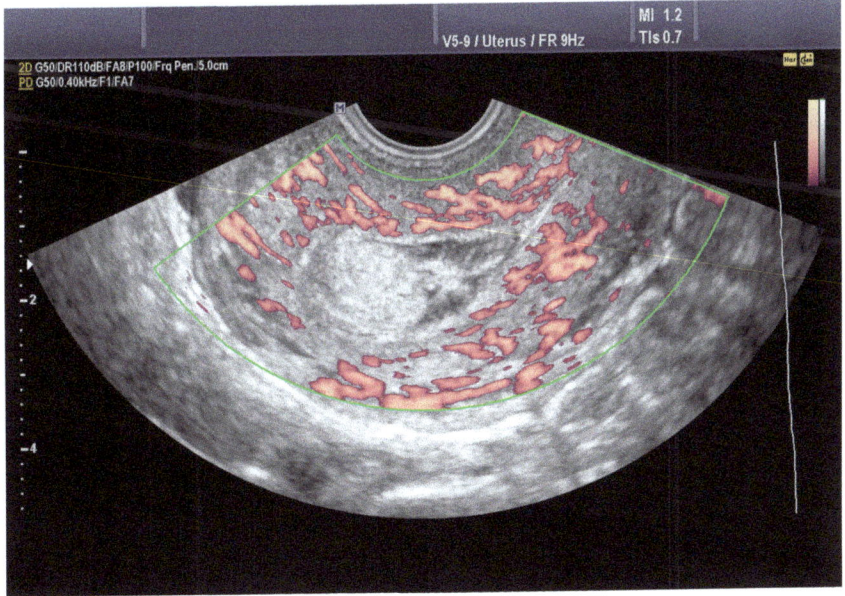

Fig. 6.7.20: Moderately vascular uterus

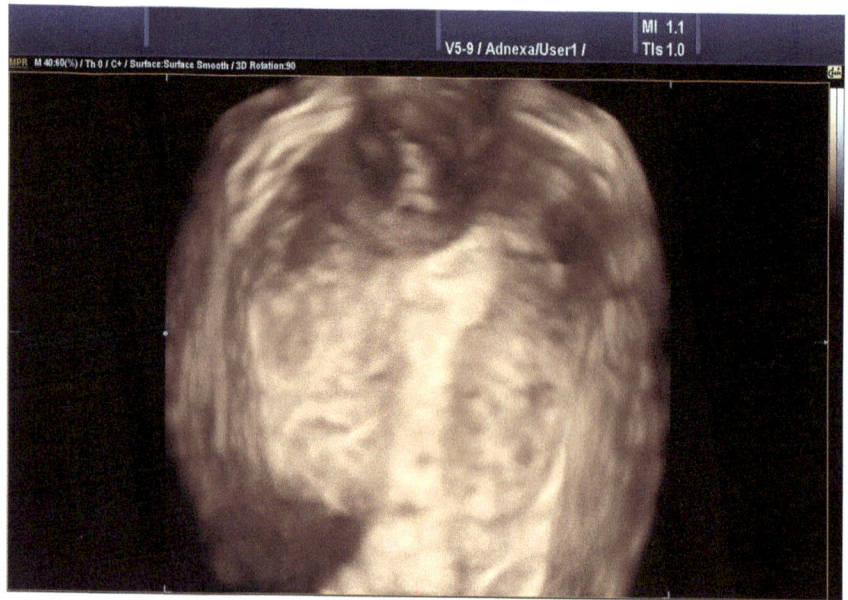

Fig. 6.7.21: Irregular endometrium on 3D

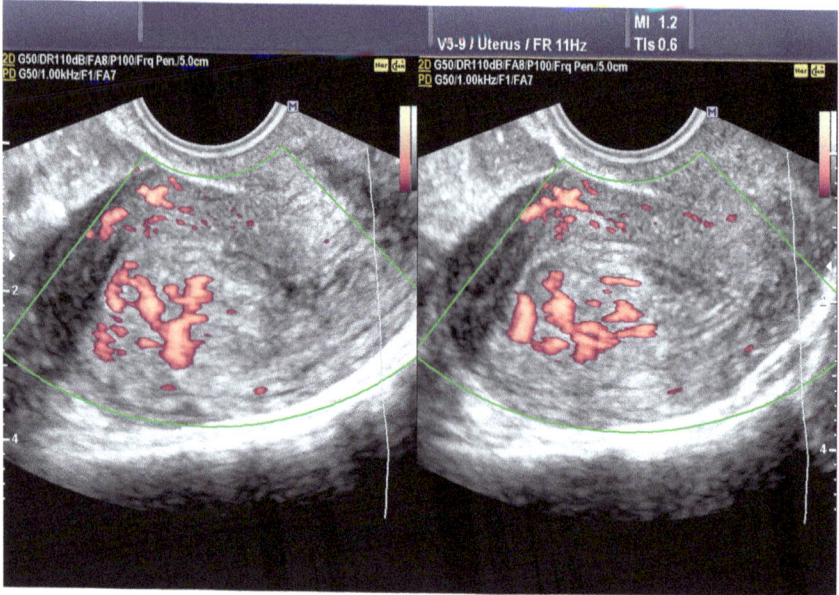

Fig. 6.7.22: Moderately vascular endometrium

6.7. Endometrium: Abnormal Thickness and Echo Pattern

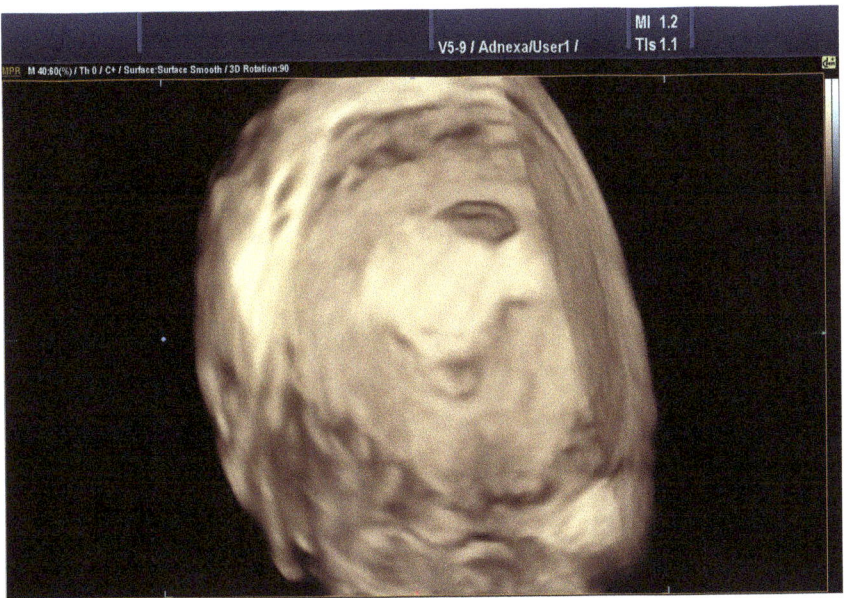

Fig. 6.7.23: As seen on 3D

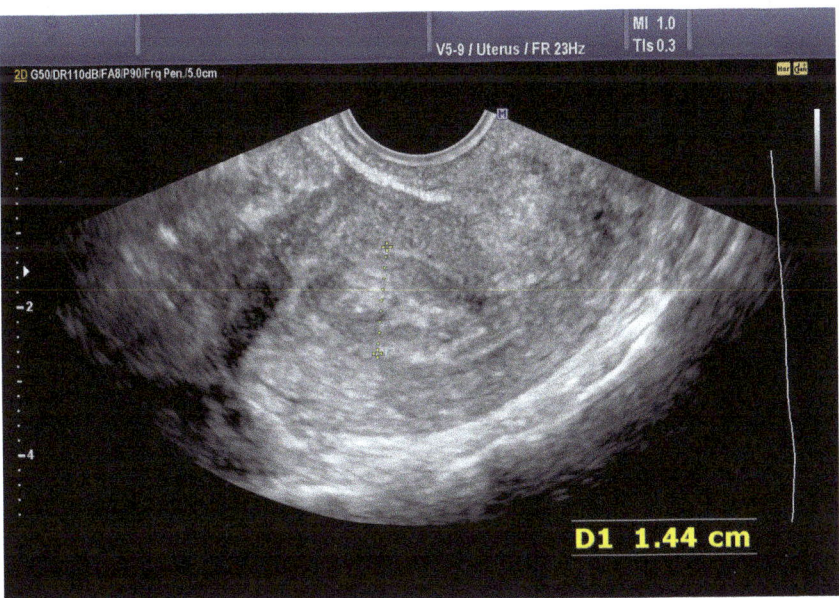

Fig. 6.7.24: 14.4 mm thick endometrium take the history carefully to evaluate possible pathology

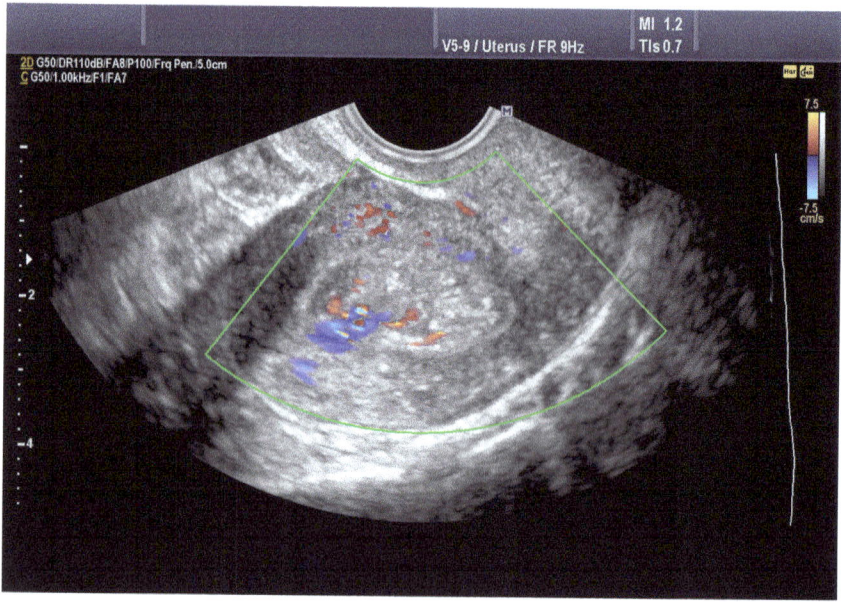

Fig. 6.7.25A: Moderate vascularity in the endometrium

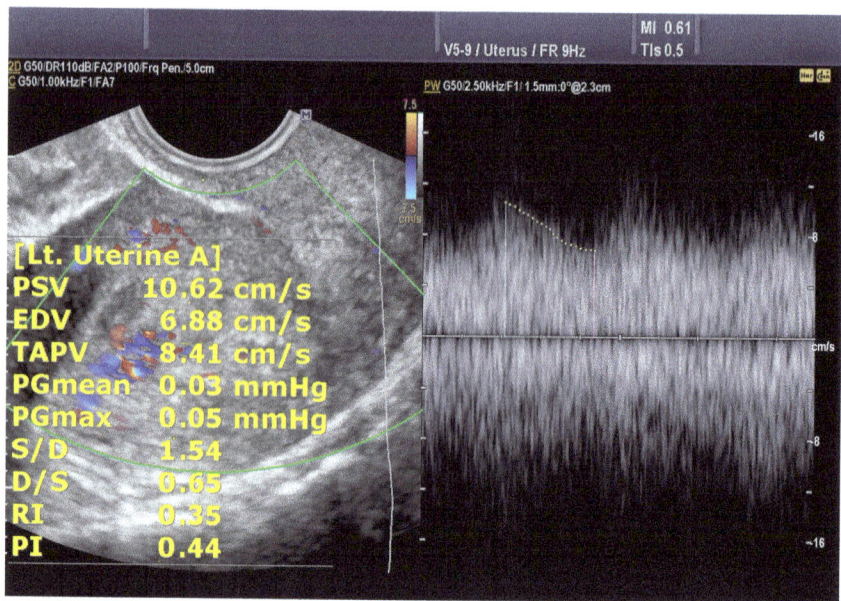

Fig. 6.7.25B: Low impedance flow seen in the endometrium

6.7. Endometrium: Abnormal Thickness and Echo Pattern

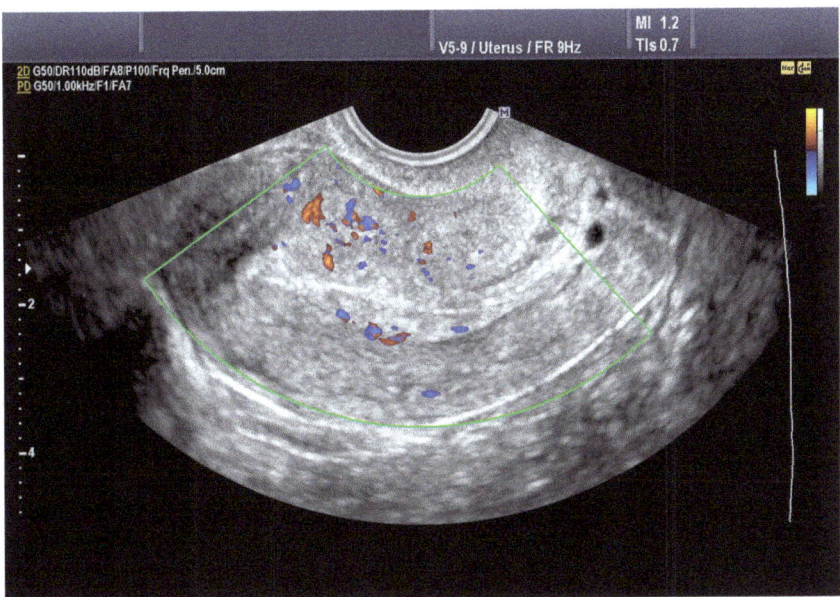

Fig. 6.7.26: Thick vascular endometrium

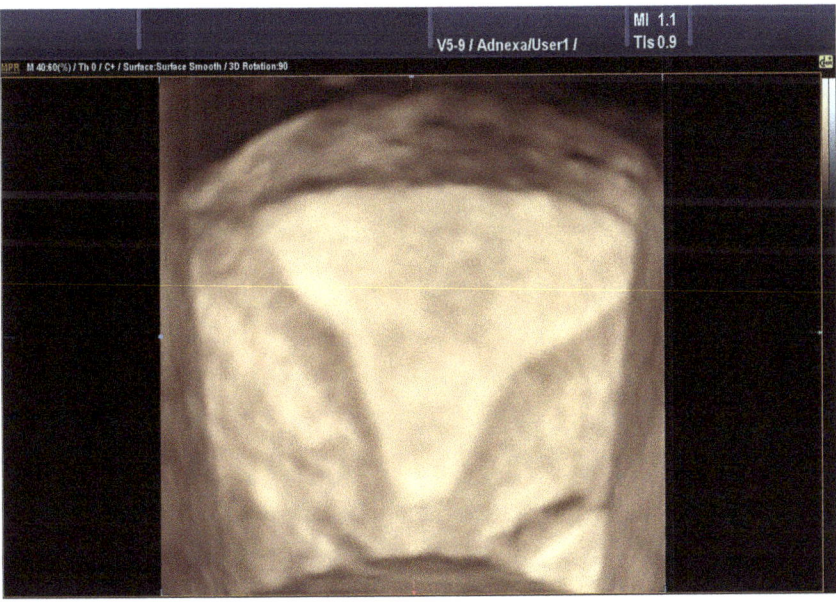

Fig. 6.7.27: Thick endometrium seen on 3D

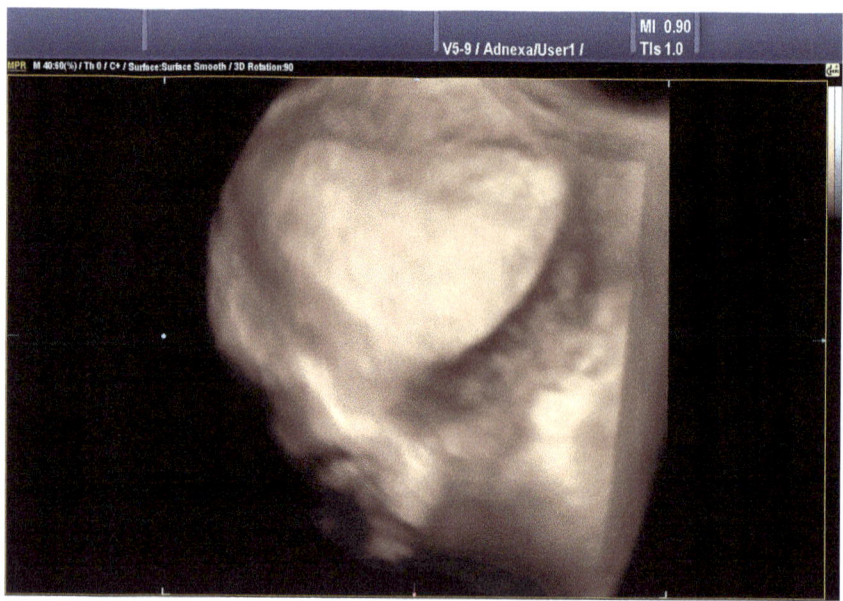

Fig. 6.7.28: Look at the endometrial-myometrial differentiation carefully on 3D as well

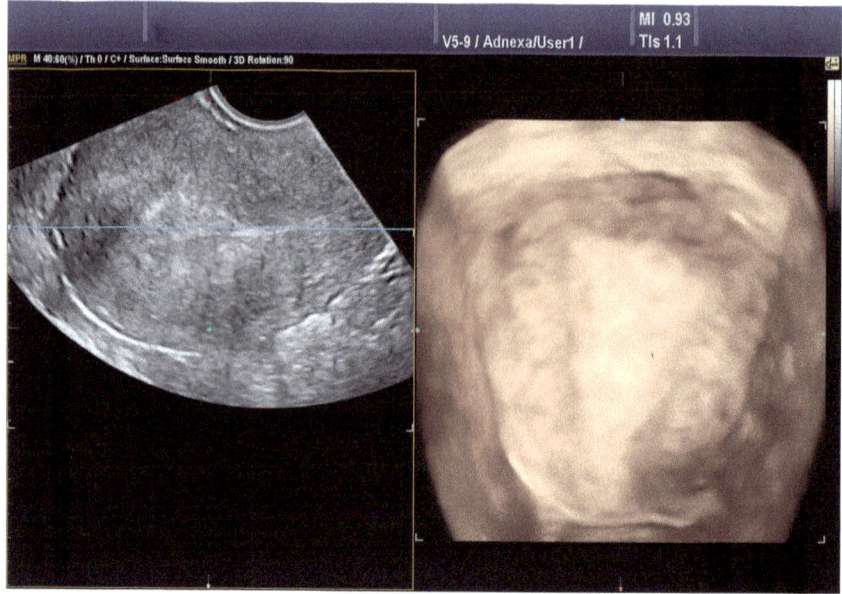

Fig. 6.7.29: Carefully evaluate the myometrial thickness and differentiation with the endometrium on all sides

6.7. Endometrium: Abnormal Thickness and Echo Pattern

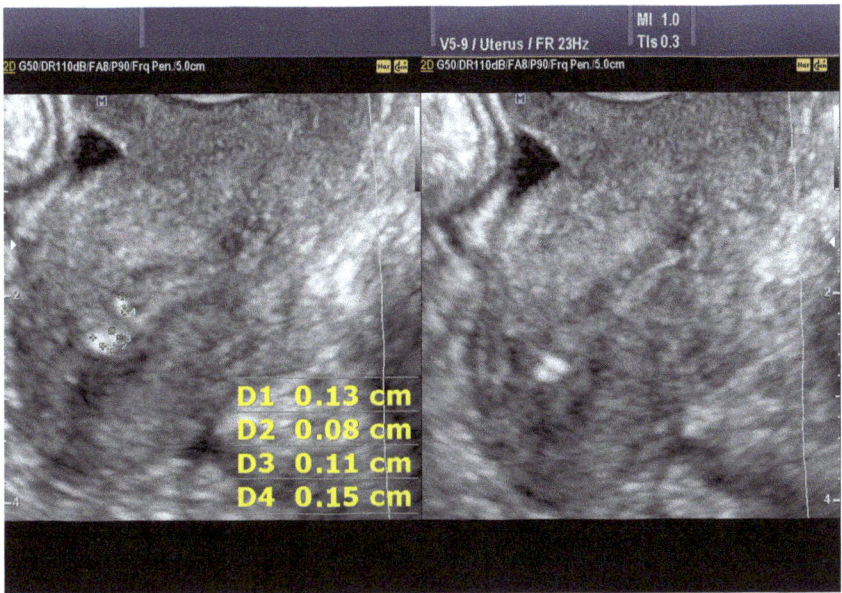

Fig. 6.7.30: Patients with infertility need to be assess for calcific foci in the endometrium and subendometrial area as well

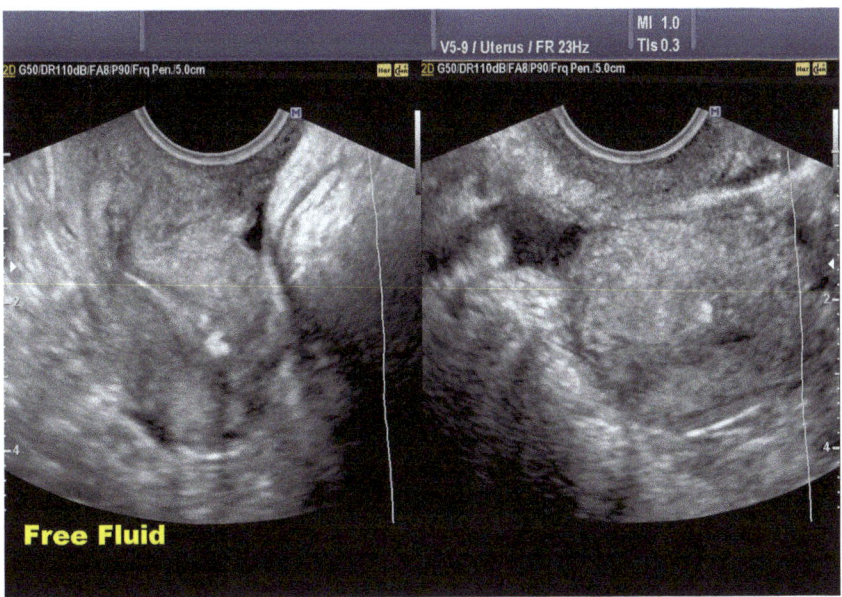

Fig. 6.7.31: Endometrium with calcific foci

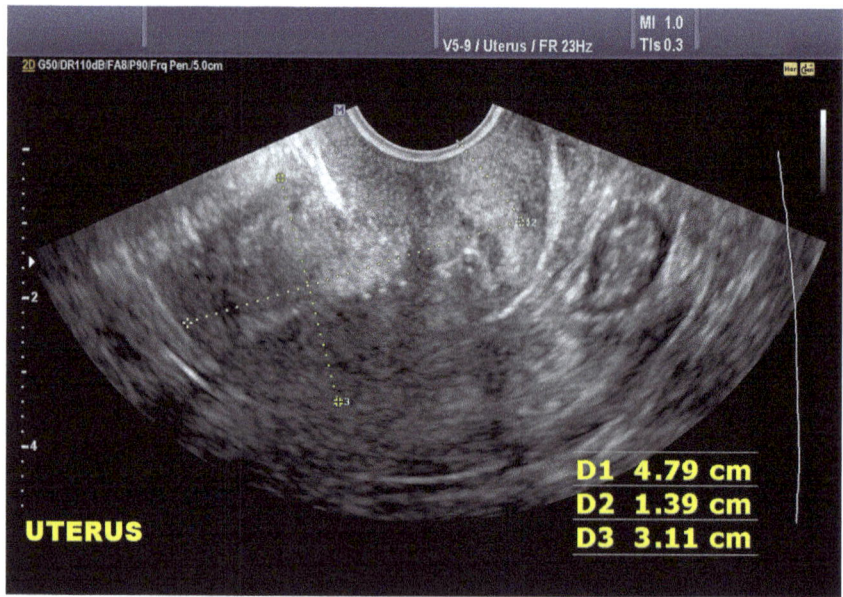

Fig. 6.7.32: Calcific foci seen in the uterine cavity

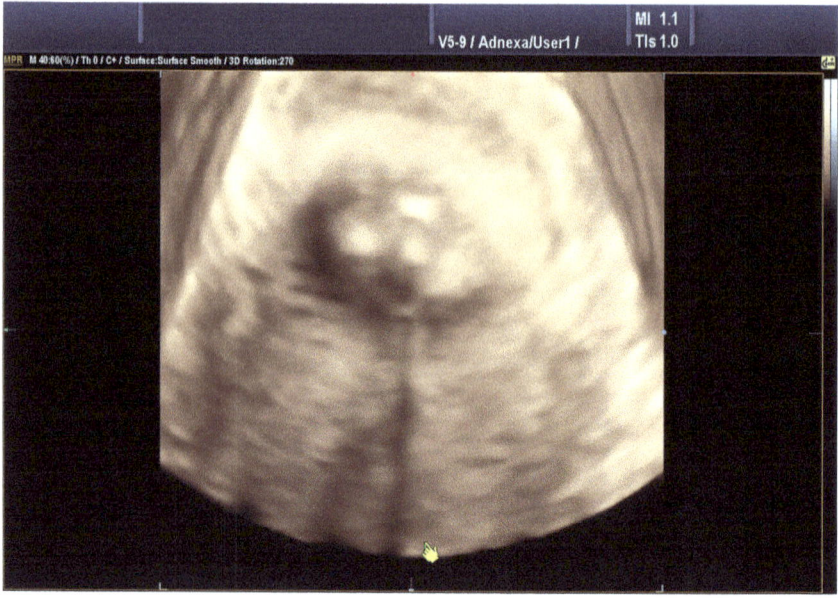

Fig. 6.7.33: As seen on 3D

6.7. Endometrium: Abnormal Thickness and Echo Pattern

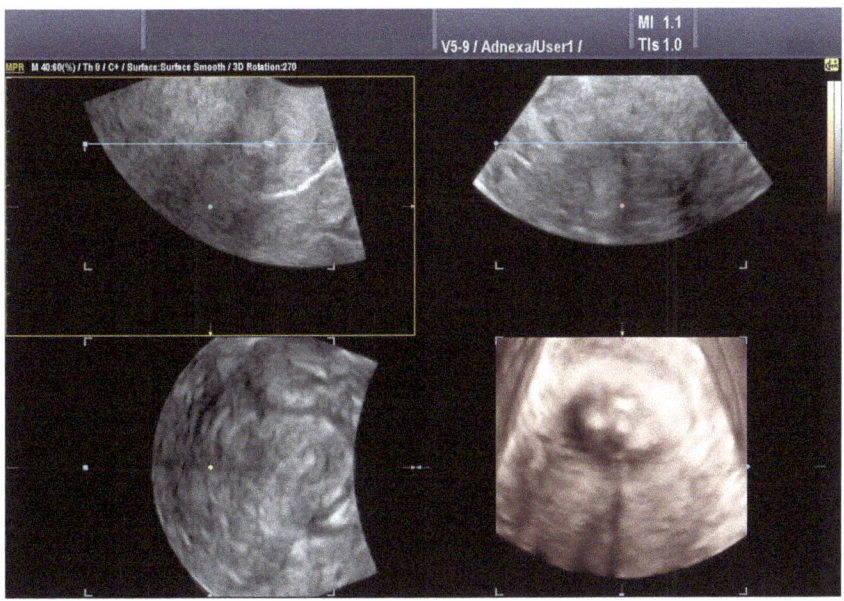

Fig. 6.7.34: As seen on MPR

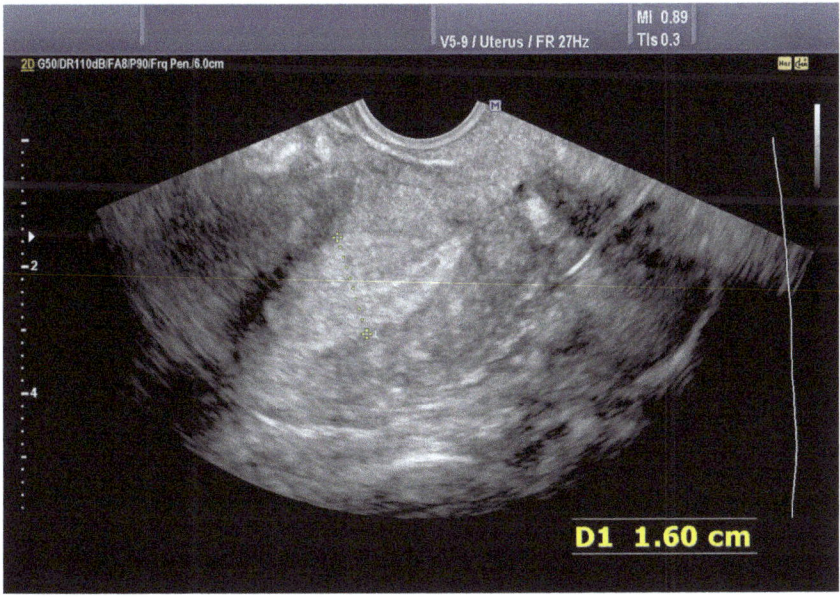

Fig. 6.7.35: Thick endometrium seen on the 33rd day of the cycle (?very early pregnancy)

6.8. CERVICAL POLYP

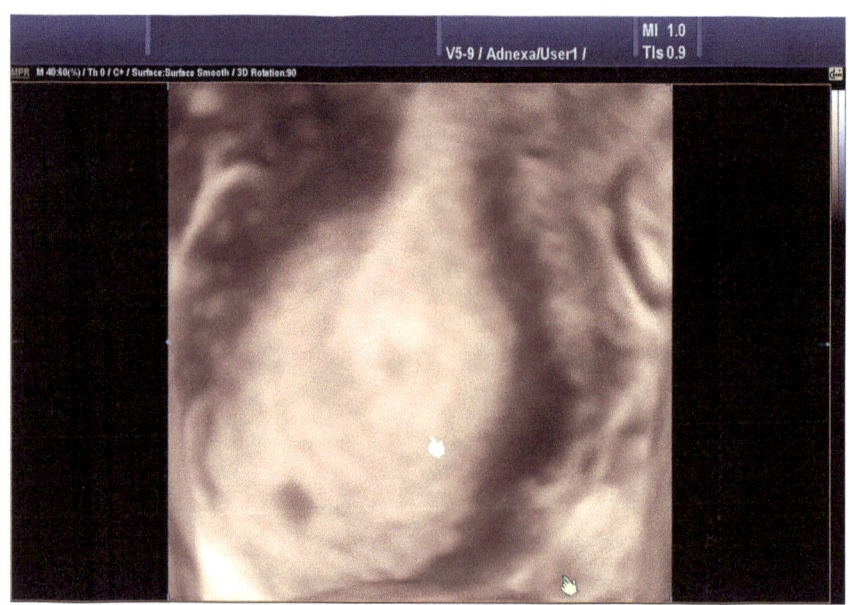

6.8. Cervical Polyp

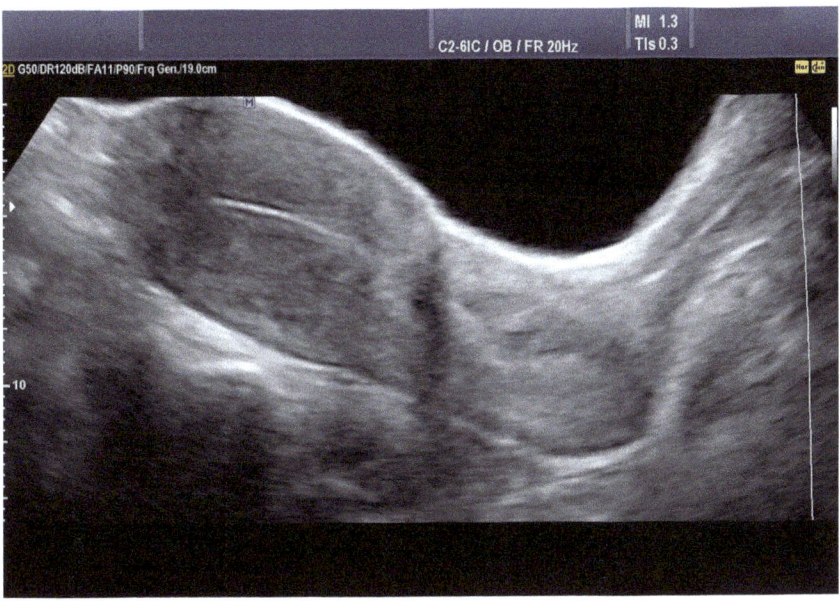

Fig. 6.8.1: Mass in the cervical canal as seen on TAS

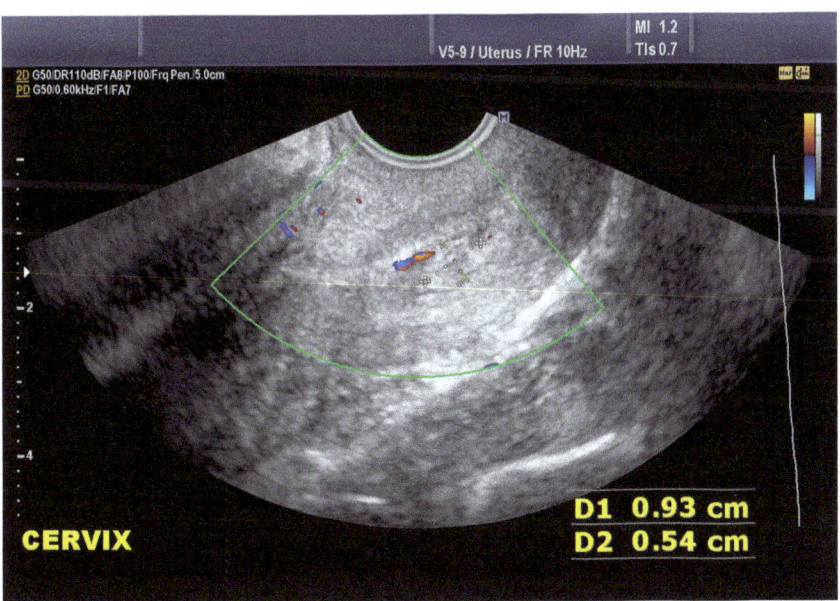

Fig. 6.8.2A: Polyp seen in the cervical canal with a vascular pedicle as seen on color flow mapping

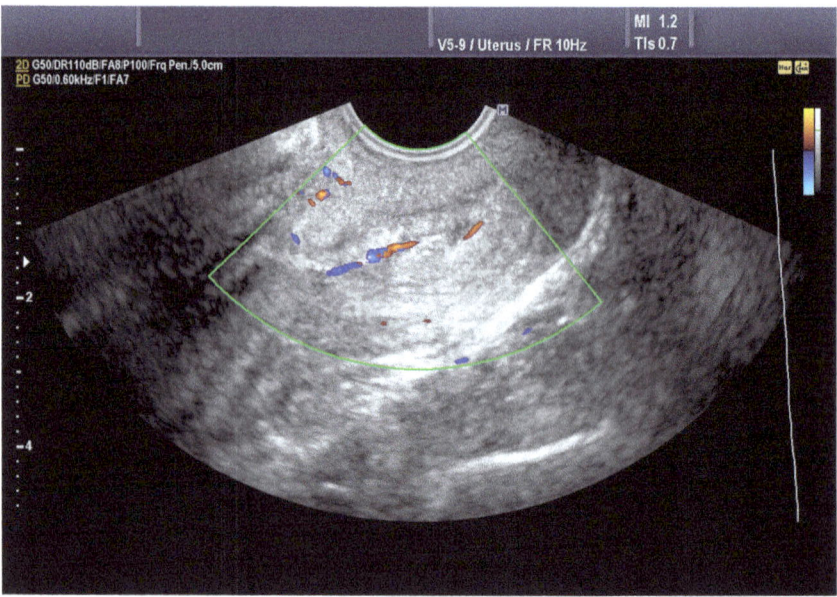

Fig. 6.8.2B: Long vascular pedicle arising from the anterior cervical wall superior position

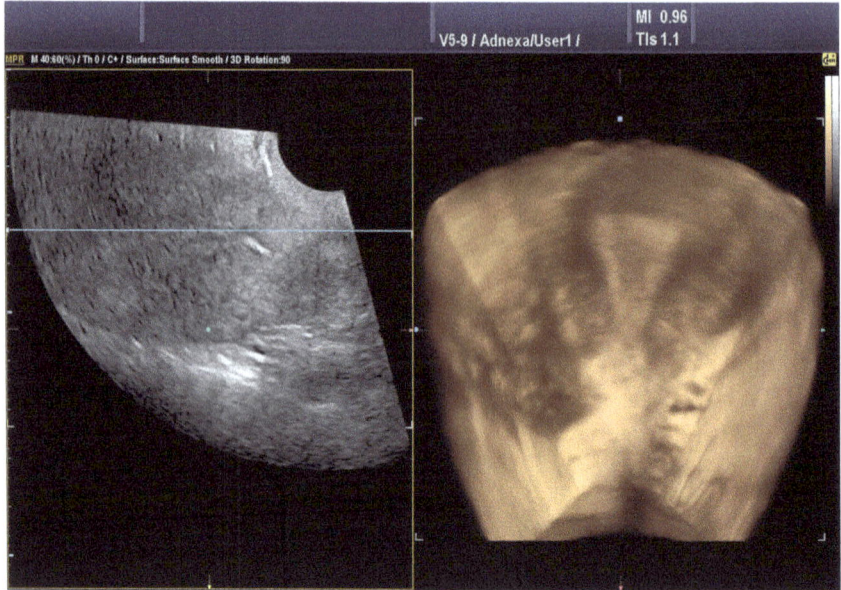

Fig. 6.8.3A: Polyp in the cervical canal as seen on 3D

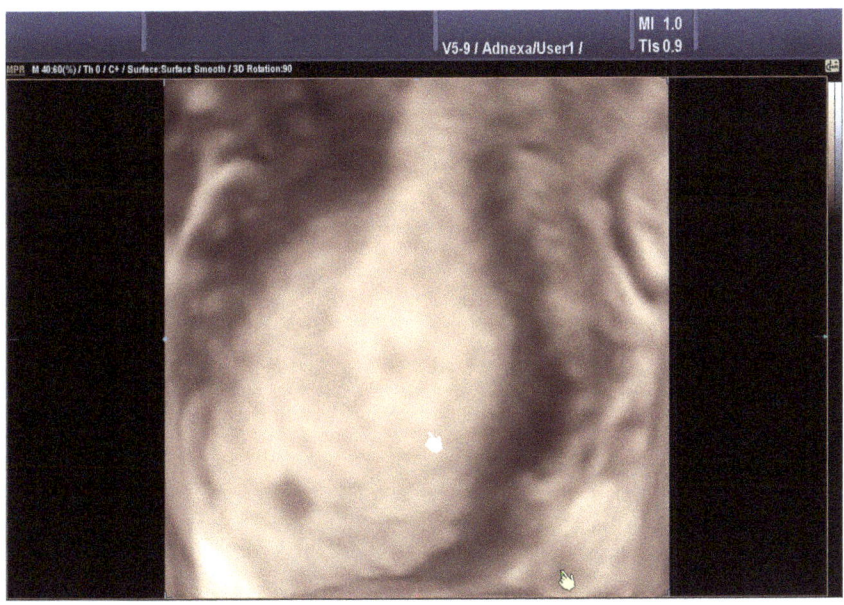

Fig. 6.8.3B: Polyp in the cervical canal on 3D reconstruction

6.9. CERVICAL MASS

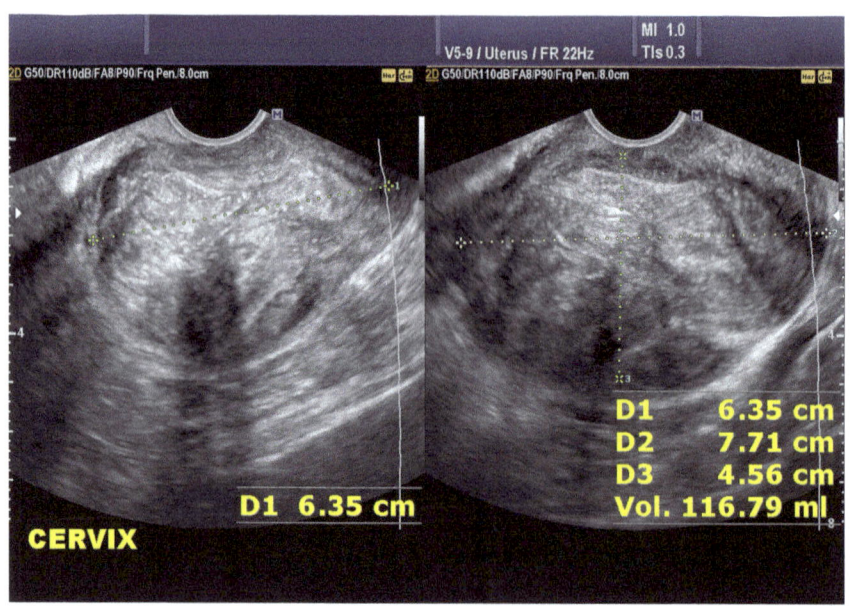

6.9. Cervical Mass

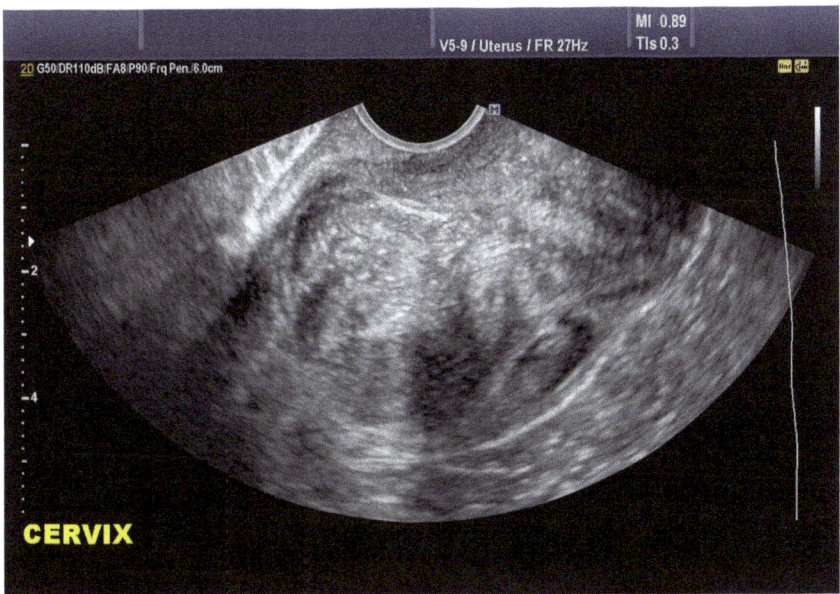

Fig. 6.9.1: Large mass seen in the cervix, inhomogeneous in echo pattern

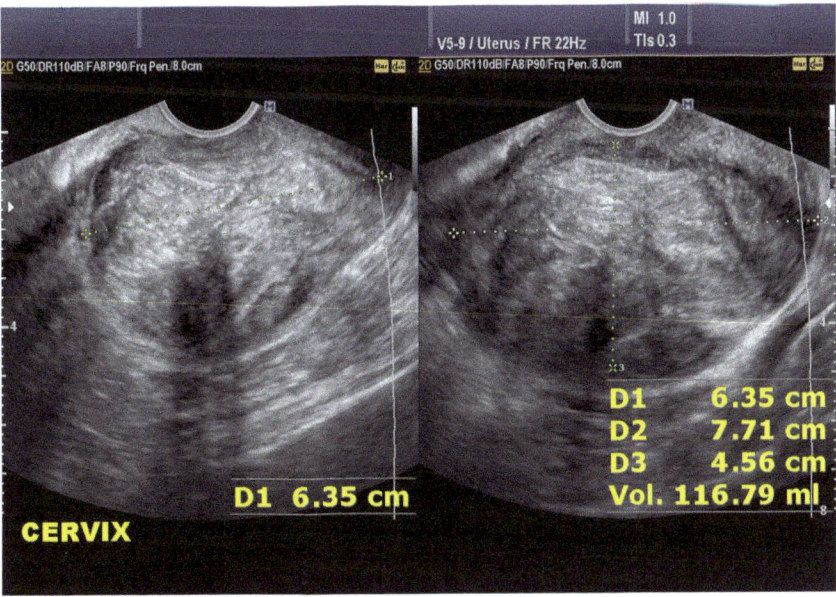

Fig. 6.9.2: Mass in the cervix, 77 mm in size, showing various inhomogeneous areas within the mass

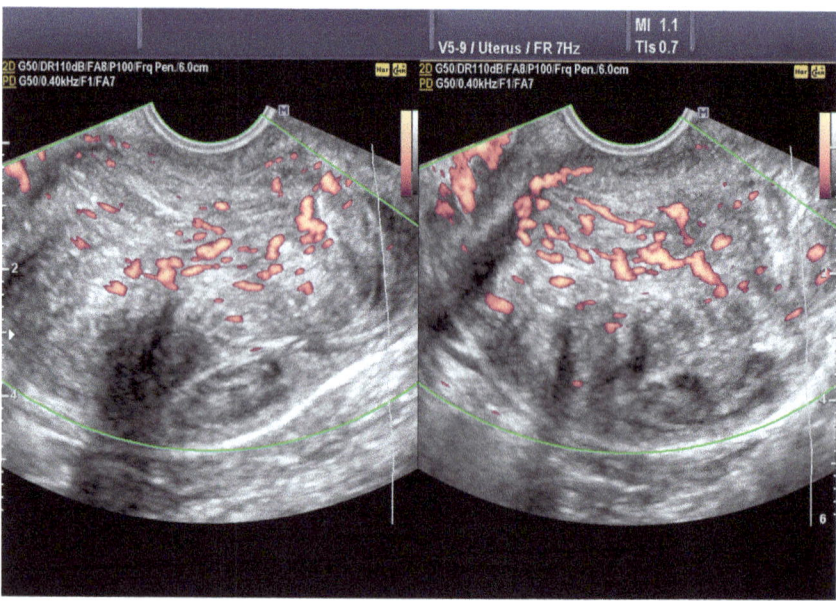

Fig. 6.9.3: On color flow mapping and power angio studies the mass is moderately vascular

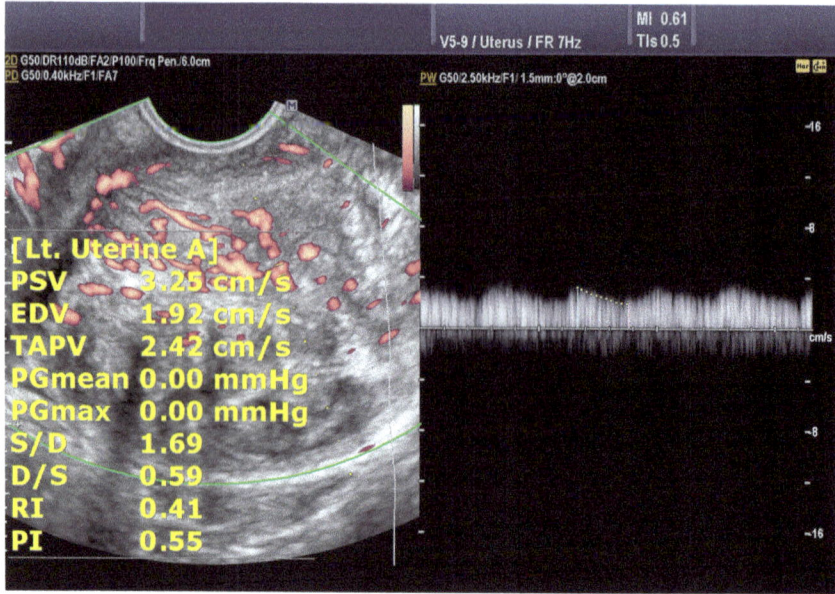

Fig. 6.9.4: On duplex Doppler evaluation the arterial flow velocity waveform shows a low impedance flow with a Resistive Index of 0.41 and a Pulsatility Index of 0.55. Re-evaluation with a CT scan is suggested

CHAPTER 7

ADNEXAL ABNORMALITIES

7.1. Small Ovaries
7.2. Dysfunctional Cysts
7.3. Hemorrhagic Cyst
7.4. Cyst with Fluid-fluid Level
7.5. Cyst with Clot
7.6. Ovarian Tumor
7.7. Dermoid
7.8. Polycystic Ovaries
7.9. Endometriosis
7.10. Adnexal Mass
7.11. Hydrosalpinx
7.12. Pouch of Douglas
7.13. Ectopic
7.14. Free Fluid

7.1. SMALL OVARIES

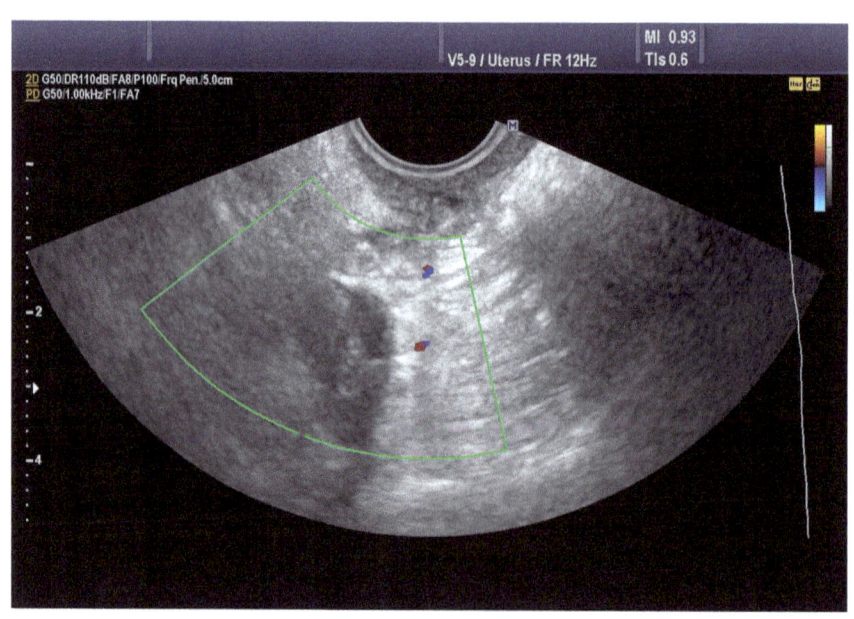

7.1. Small Ovaries

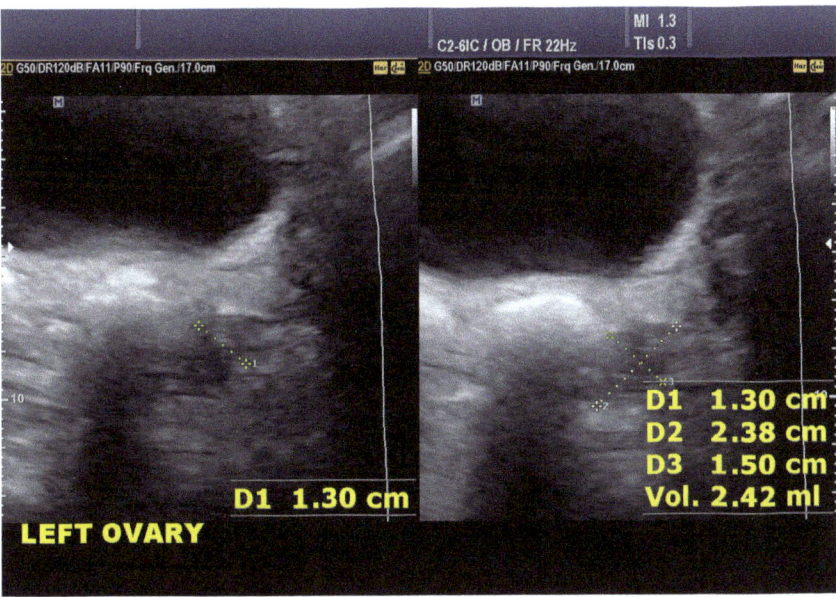

Fig. 7.1.1: Ovaries which are small in size can be difficult to visualize on a TVS. Always distend the bladder and measure the ovarian volume

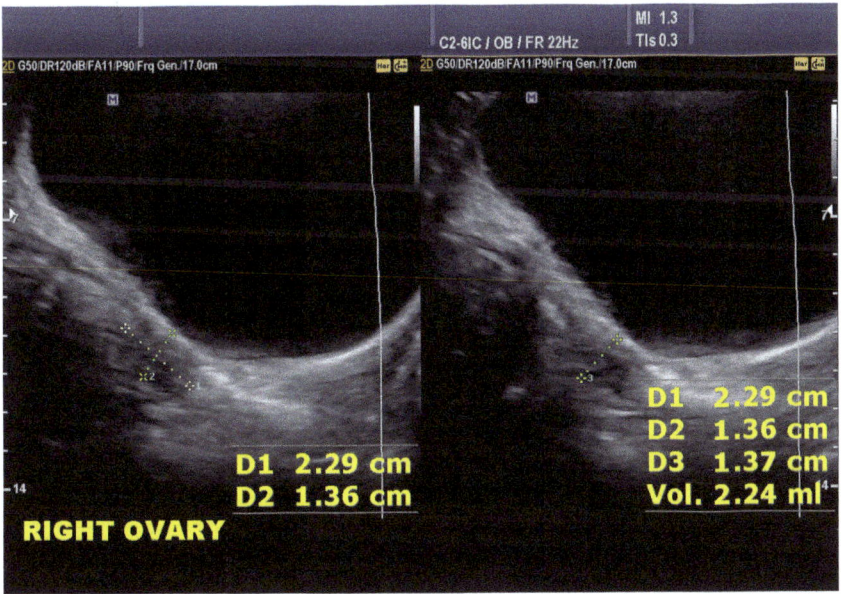

Fig. 7.1.2: The patient could complain of irregular cycles or a problem in conceiving

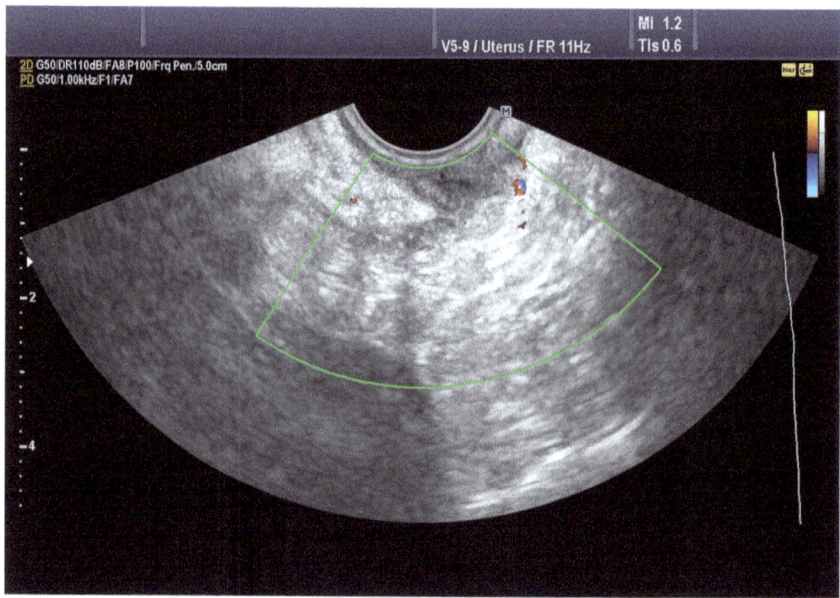

Fig. 7.1.3: On a TVS, visualize the vessel and the ovary adjacent to it

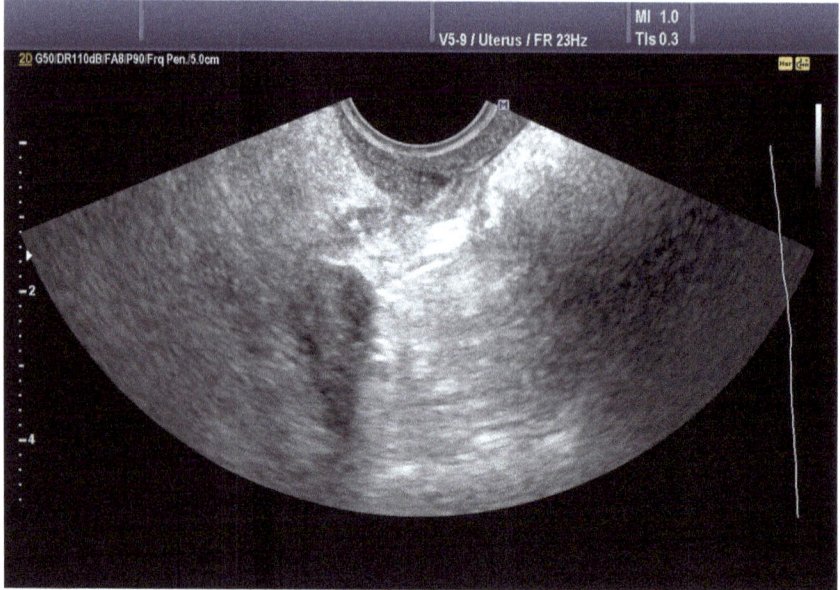

Fig. 7.1.4: Once the ovary is visualized, look for immature follicles and mention if there is a paucity of immature follicles

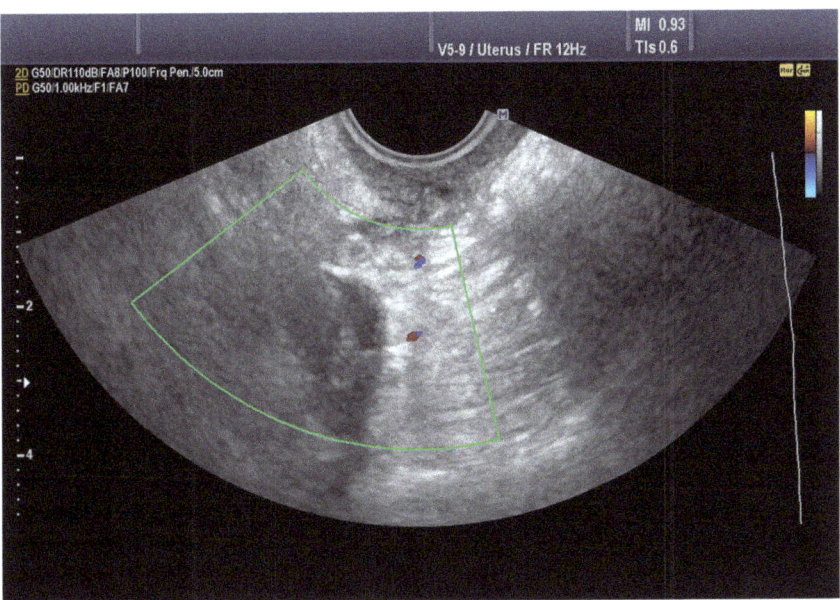

Fig. 7.1.5: Vascularity within the ovary, ovarian volume and appearance of follicles along with the patients age and hormonal profile can give a fair idea of a perimenopausal phase for the patient

7.2. DYSFUNCTIONAL CYSTS

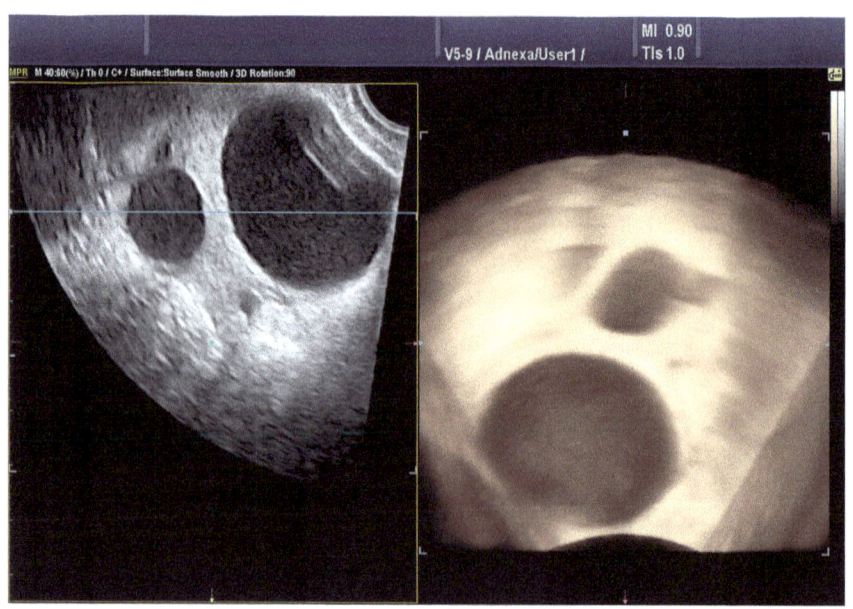

7.2. Dysfunctional Cysts

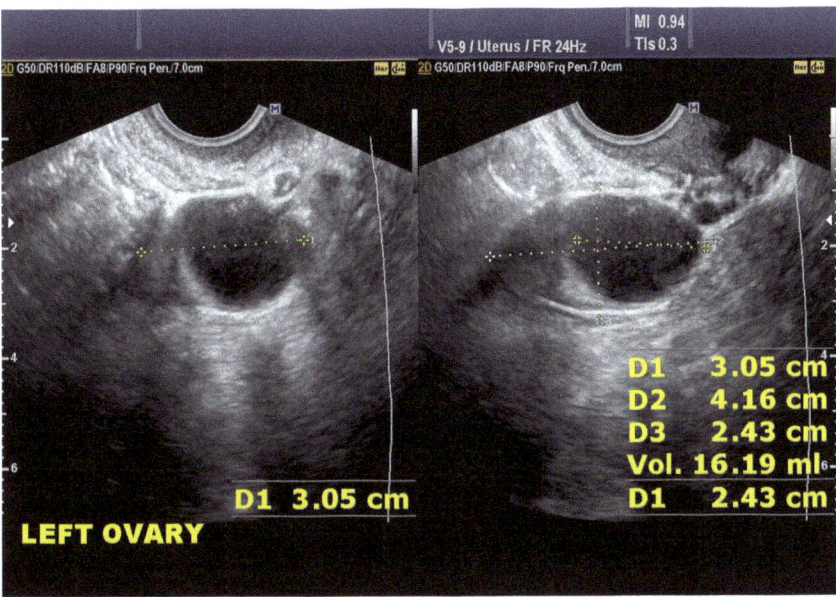

Fig. 7.2.1: For functional ovarian cysts always check for previous scan, and check for phase of the cycle

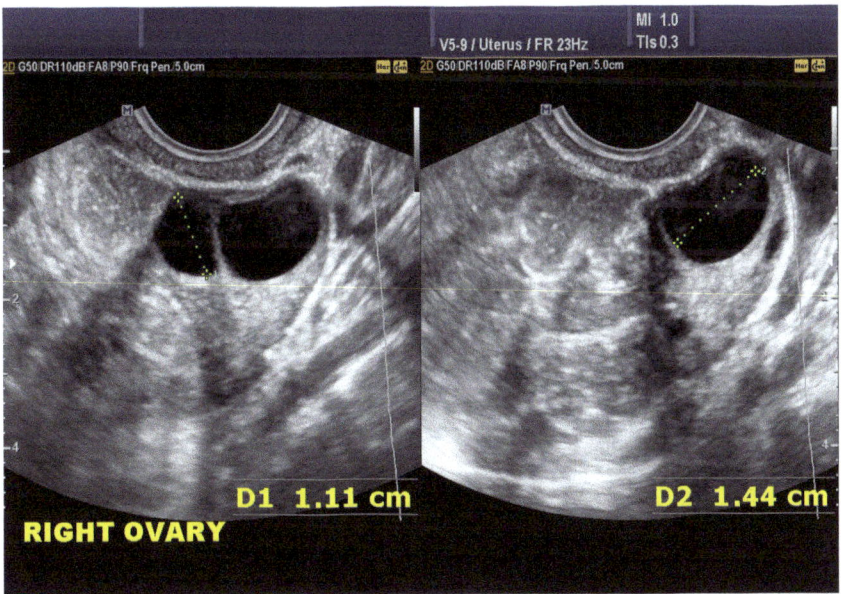

Fig. 7.2.2: Cysts can be follicular or luteal cyst

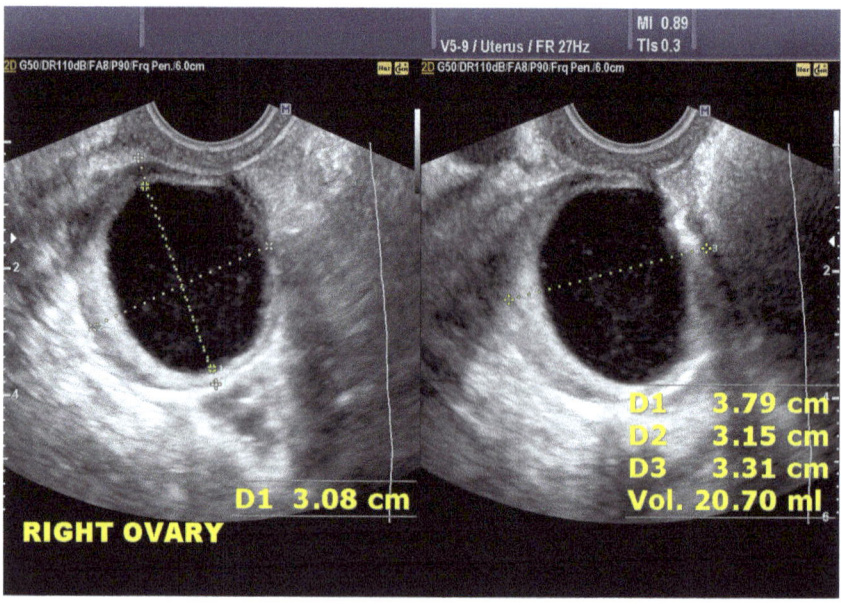

Fig. 7.2.3: Cysts can be small or large but should always be evaluated immediate postmenstrual to see whether they are persisting

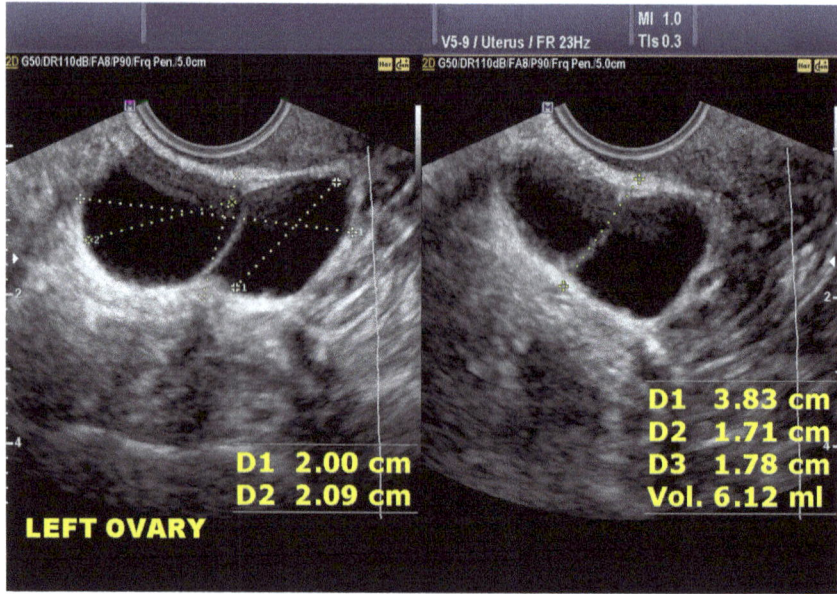

Fig. 7.2.4: Multiple cysts can be seen if one is on infertility treatment and is being stimulated

7.2. Dysfunctional Cysts

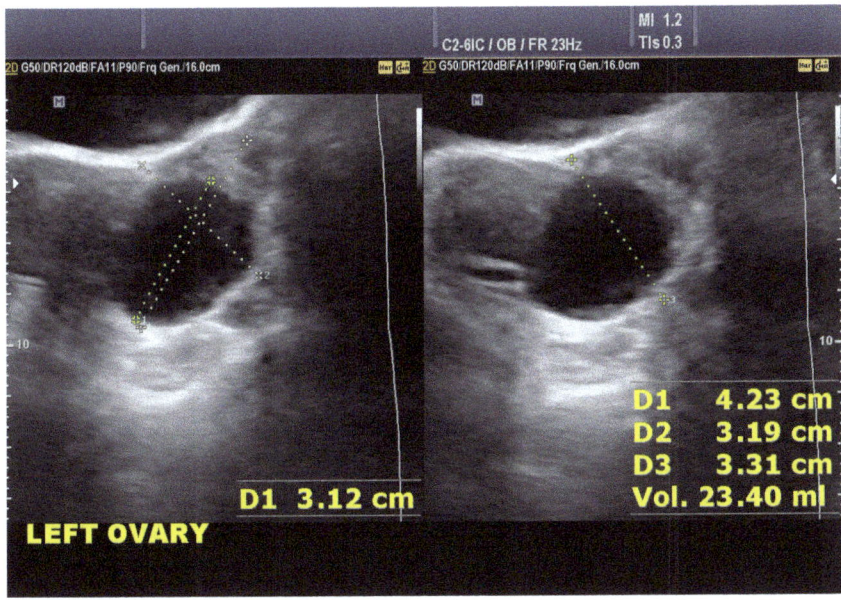

Fig. 7.2.5: Look for cyst wall and any focal thickening, solid areas or septae

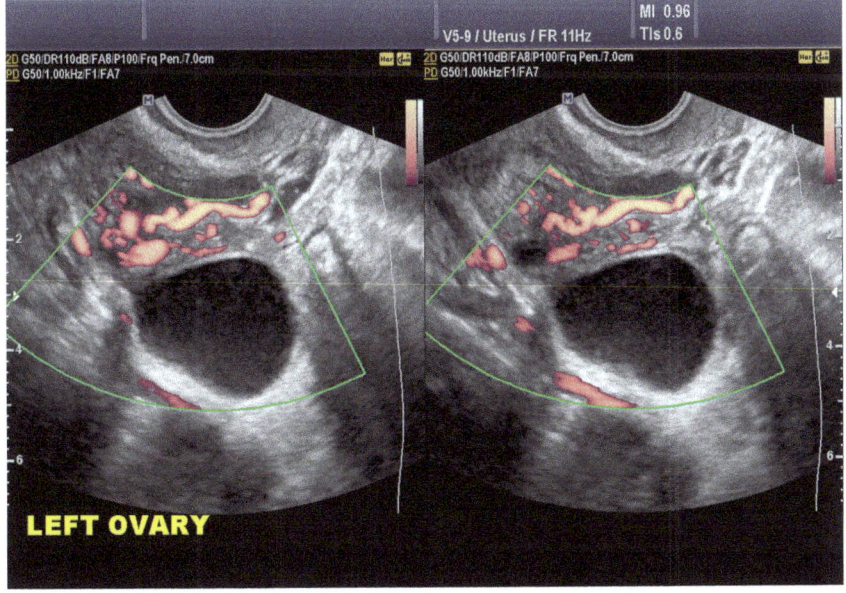

Fig. 7.2.6: Look for vascularity of these cysts

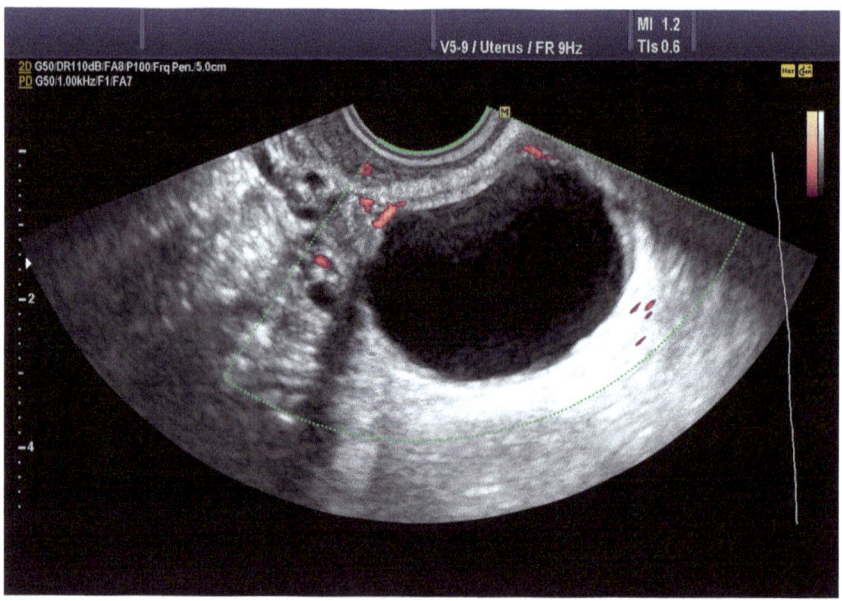

Fig. 7.2.7: Look for any torsion of these cysts

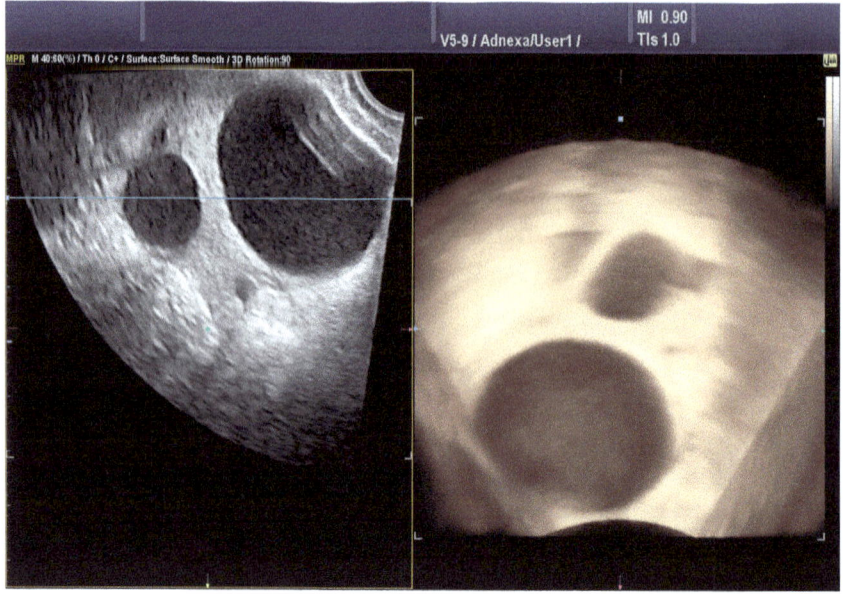

Fig. 7.2.8: Functional cyst as seen on 3D

7.2. Dysfunctional Cysts

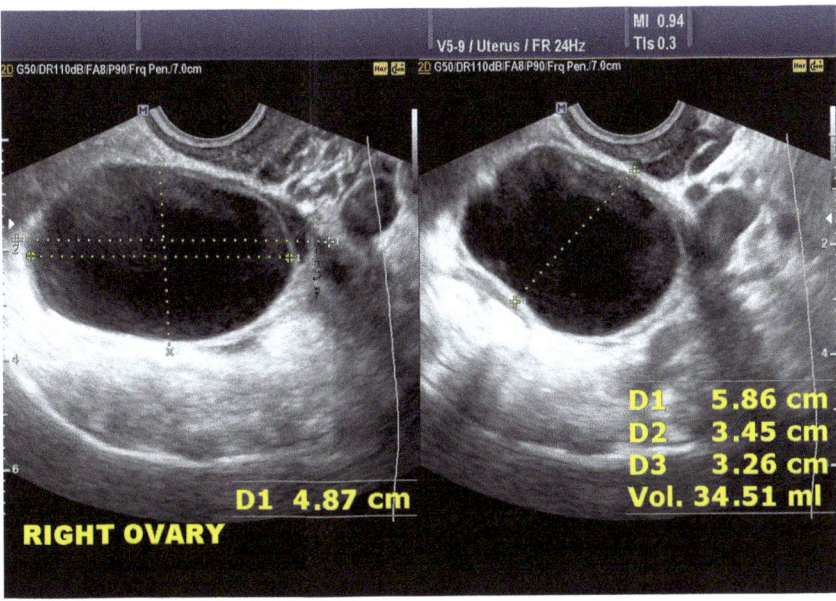

Fig. 7.2.9: Large cysts sometimes regress/disappear after the next cycle. If the patient is asymptomatic can be checked again after 1 or 2 cycles

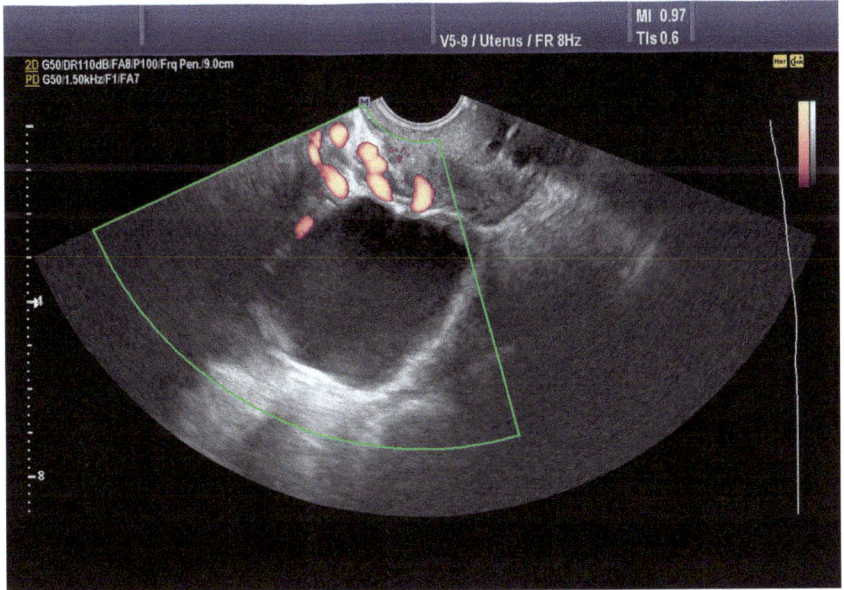

Fig. 7.2.10: Cyst as seen on color flow mapping

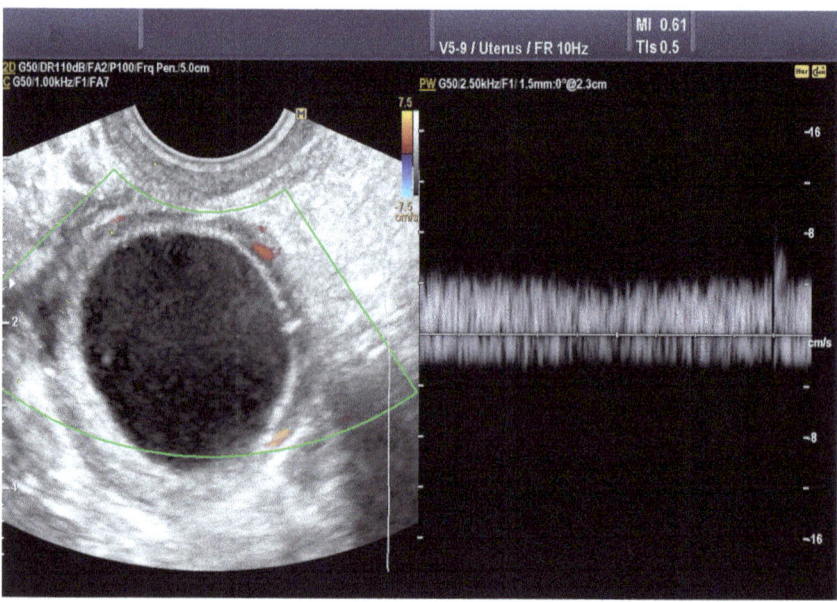

Fig. 7.2.11: Duplex Doppler evaluation of the cyst

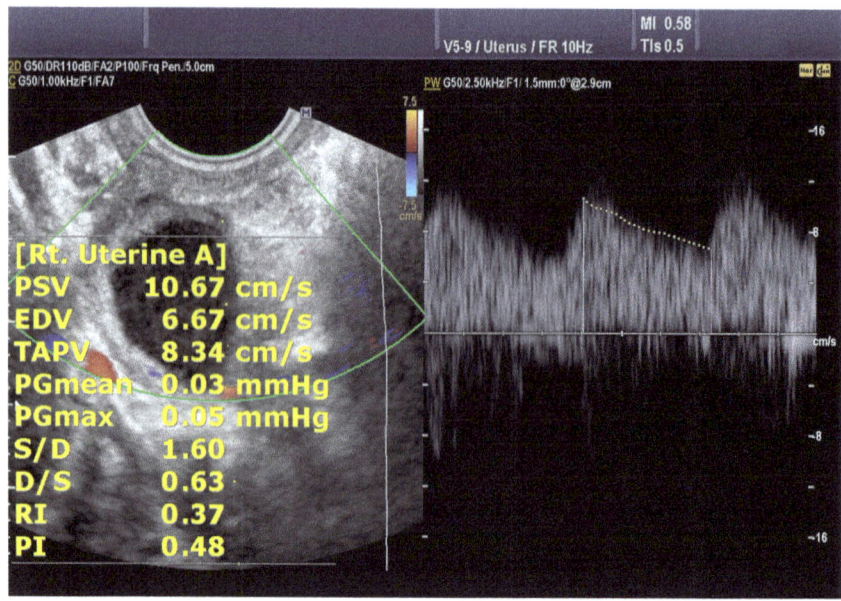

Fig. 7.2.12: On duplex Doppler evaluation low impedance flow seen, suggesting a corpus luteal cyst

7.3. HEMORRHAGIC CYST

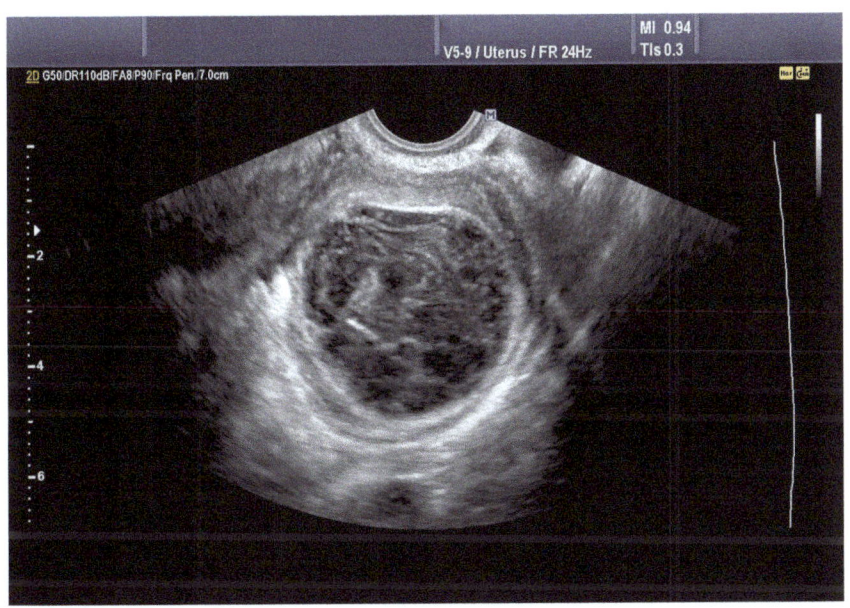

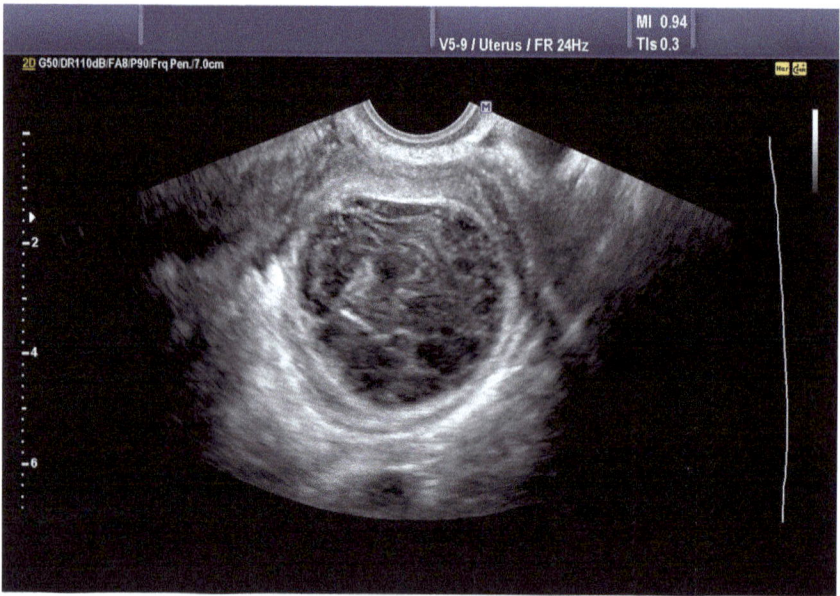

Fig. 7.3.1: Patient can present with sudden onset pelvic pain, or pelvic mass or can be asymtomatic

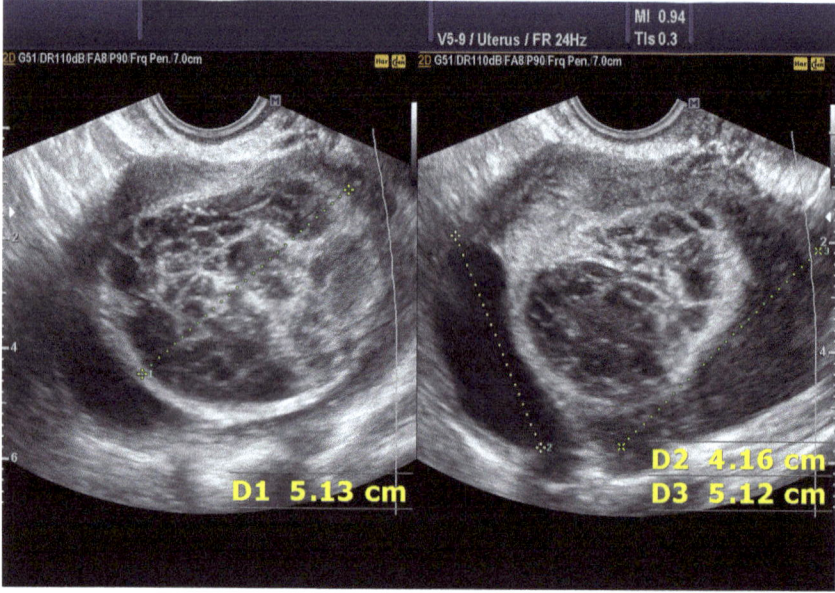

Fig. 7.3.2: Hemorrhagic ovarian cyst can be seen as a lace like reticular pattern in a cyst

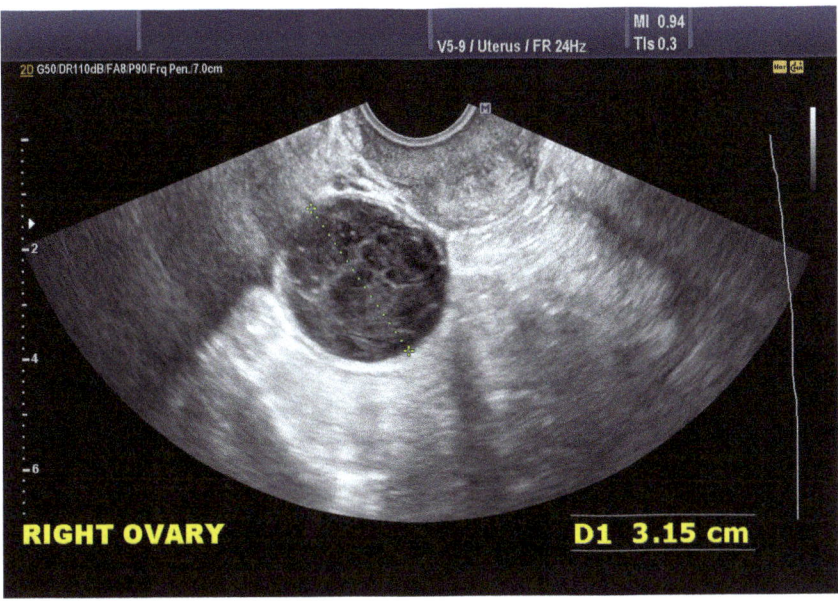

Fig. 7.3.3: Diffuse reticular pattern seen within the cyst

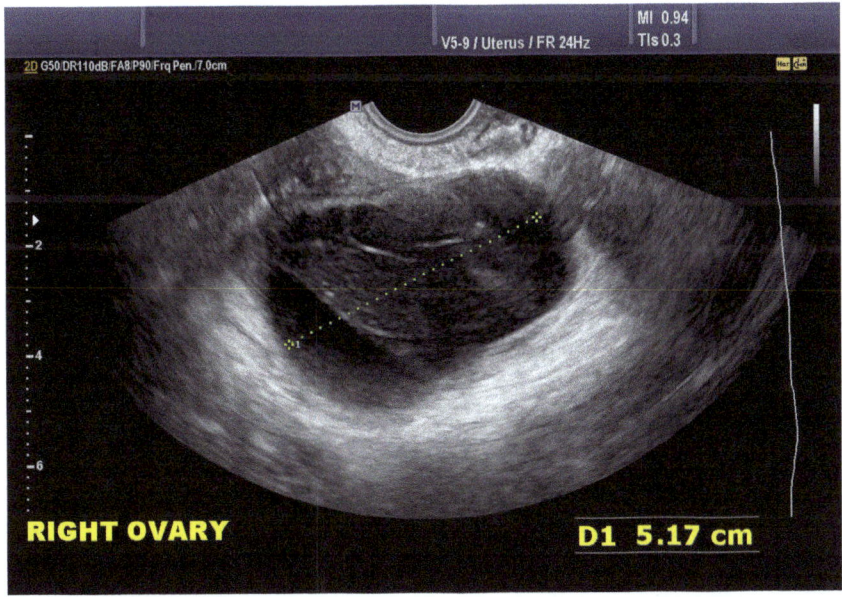

Fig. 7.3.4: Hemorrhage can be seen as a solid mass within the cyst, but does not show any vascularity within the clot

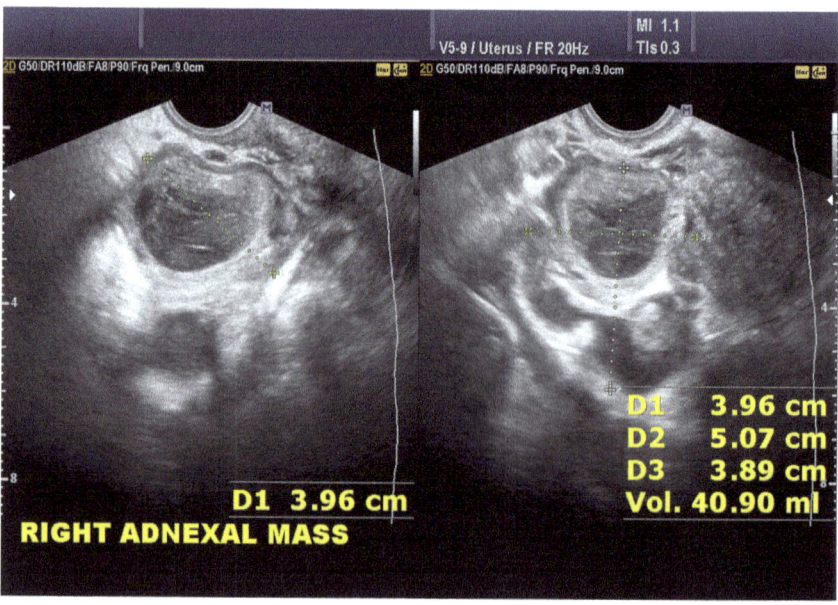

Fig. 7.3.5: Fluid-fluid level can also be seen in a hemorrhagic cyst

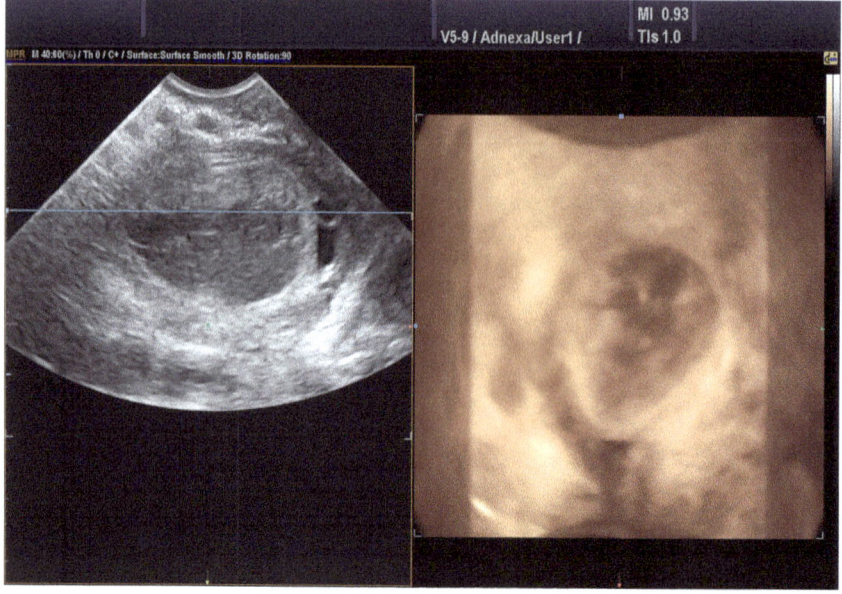

Fig. 7.3.6: As seen on MPR

7.3. Hemorrhagic Cyst

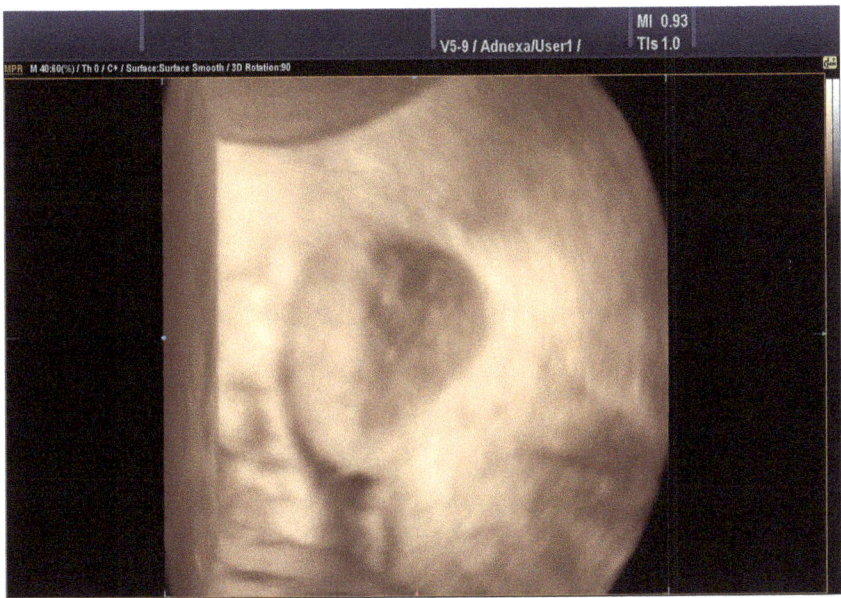

Fig. 7.3.7: Hemorrhagic cyst as seen on 3D

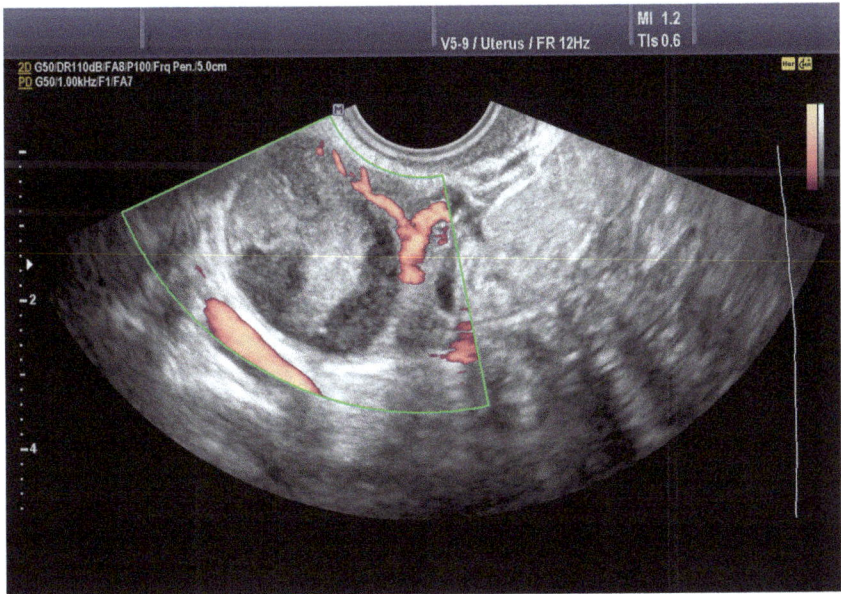

Fig. 7.3.8: Clot can be seen within the cyst

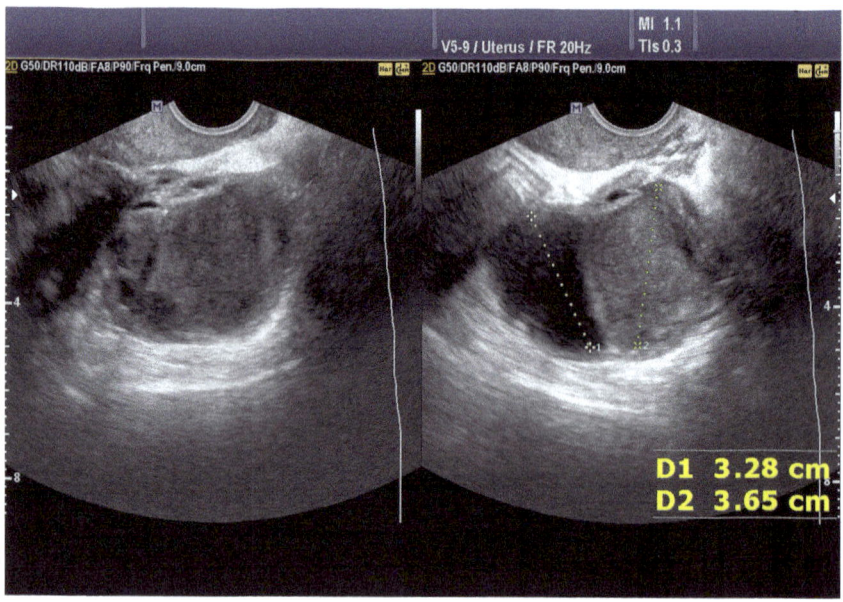

Fig. 7.3.9: Two cysts, one with hemorrhage and the other nonhemorrhagic

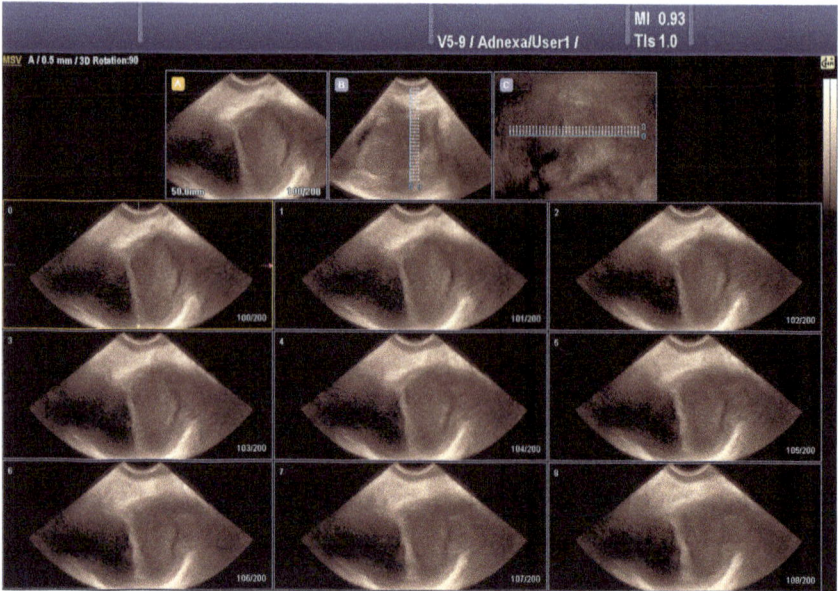

Fig. 7.3.10: Both cysts seen on MSV

7.3. Hemorrhagic Cyst

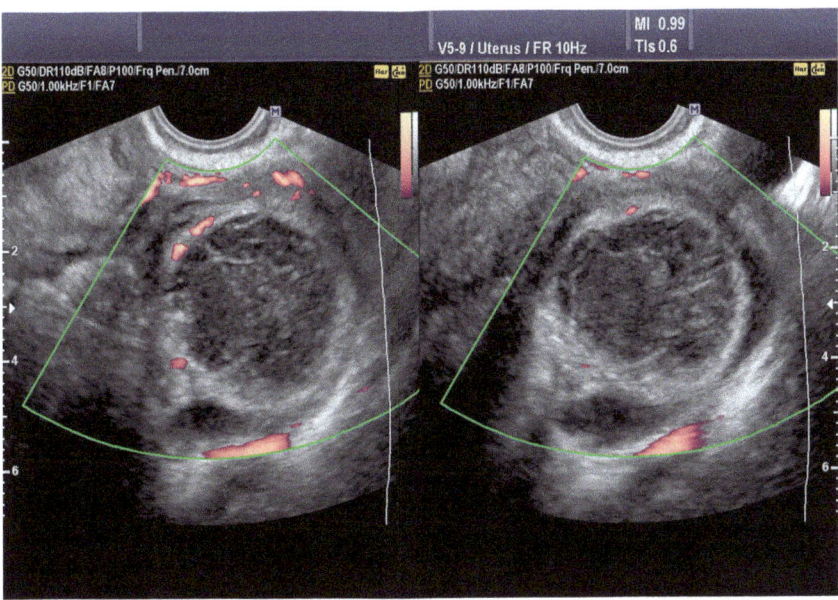

Fig. 7.3.11: Always take the patient's menstrual history to see if she is in the postovulatory phase

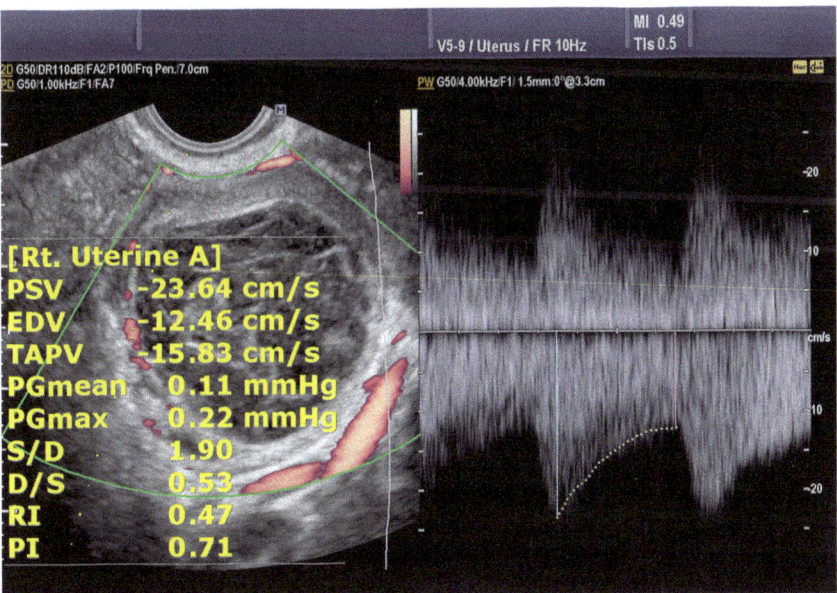

Fig. 7.3.12: On duplex Doppler the arterial flow velocity waveform shows a low impedance flow suggesting a hemorrhagic corpus luteum

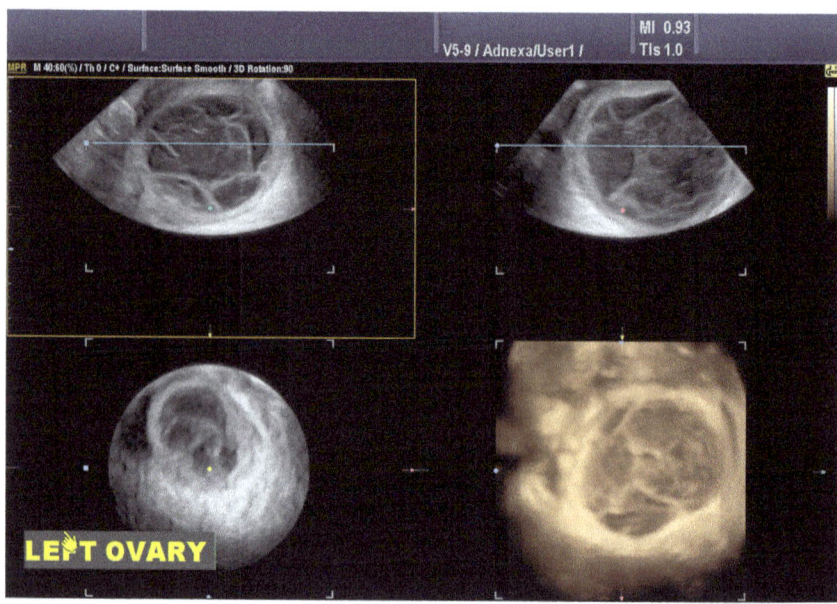

Fig. 7.3.13: Hemorrhagic corpus luteum as seen on MPR

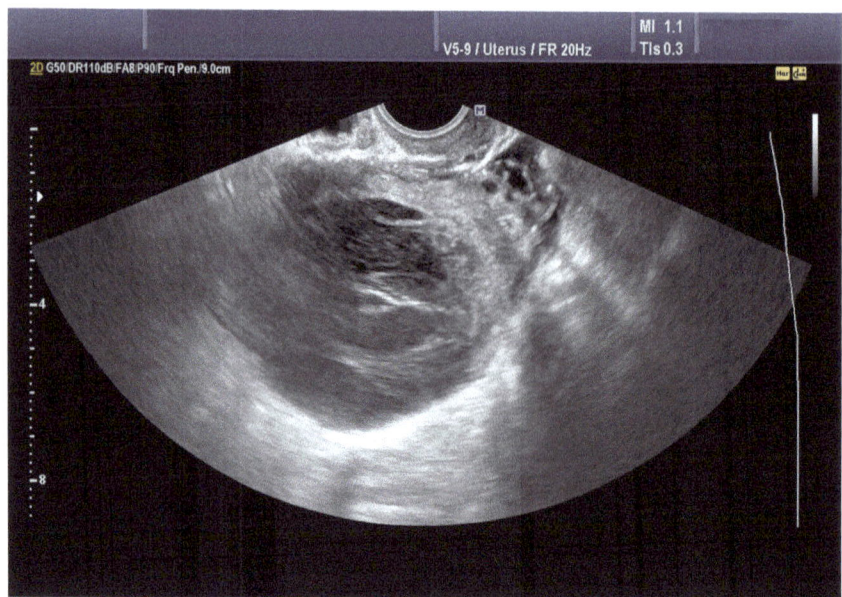

Fig. 7.3.14: Large hemorrhagic cyst seen. Look for any other adnexal mass and free fluid

7.3. Hemorrhagic Cyst

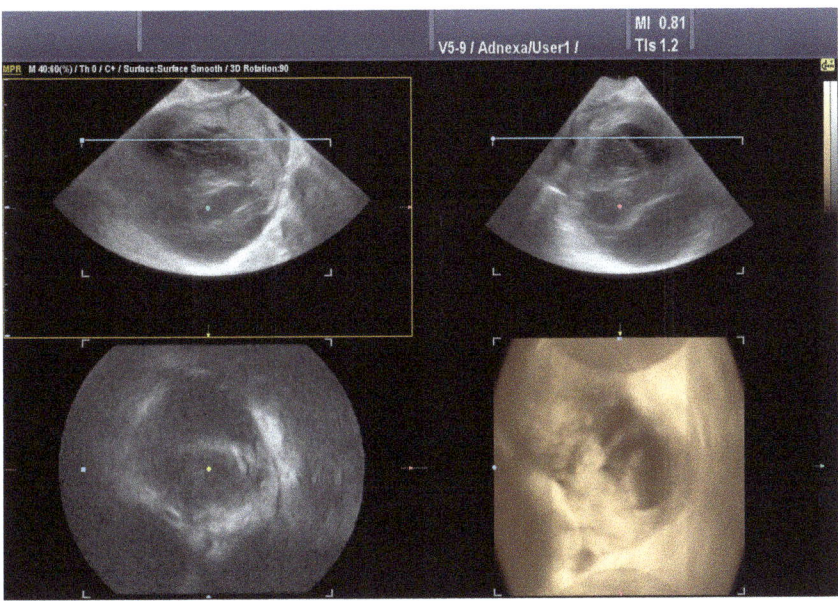

Fig. 7.3.15: Hemorrhagic cyst as seen on MPR

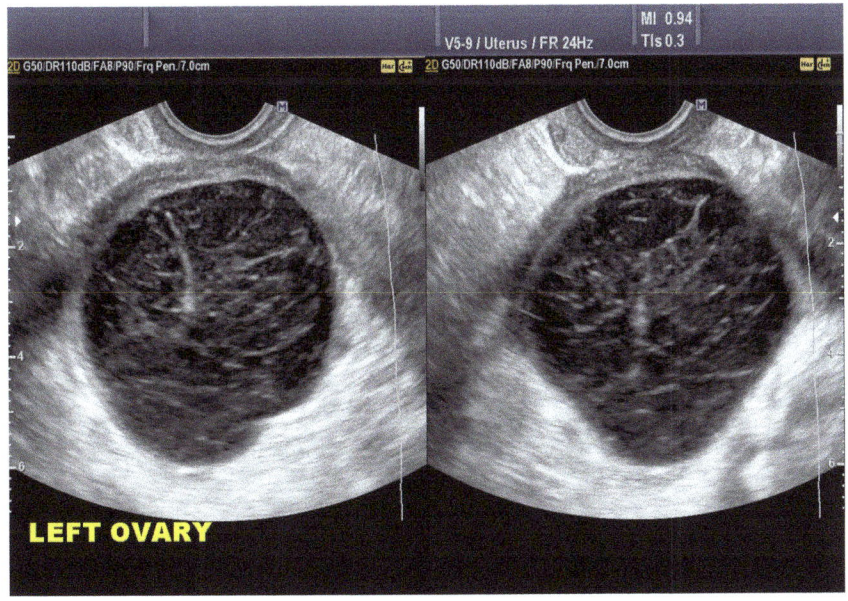

Fig. 7.3.16: Multiple strands seen within the cyst

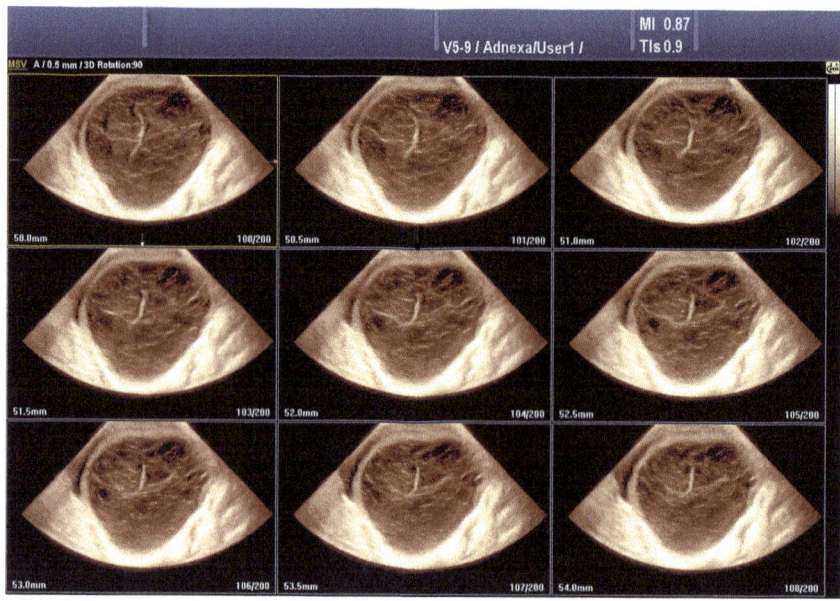

Fig. 7.3.17: Hemorrhagic cyst as seen on MSV

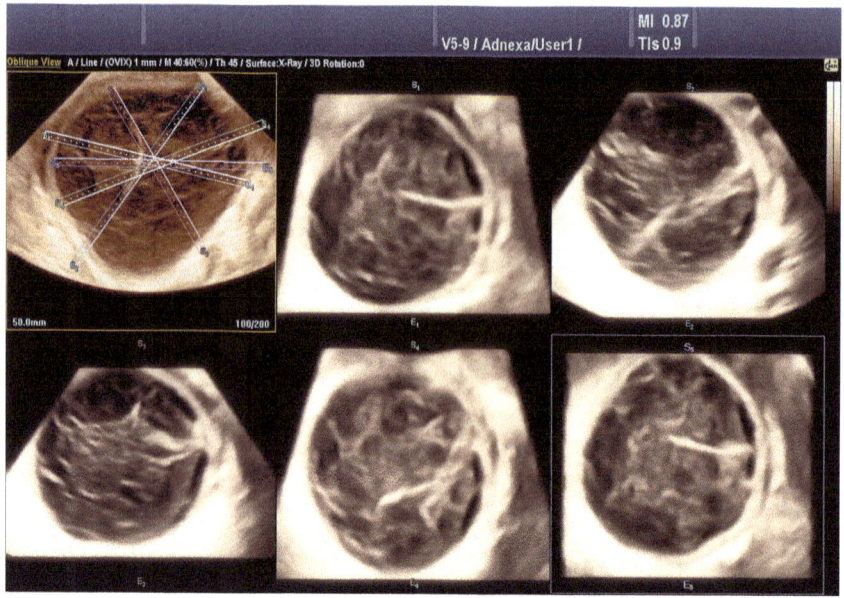

Fig. 7.3.18: As seen on MSV OVIX mode

7.3. Hemorrhagic Cyst

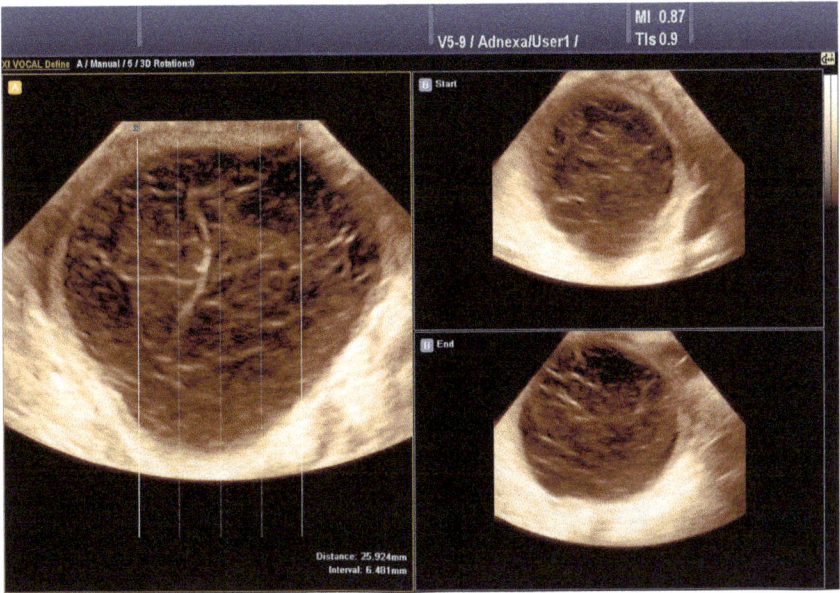

Fig. 7.3.19: As seen on 3D Vocal

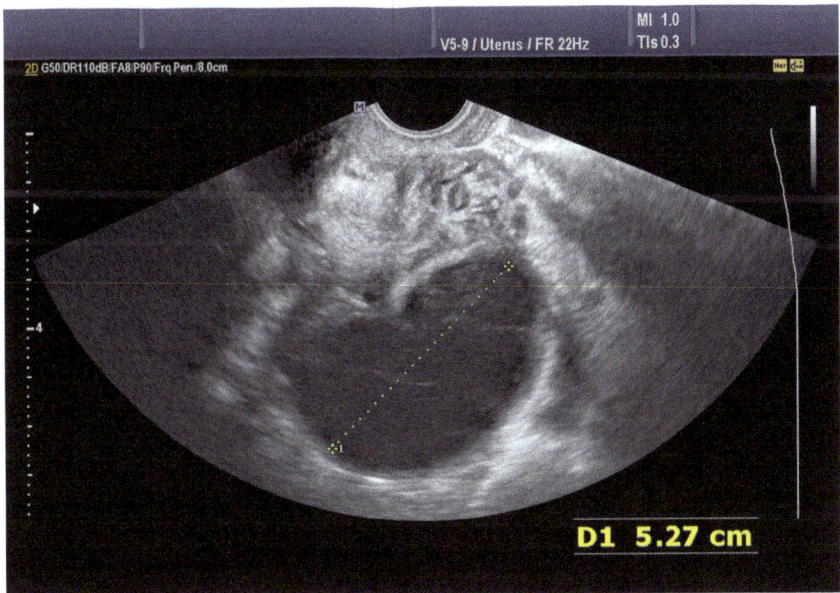

Fig. 7.3.20: In a premenopausal patient any cyst >5 cm in diameter should be followed up

7.4. CYST WITH FLUID-FLUID LEVEL

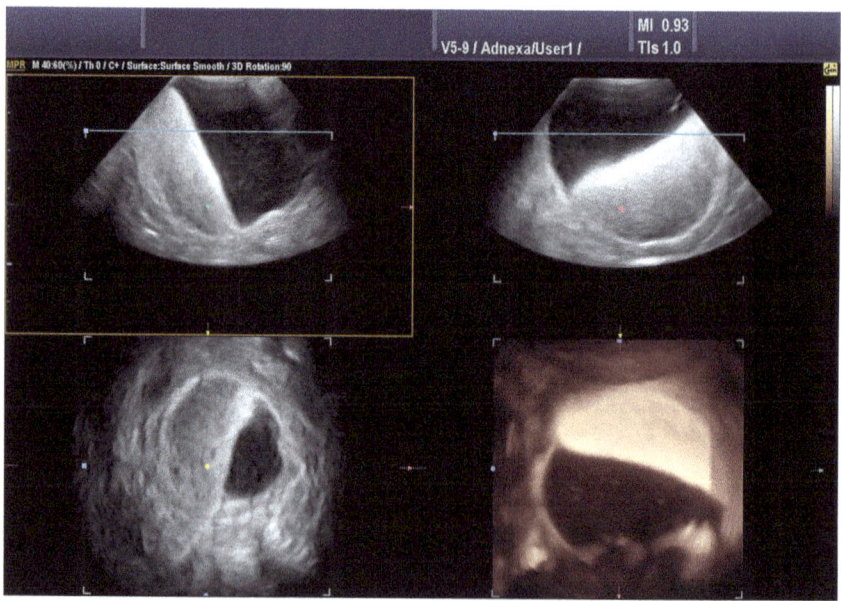

7.4. Cyst with Fluid-fluid Level

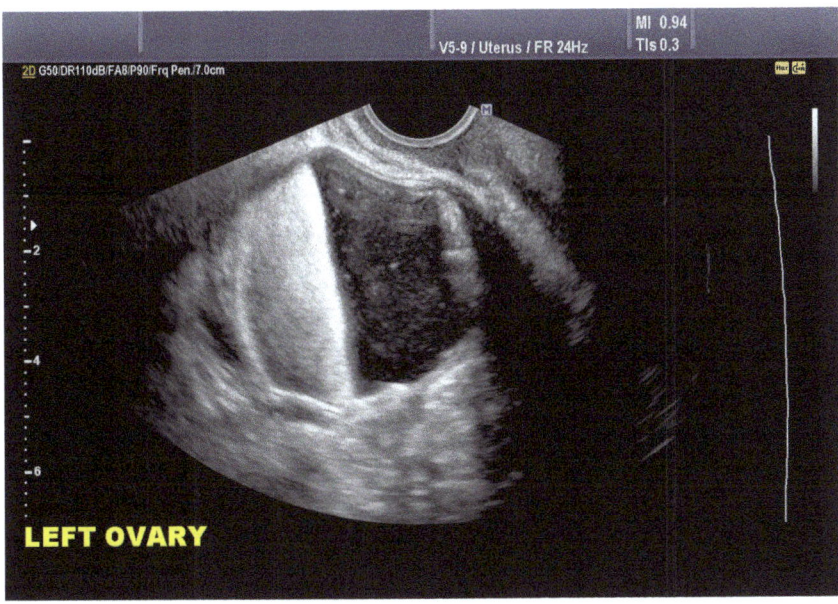

Fig. 7.4.1: Thin-walled cystic area with a fluid-fluid level

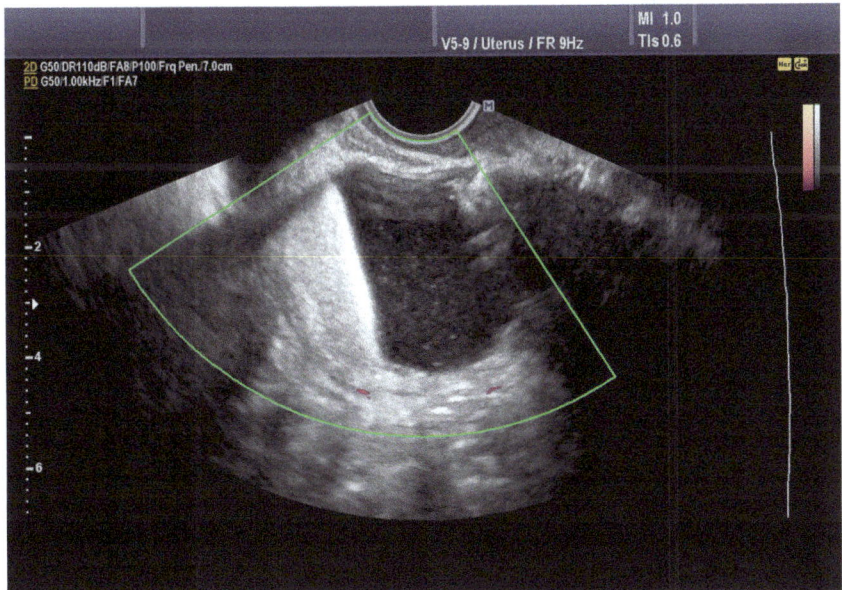

Fig. 7.4.2: The cyst as seen on color flow mapping

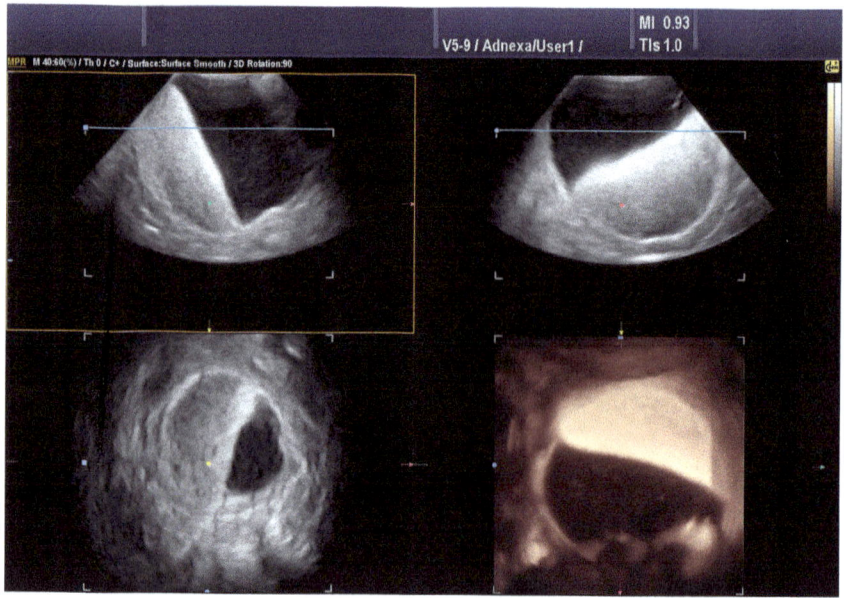

Fig. 7.4.3: Fluid-fluid level in the cyst as seen on MPR

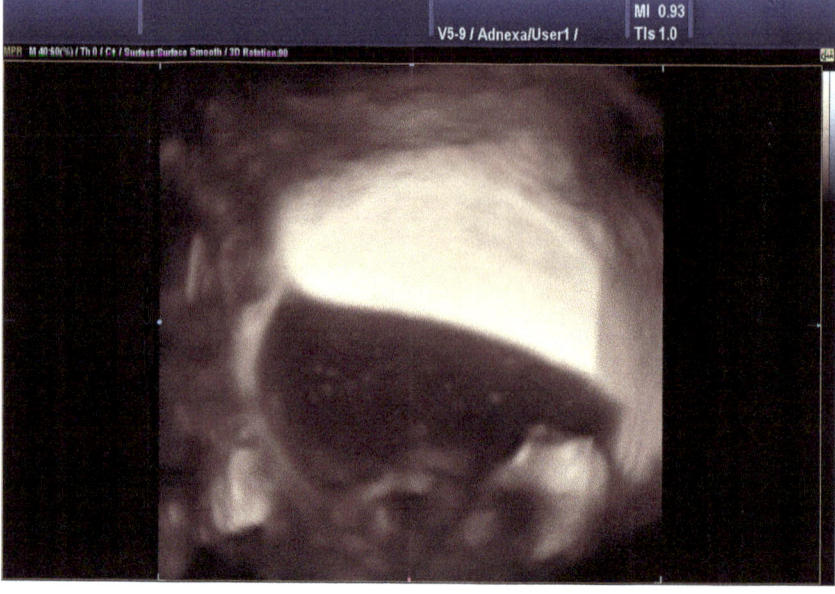

Fig. 7.4.4: As seen on 3D

7.5. CYST WITH CLOT

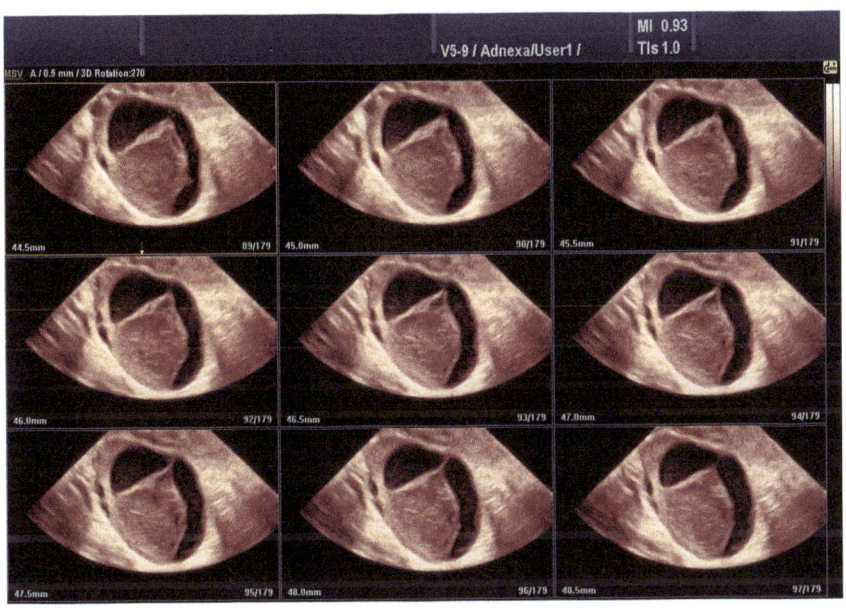

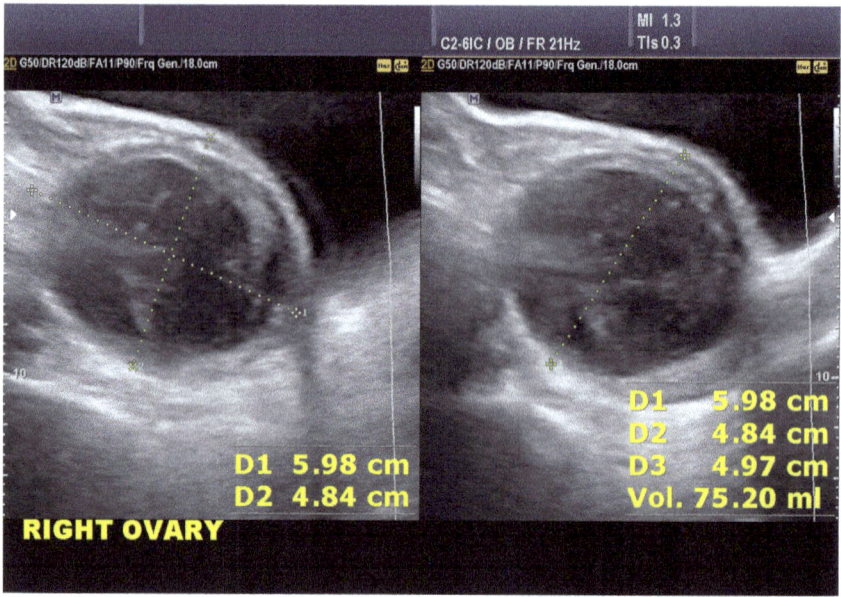

Fig. 7.5.1: Thin-walled cyst with multiple internal echoes as seen on TAS

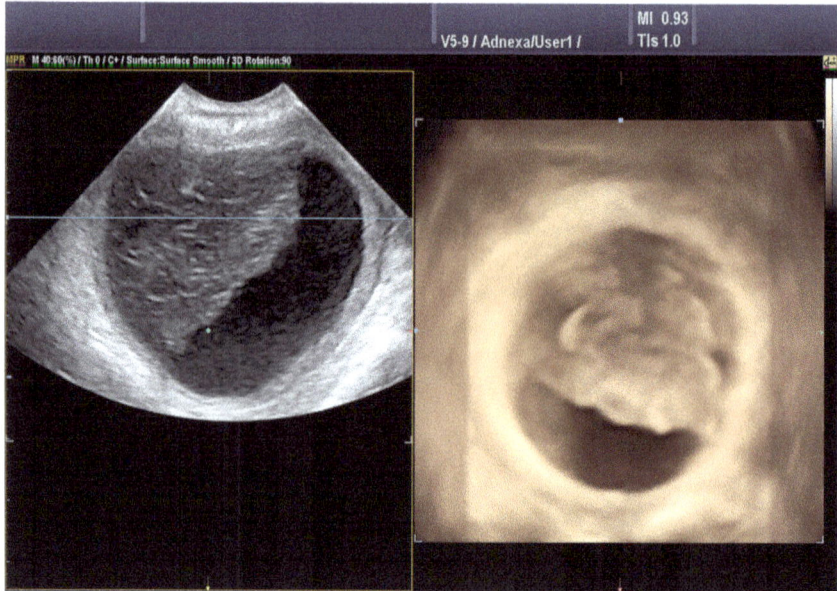

Fig. 7.5.2: The cyst as seen on TVS, 3D studies shows a clot within the cyst

7.5. Cyst with Clot

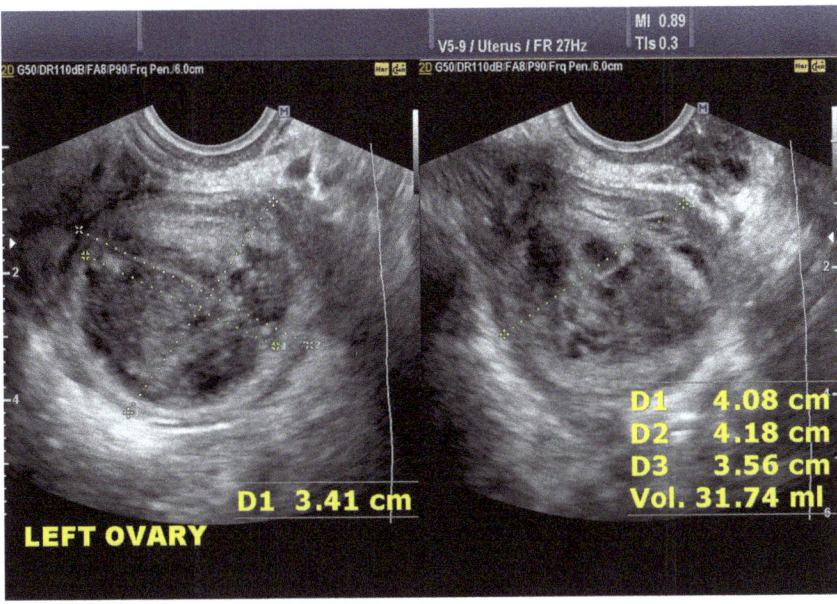

Fig. 7.5.3: 4 cm thin-walled cyst with multiple internal echoes as seen on TVS

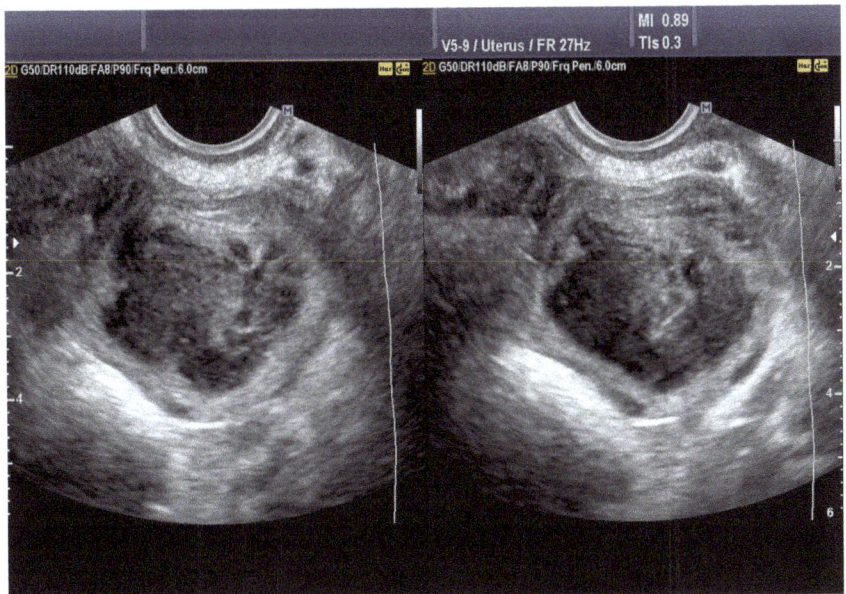

Fig. 7.5.4: On moving the probe one can see a clot within the cyst

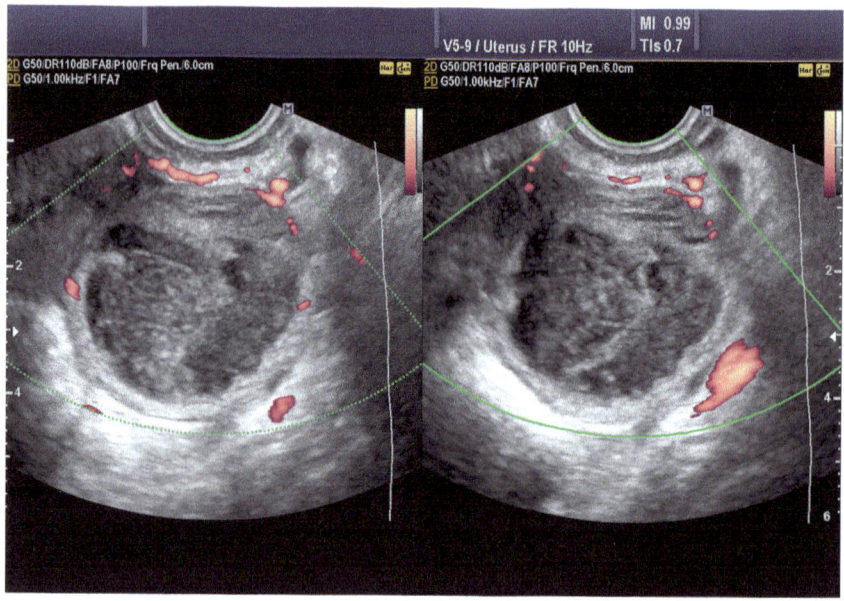

Fig. 7.5.5: Mildly vascular as seen on color flow mapping

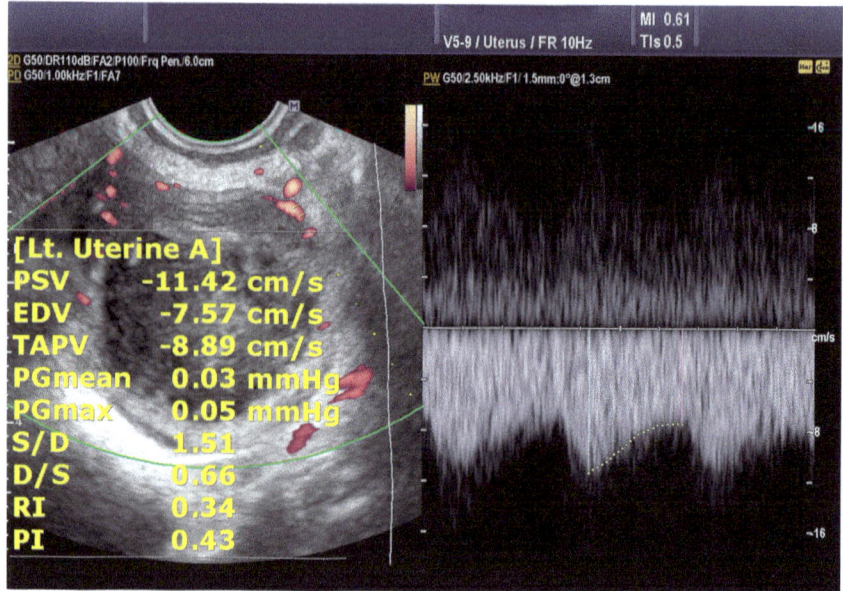

Fig. 7.5.6: On duplex Doppler evaluation, the arterial flow velocity waveform shows a low impedance flow with a resistive index of 0.34 and a pulsatility index of 0.43

7.5. Cyst with Clot

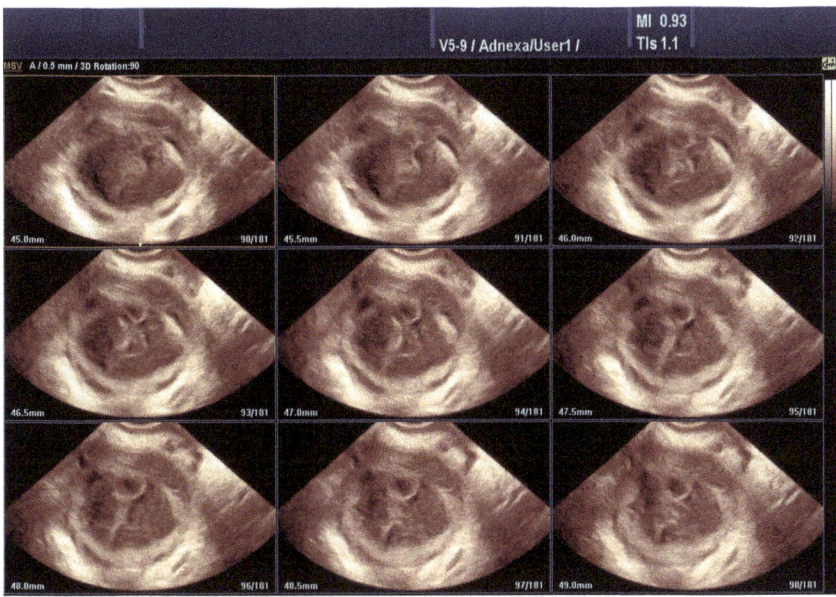

Fig. 7.5.7: The cyst with the clot margins as seen on MSV

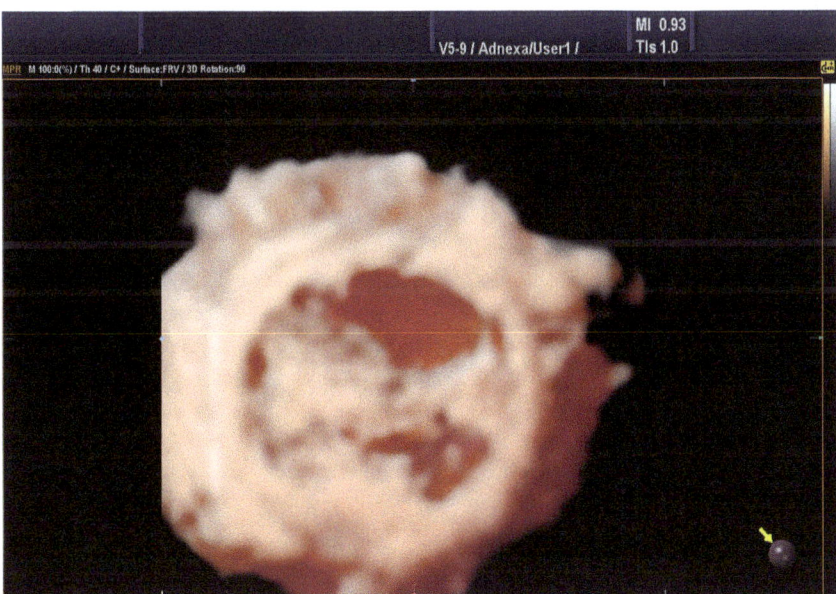

Fig. 7.5.8: Cyst as seen on 3D

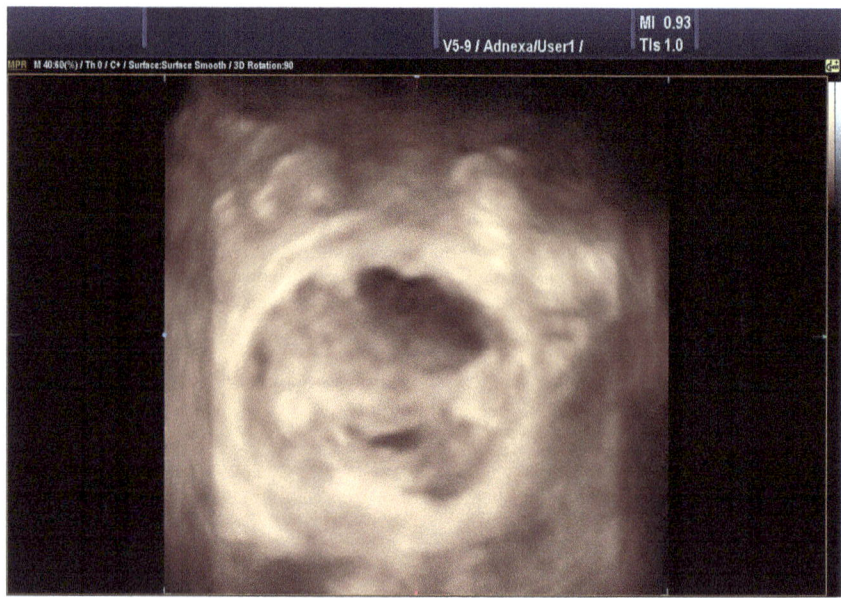

Fig. 7.5.9: The cyst as seen on 3D

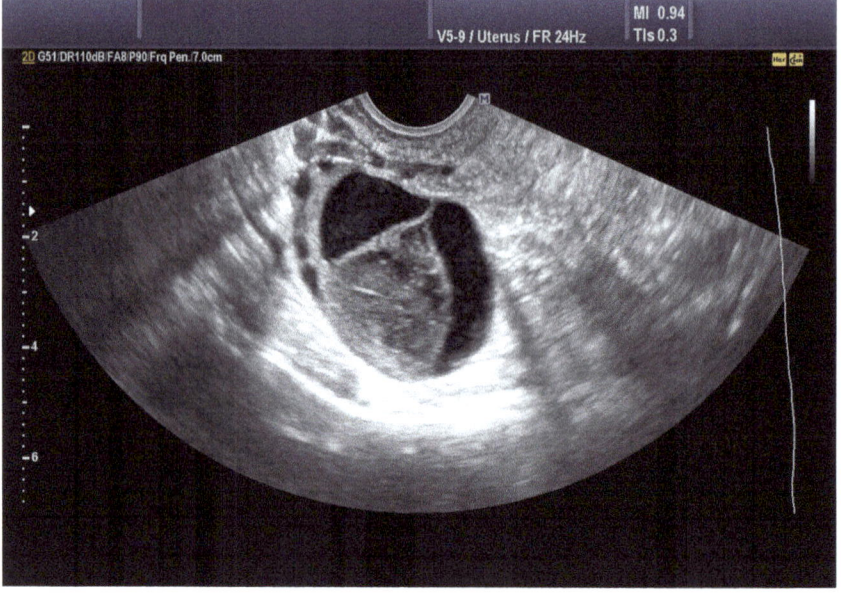

Fig. 7.5.10: Look at the margins of the retractile clot as seen on TVS

7.5. Cyst with Clot

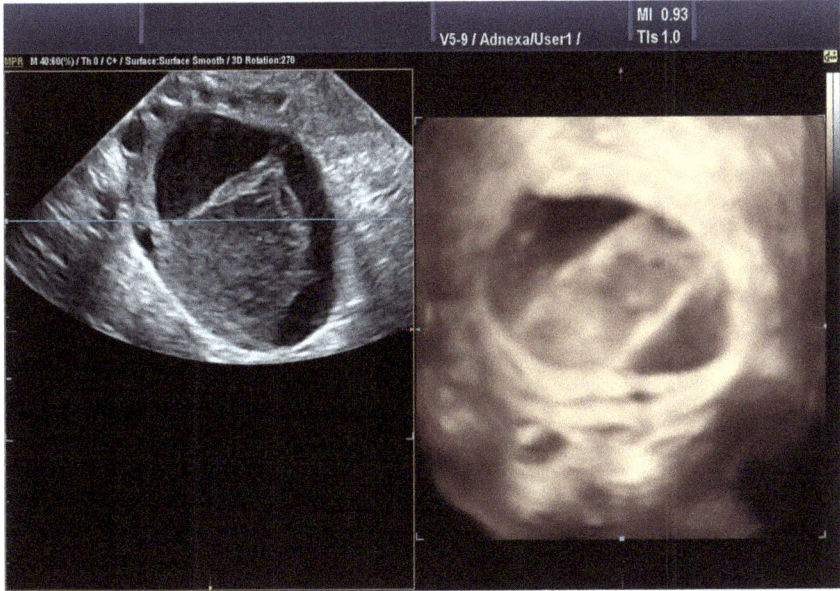

Fig. 7.5.11: The cyst as seen on 3D with the clot

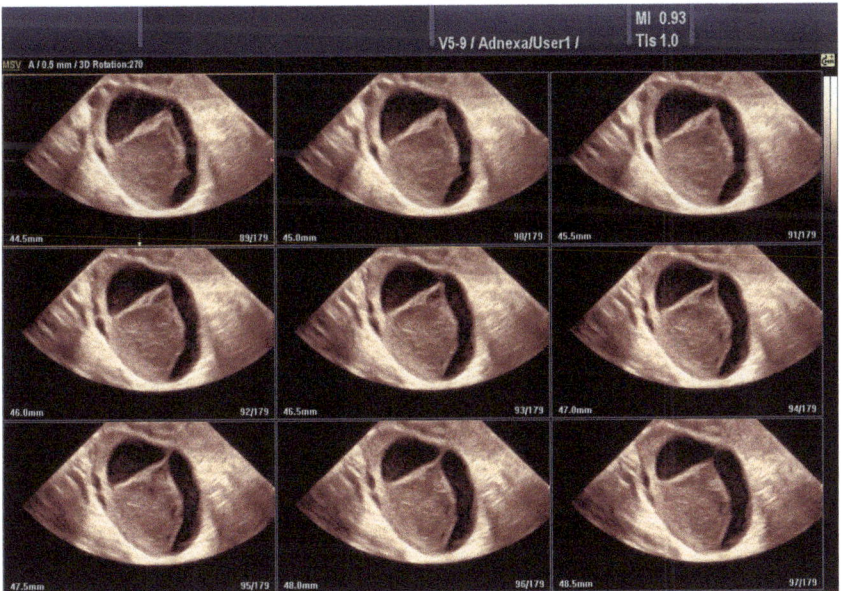

Fig. 7.5.12: Margins of the clot clearly delineated on MSV

7.6. OVARIAN TUMOR

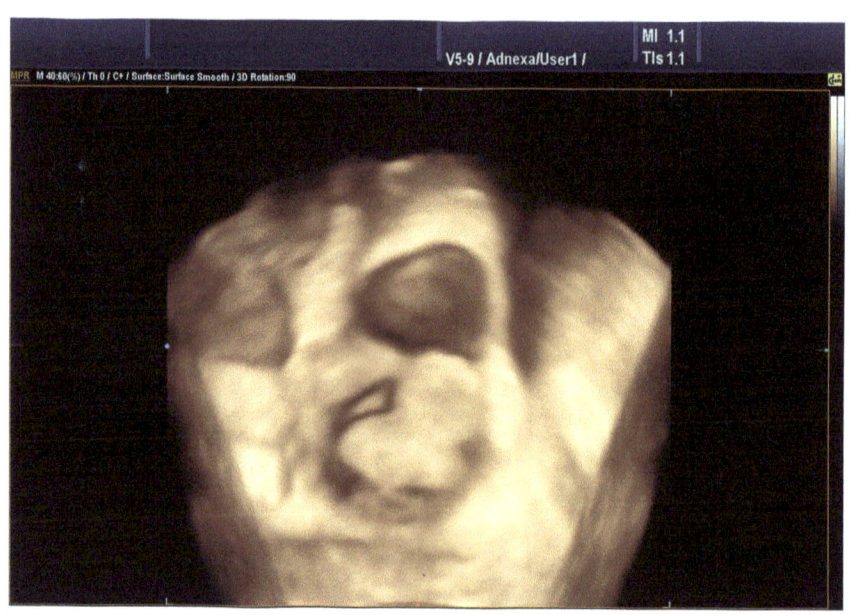

7.6. Ovarian Tumor

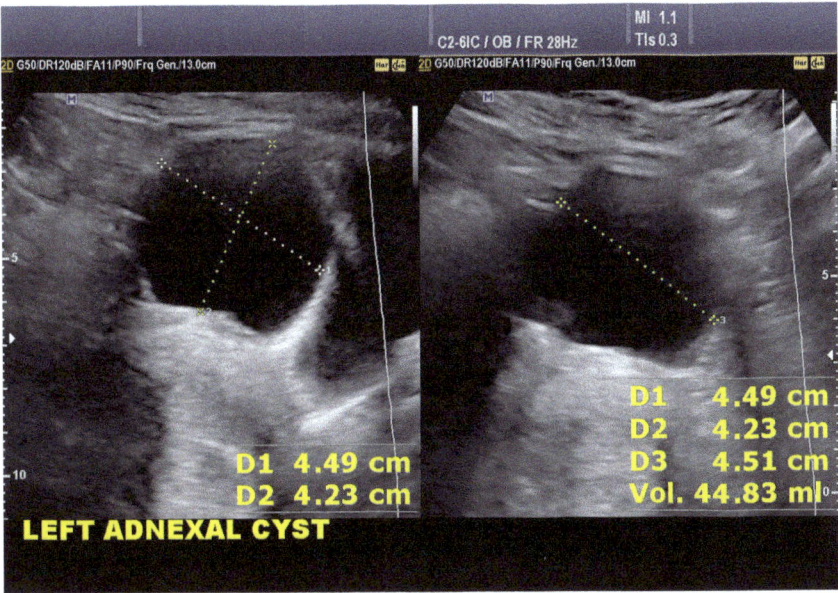

Fig. 7.6.1: Ovarian tumor can present as cystic, complex or solid

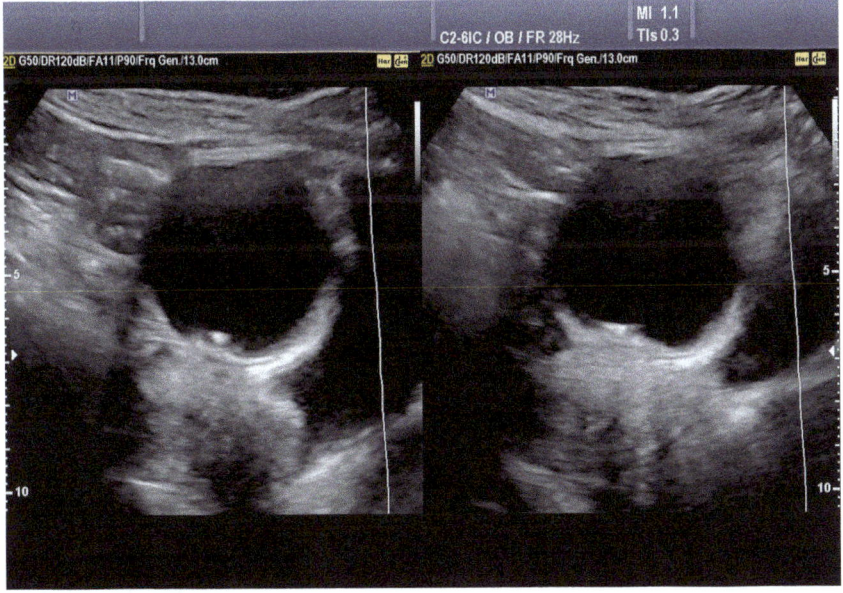

Fig. 7.6.2: On ultrasound especially TVS one needs to evaluate wall thickness

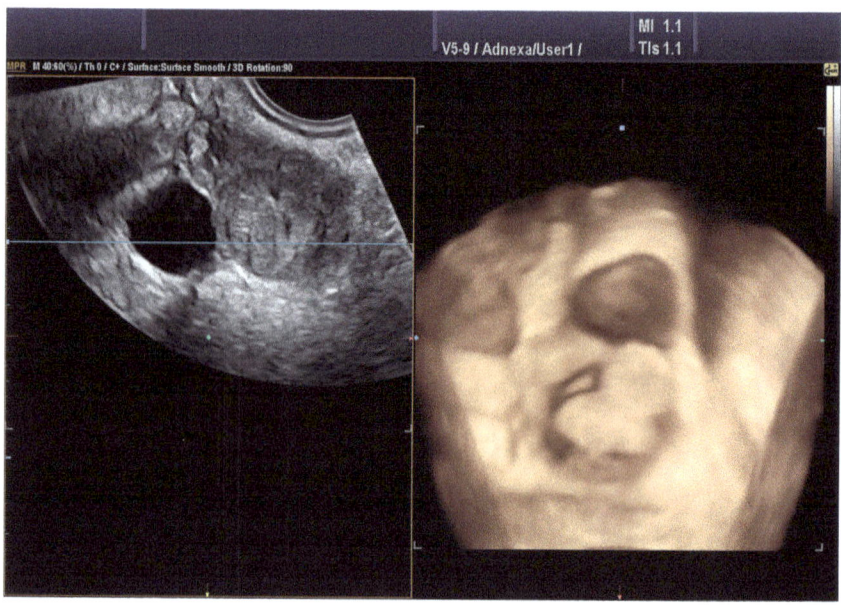

Fig. 7.6.3: One should evaluate the appearance of inner wall: smooth, simple or papillomas

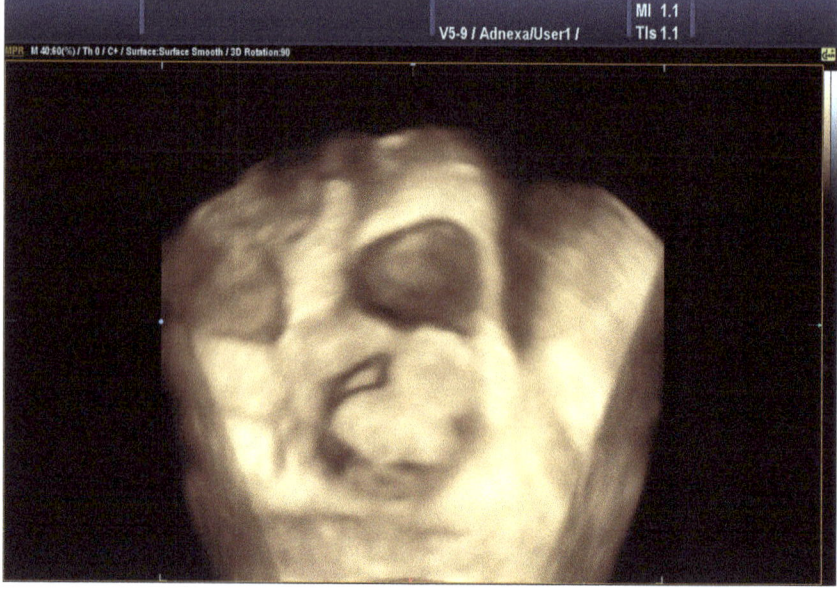

Fig. 7.6.4: As seen on 3D

7.6. Ovarian Tumor

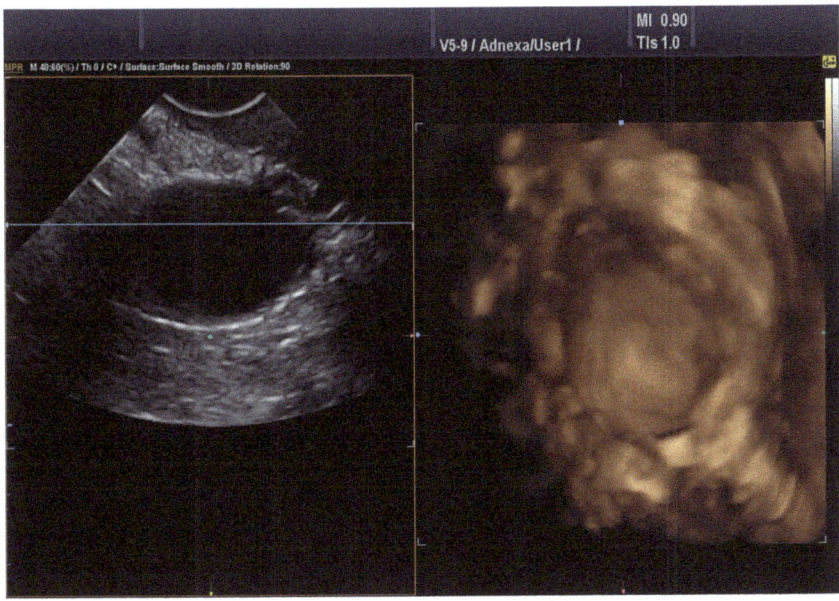

Fig. 7.6.5: Irregular thickening of the ovarian cyst. Be careful and do a complete workup

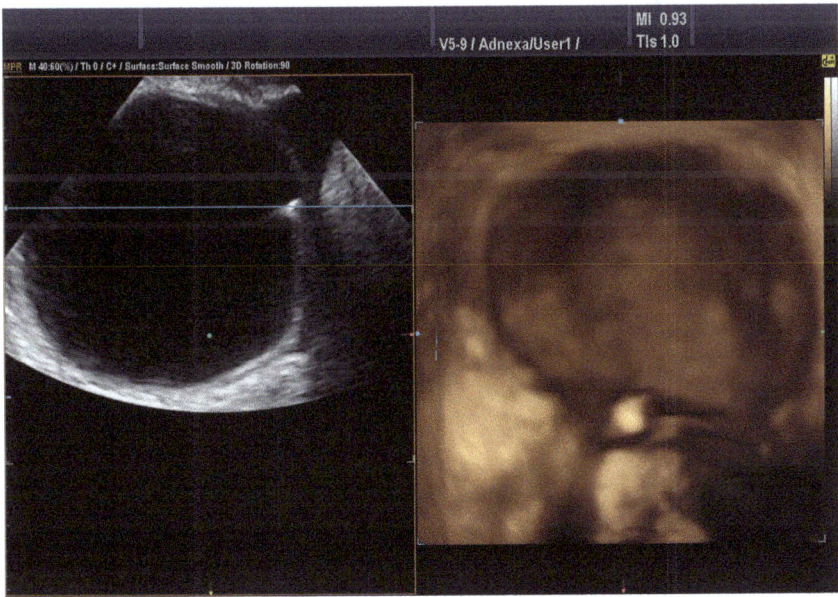

Fig. 7.6.6: Focal projection in the cyst as seen on 3D

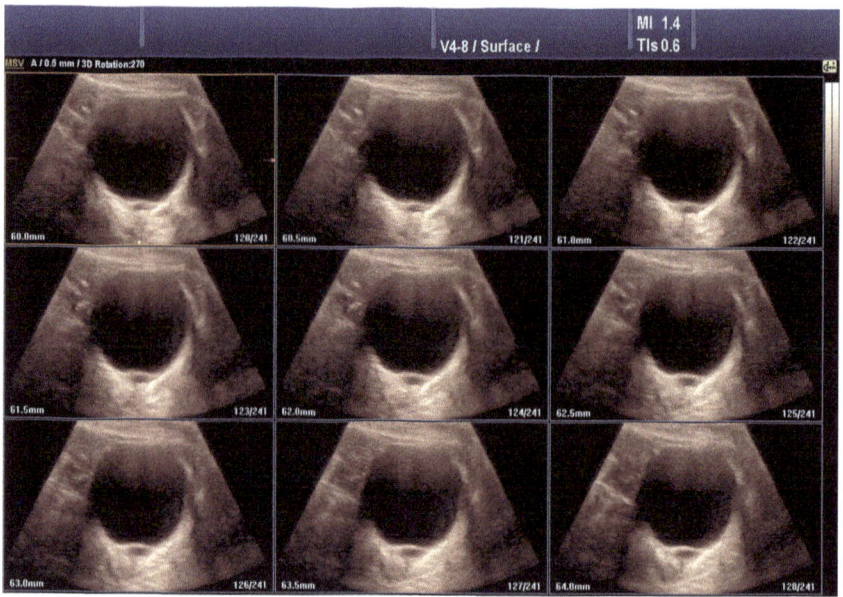

Fig. 7.6.7: Ovarian cyst as seen on MSV

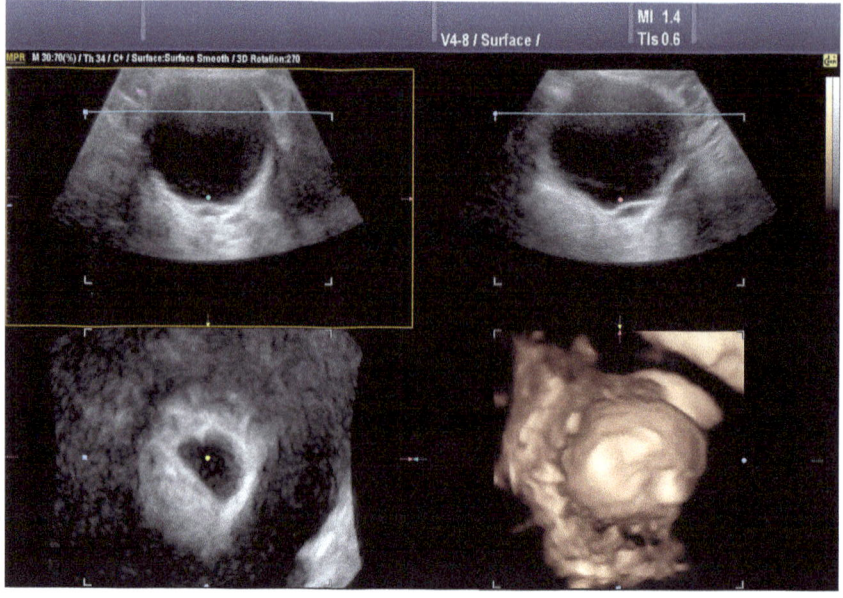

Fig. 7.6.8: As seen on 3D

7.6. Ovarian Tumor

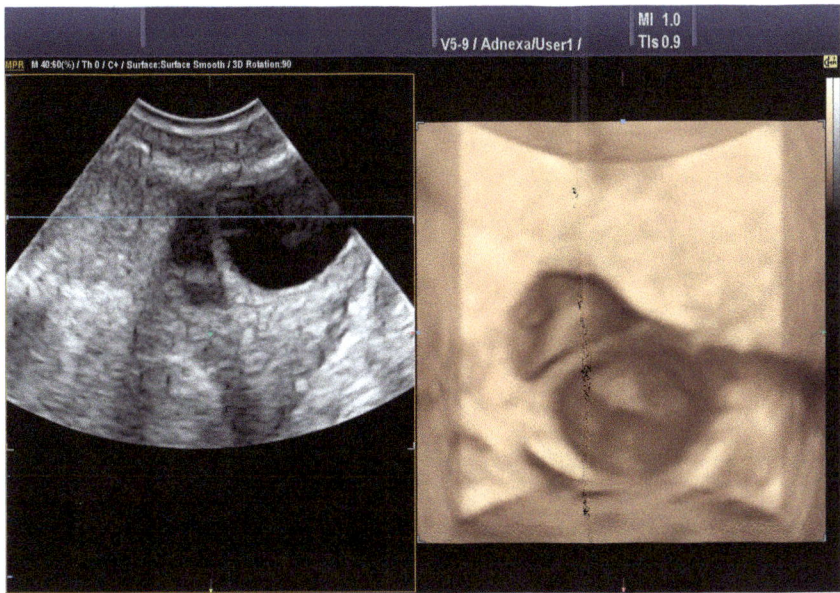

Fig. 7.6.9: Carefully evaluate the cyst for septation in the ovary

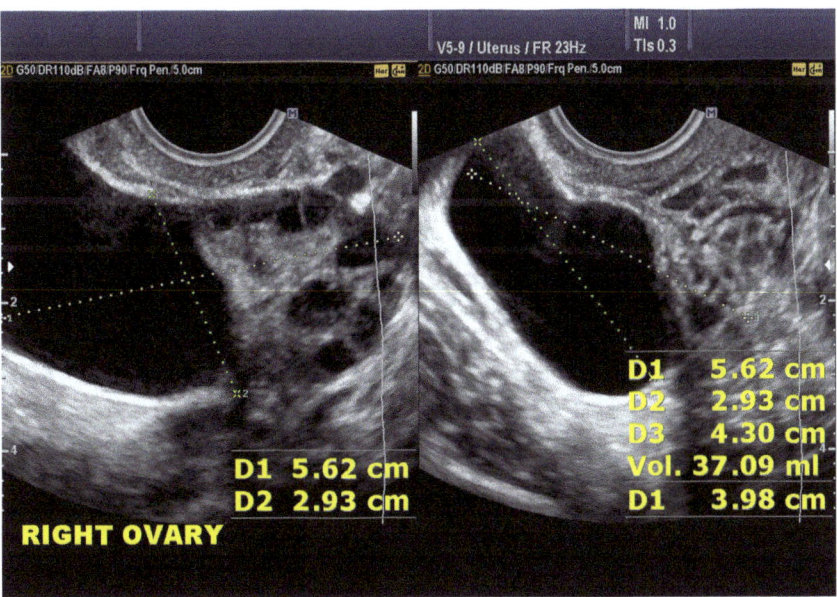

Fig. 7.6.10: If the biochemical markers are also positive evaluate the cyst with greater detail

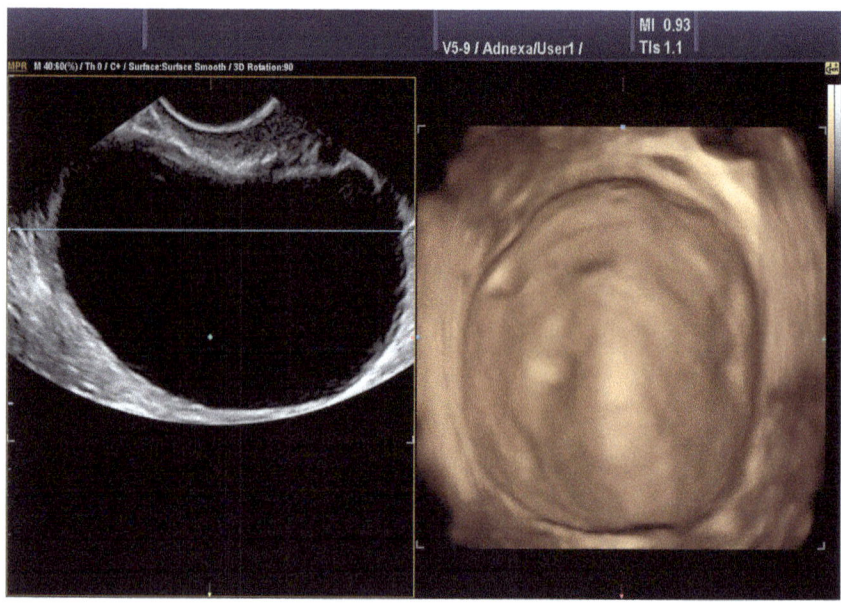

Fig. 7.6.11: Evaluate the cyst wall for any focal thickening or projection

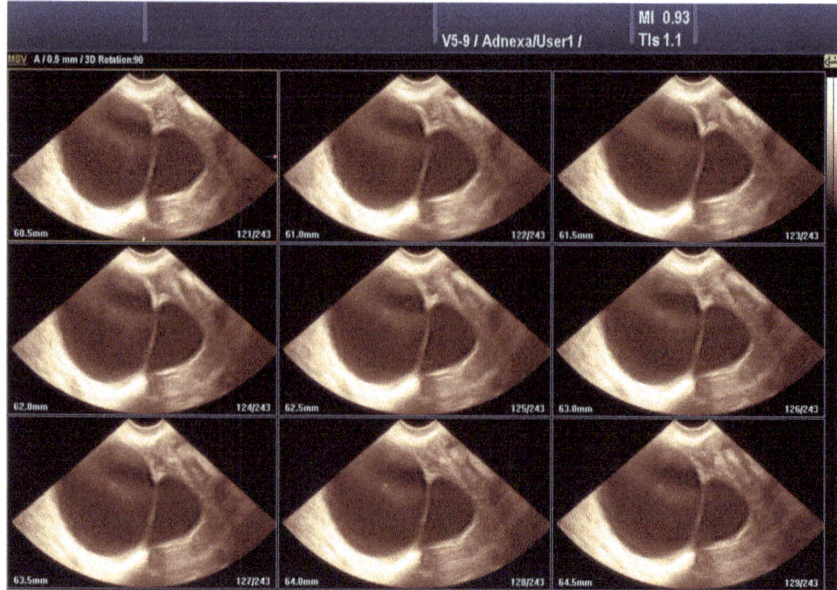

Fig. 7.6.12: Look for the thickness of the septa and any vascularity in the septa

7.6. Ovarian Tumor

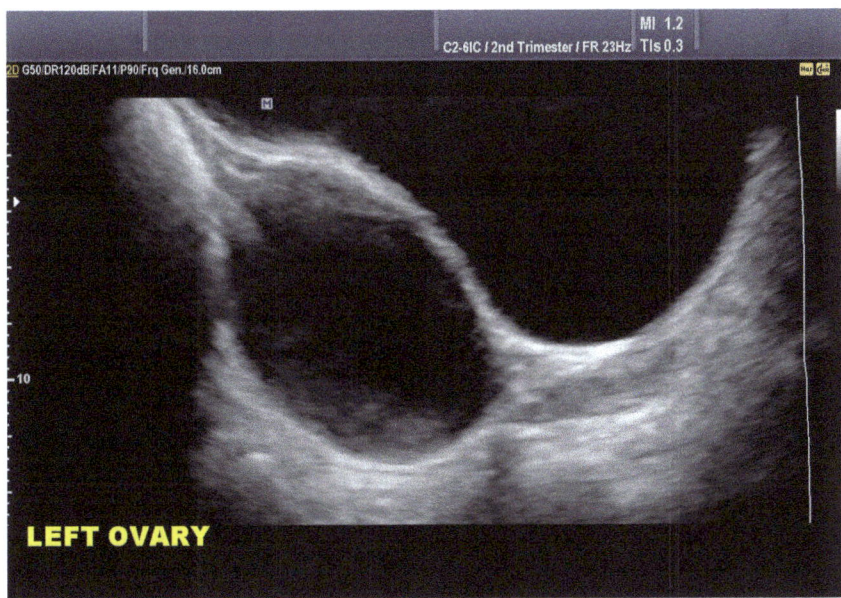

Fig. 7.6.13: An anechoic area which is thin-walled is likely to be benign and should be evaluated immediate postmenstrual

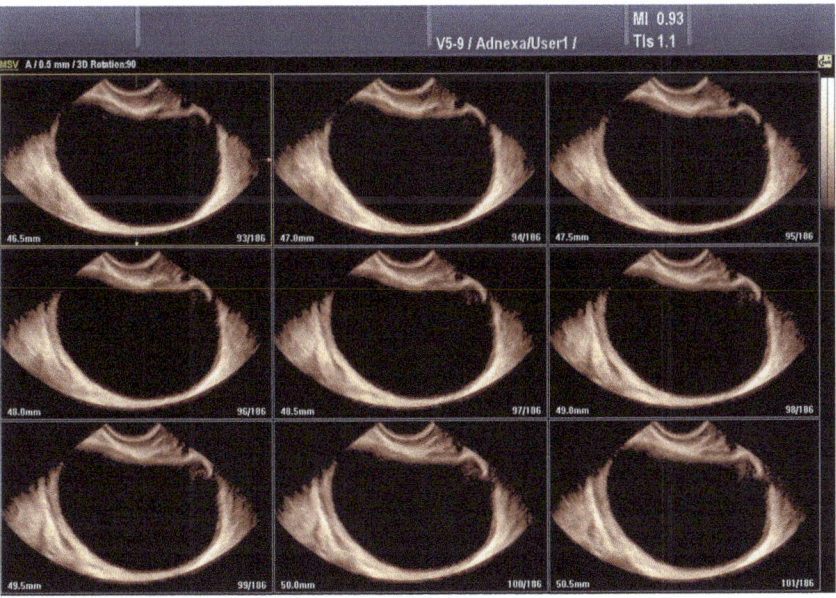

Fig. 7.6.14: Cyst as seen on MSV

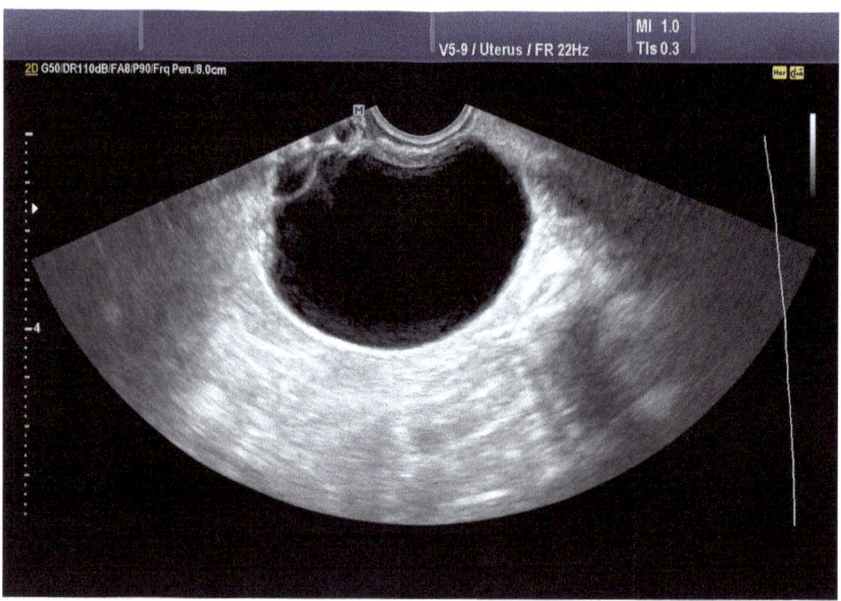

Fig. 7.6.15: Small daughter cyst should not be confused with septae

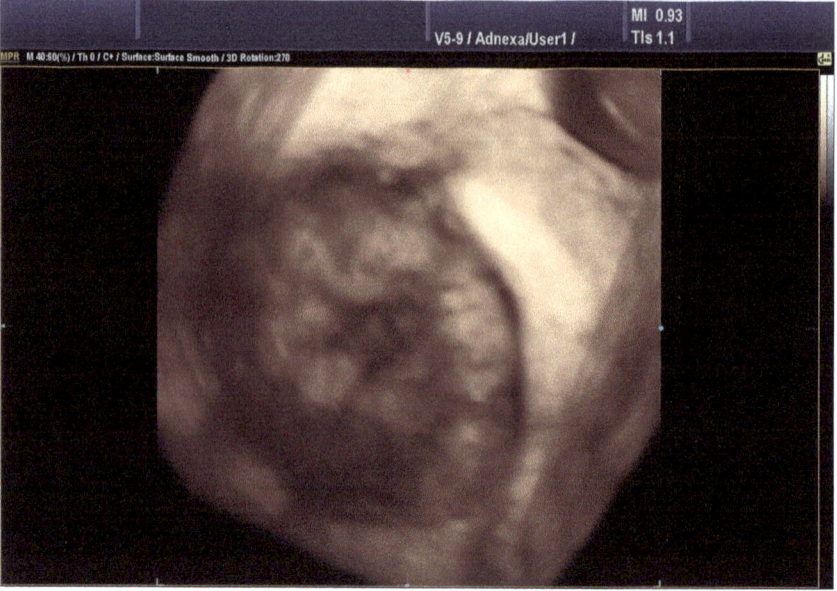

Fig. 7.6.16: Ovarian mass. Be careful to evaluate the markers of malignancy

7.6. Ovarian Tumor

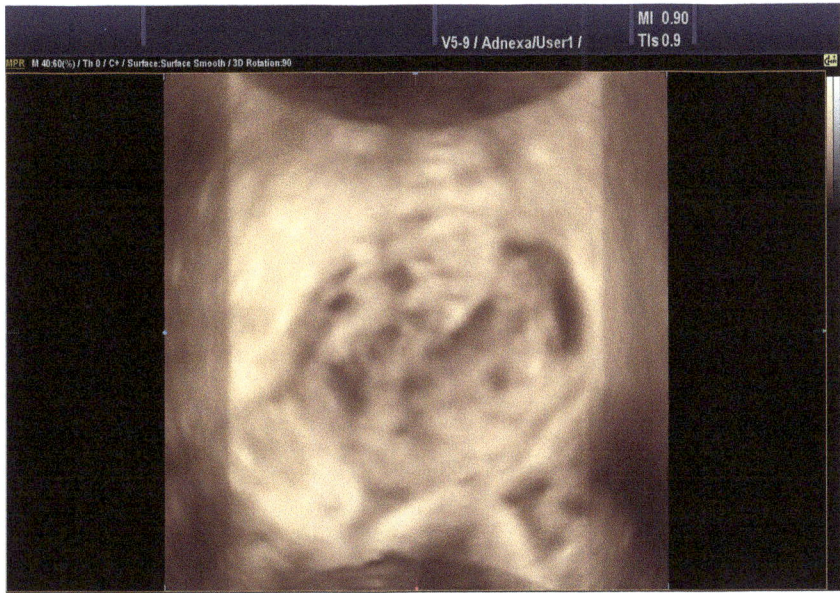

Fig. 7.6.17: Solid ovarian mass as seen on 3D

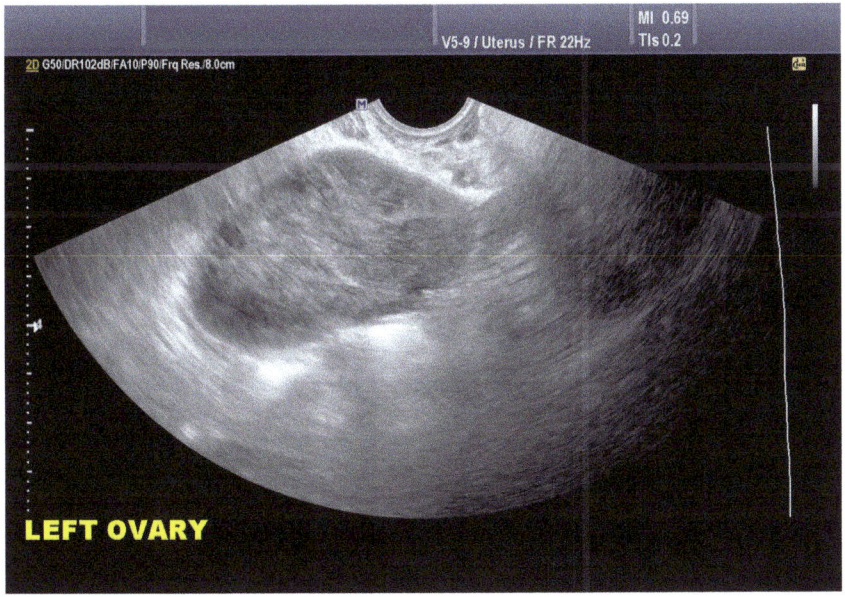

Fig. 7.6.18: Solid ovarian mass

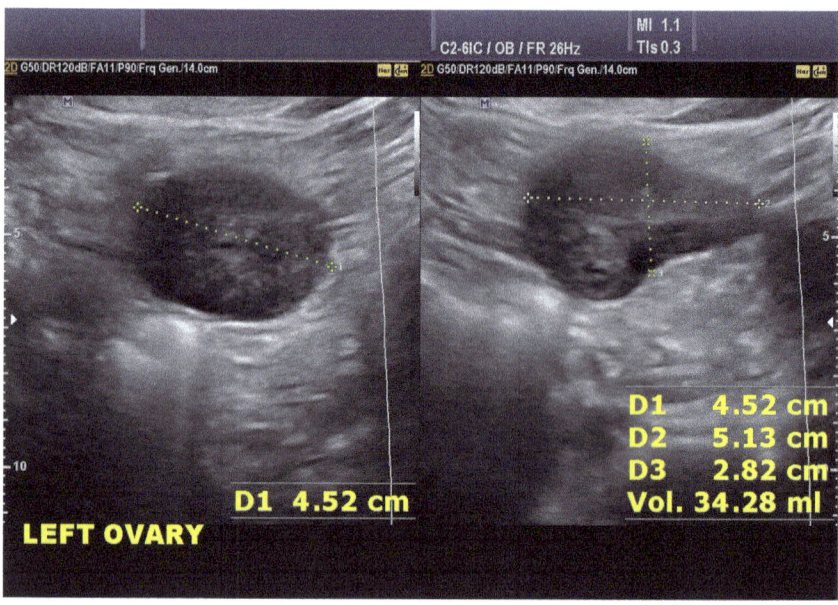

Fig. 7.6.19: Solid ovarian mass evaluate carefully for vascularity and biochemical markers of malignancy

7.7. DERMOID

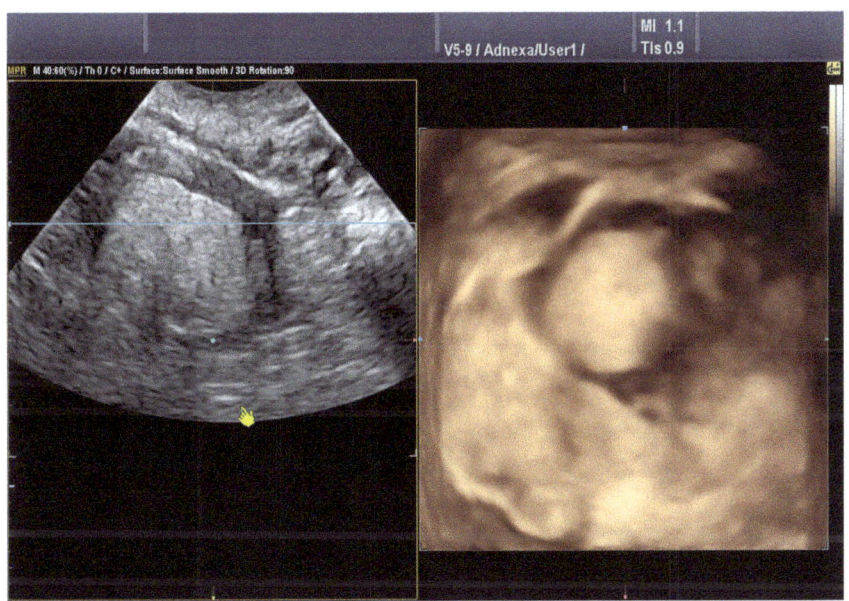

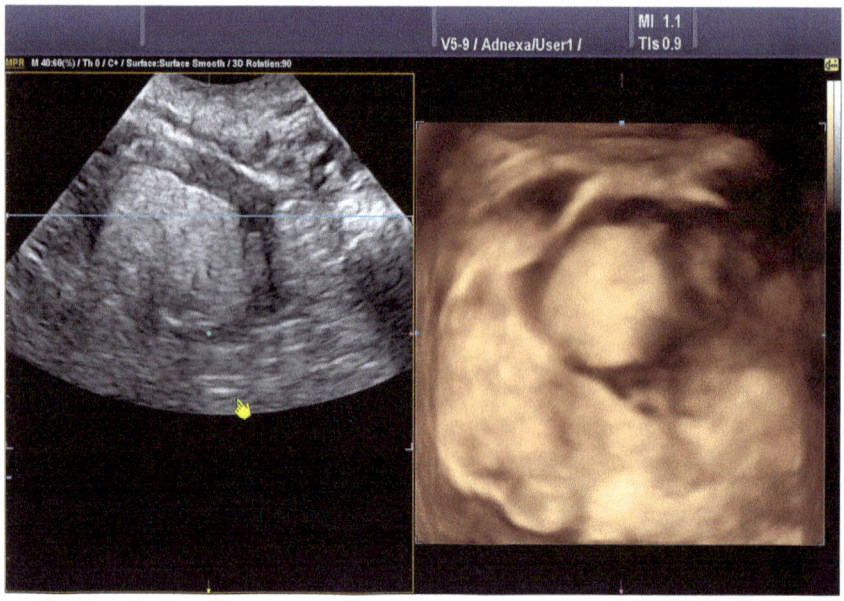

Fig. 7.7.1: Dermoid is a bizarre tumor, usually benign in the ovary that typically contains diversity of tissues

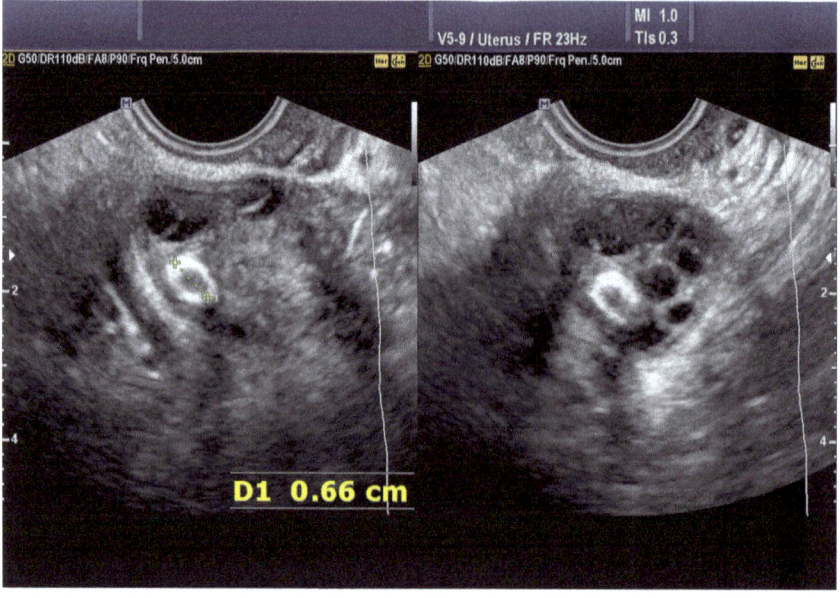

Fig. 7.7.2: Can contain hair, teeth, bone, etc

7.7. Dermoid

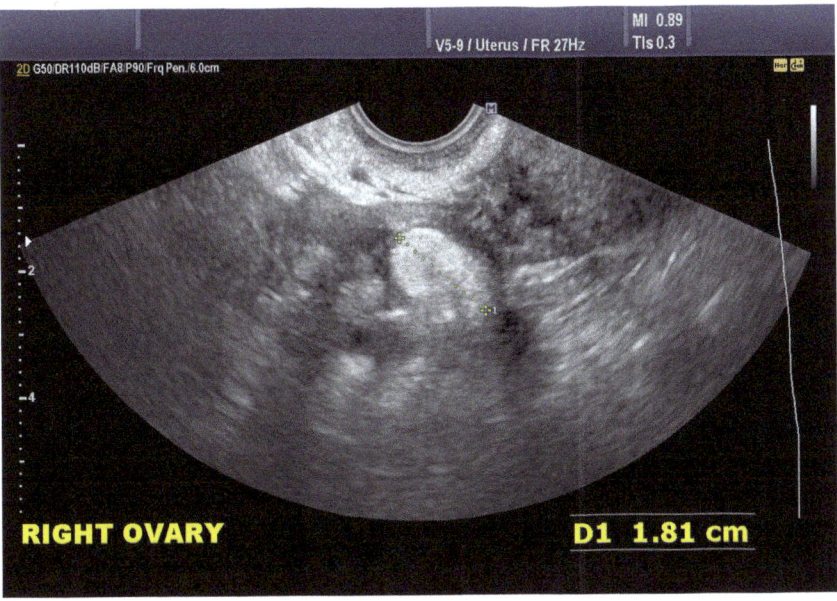

Fig. 7.7.3: Can show as a echogenic, calcific or tooth components

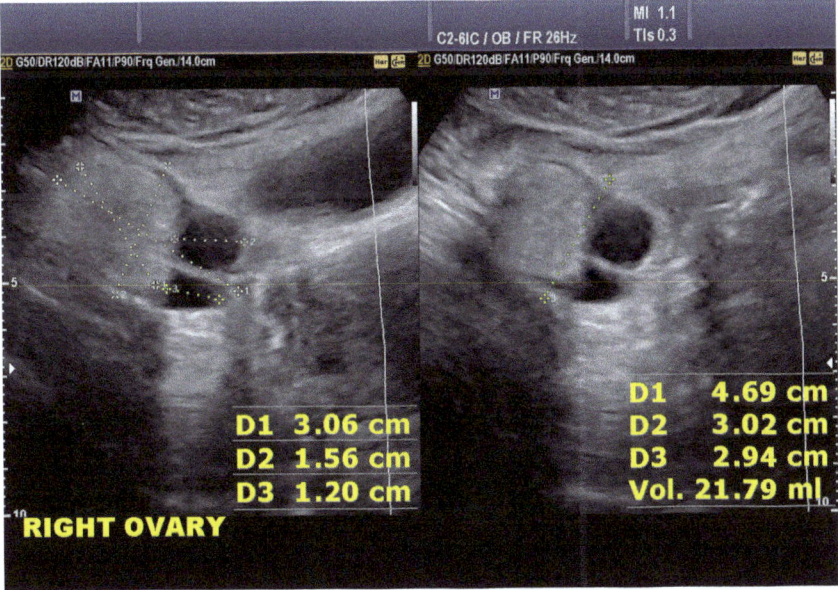

Fig. 7.7.4: Dermoid can show as a partially echogenic mass with posterior sound attenuation

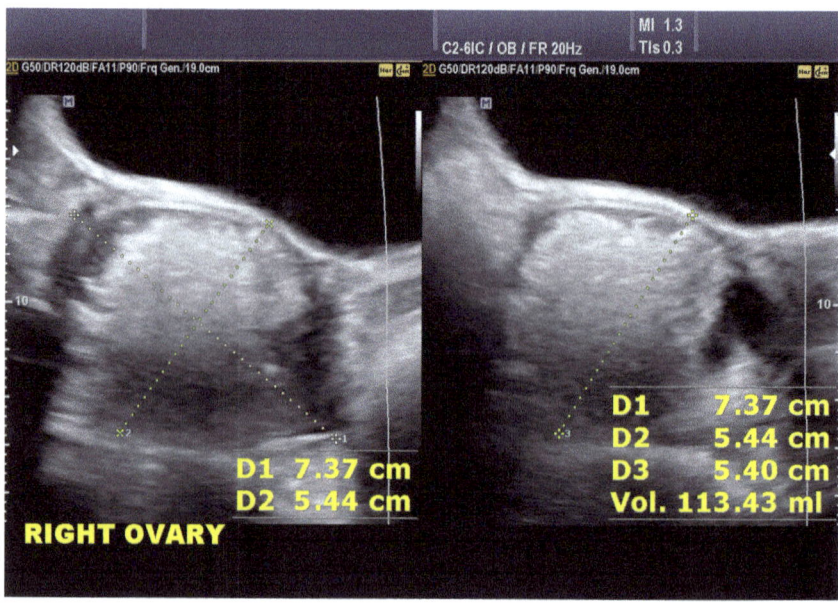

Fig. 7.7.5: Complete ovary can be seen replaced by dermoid

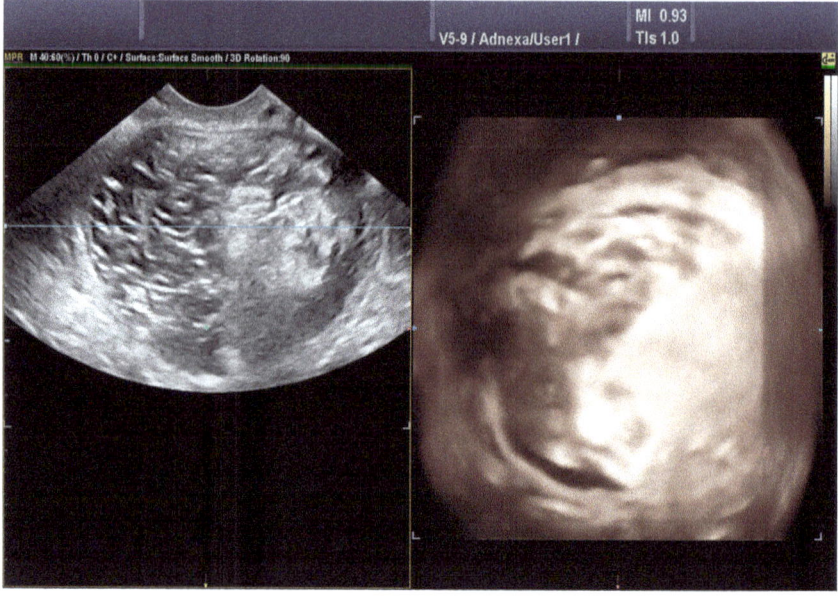

Fig. 7.7.6: Multiple thin echogenic bands caused by hair can be seen

7.7. Dermoid

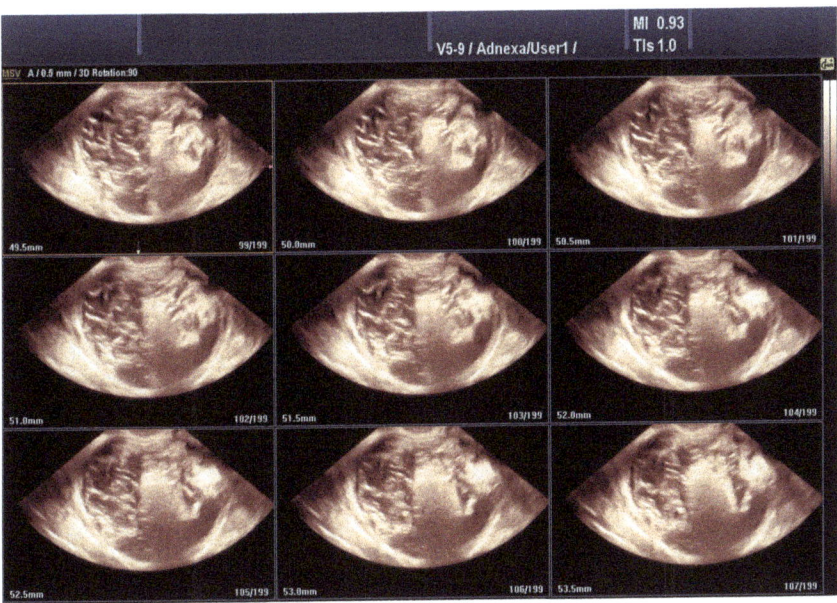

Fig. 7.7.7: Dermoid as seen on MSV

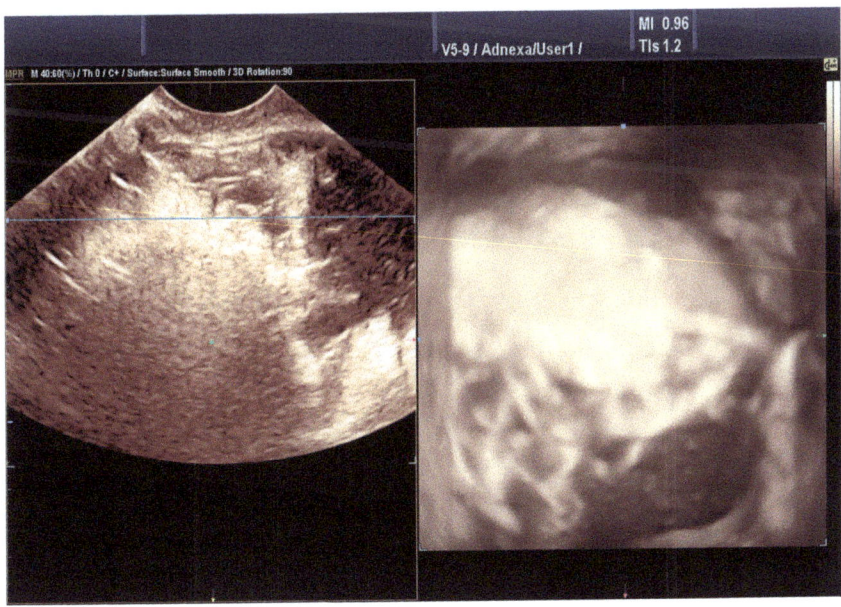

Fig. 7.7.8: Dermoid as seen on 3D

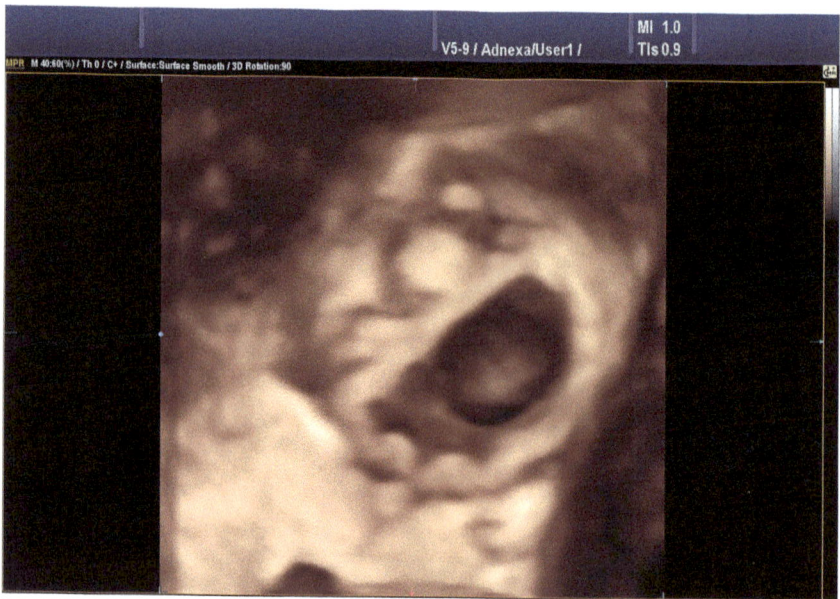

Fig. 7.7.9: Ovary shows a dysfunctional cyst and a dermoid with echogenic areas as well

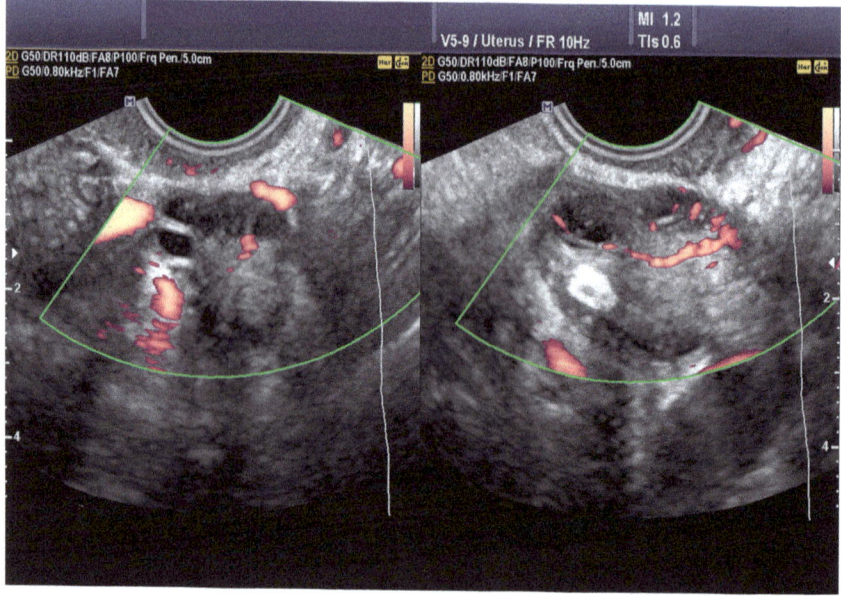

Fig. 7.7.10: On color flow mapping usually no abnormal vascularity is delineated

7.7. Dermoid

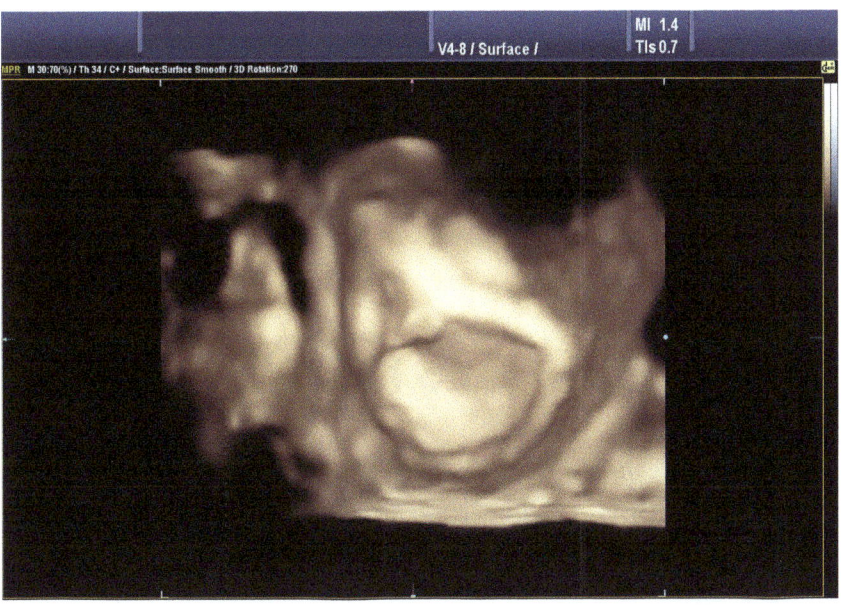

Fig. 7.7.11: Dermoid can show presence of a fluid-fluid level

7.8. POLYCYSTIC OVARIES

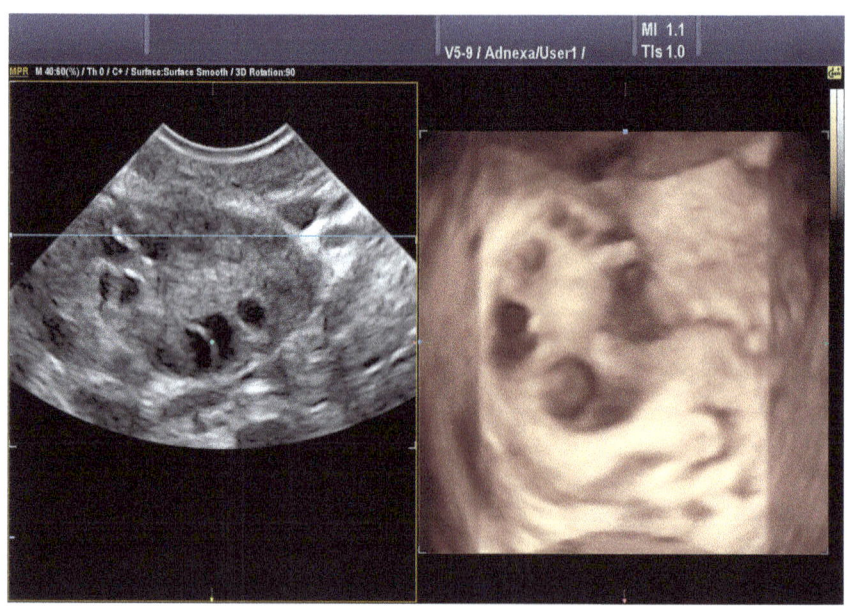

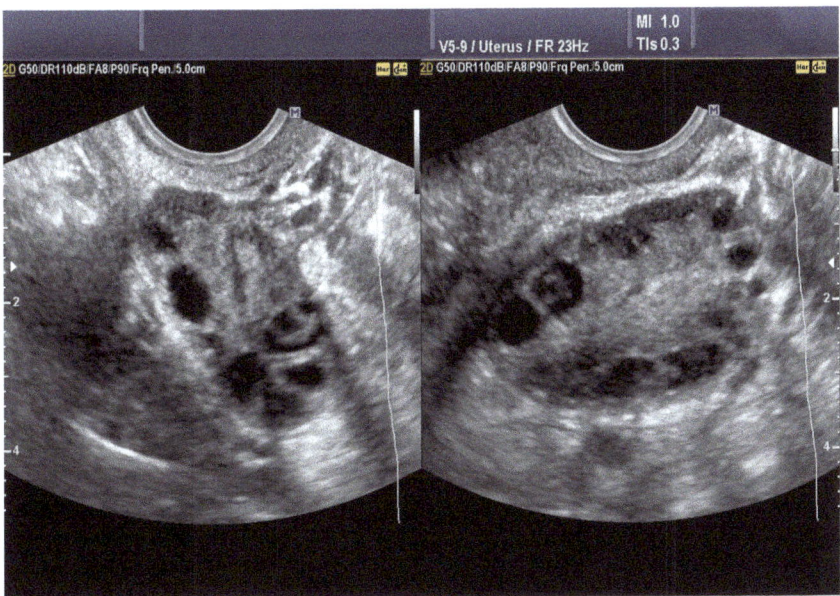

Fig. 7.8.1: Patients with polycystic ovaries have the usual triad of Stein-Leventhal: oligomenorrhea, hirsutism and obesity

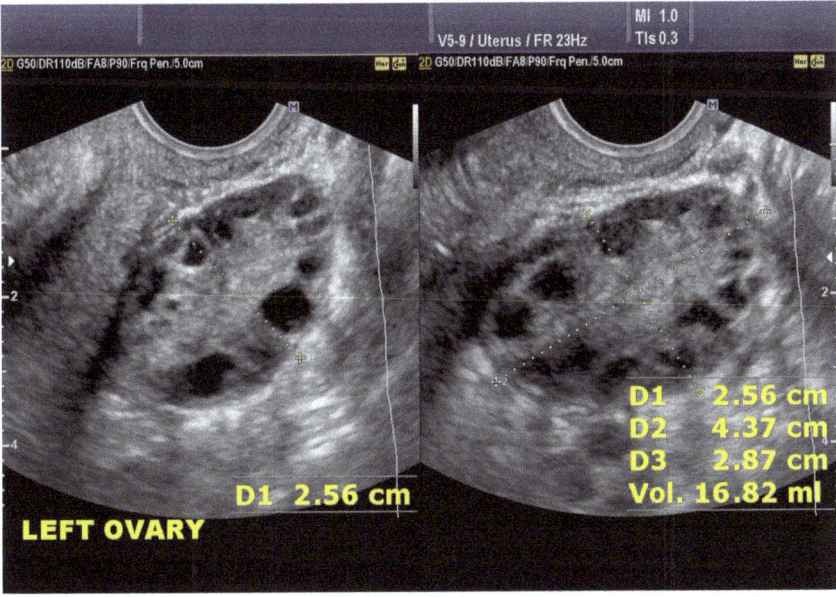

Fig. 7.8.2: In addition they can have infertility, acne or biochemically show increased androgen levels

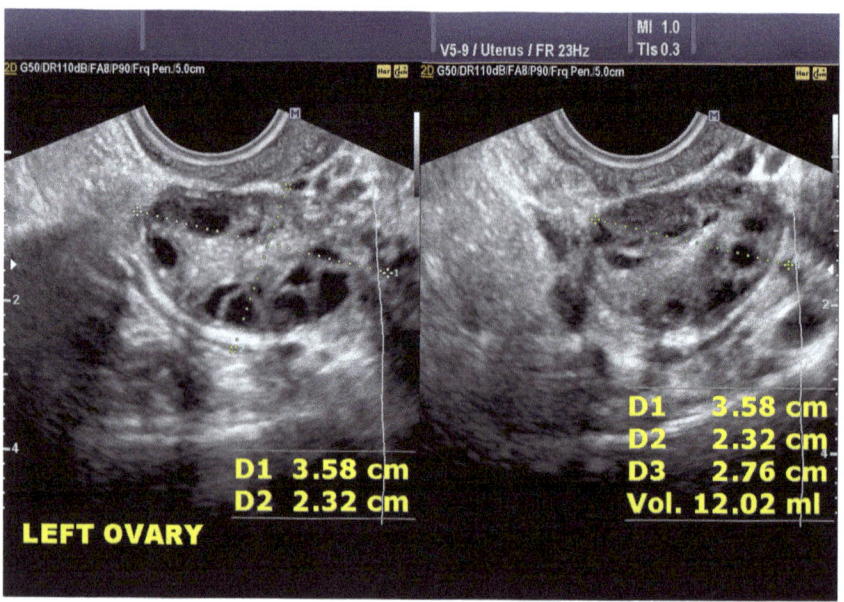

Fig. 7.8.3: Sonographic features of polycystic ovaries are bilateral enlarged ovaries with multiple small follicles

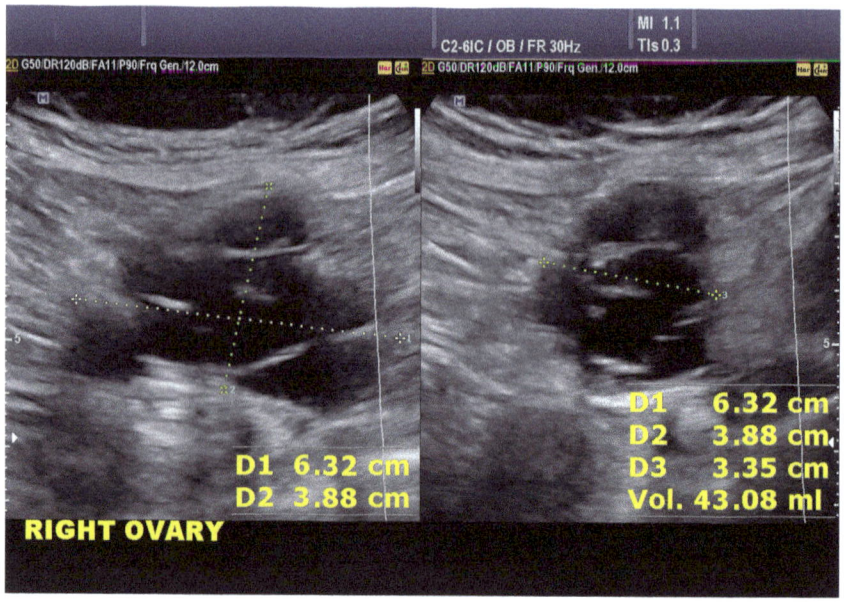

Fig. 7.8.4: Increased ovarian size (>10 ml)

7.8. Polycystic Ovaries

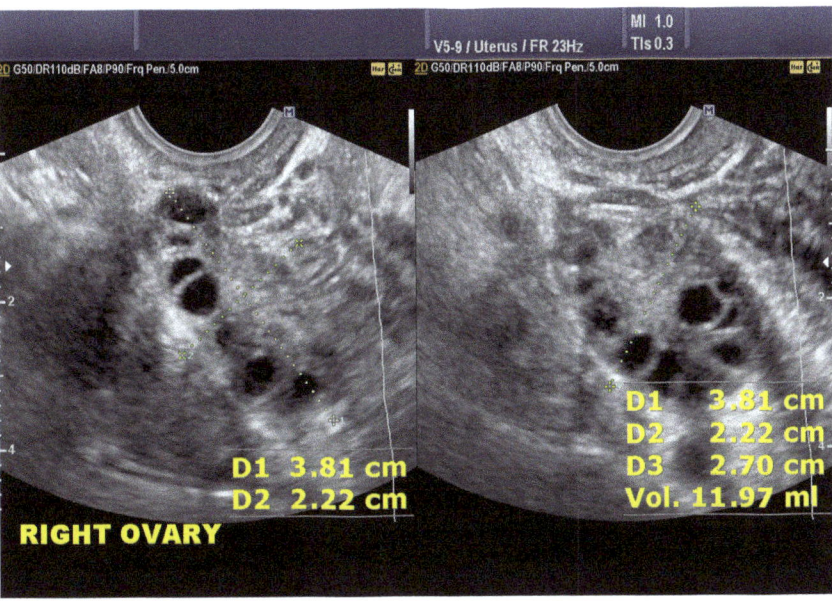

Fig. 7.8.5: Twelve or more follicles measuring 2-9 mm, peripheral location of follicles giving a string of pearl appearance

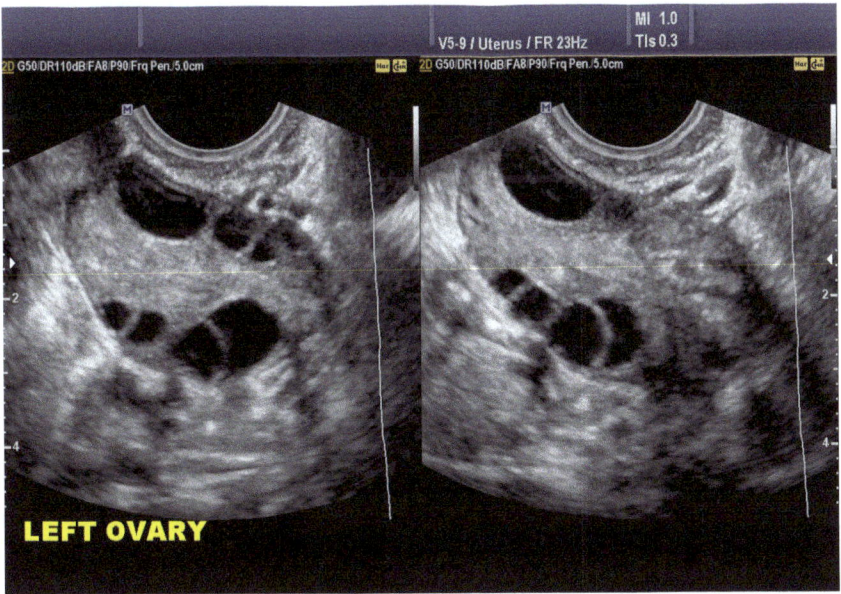

Fig. 7.8.6: Hyperechoic central stroma

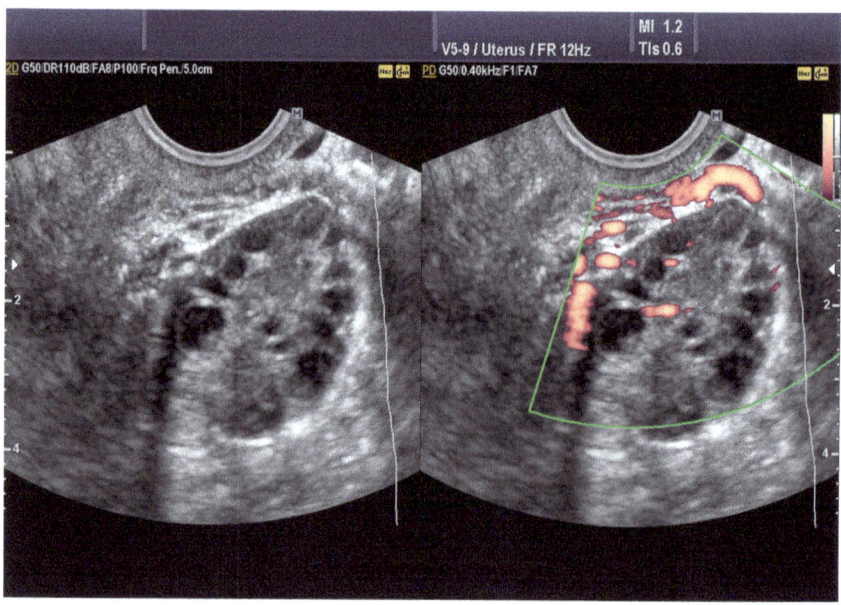

Fig. 7.8.7: Peripheral distribution of cysts with echogenic stroma

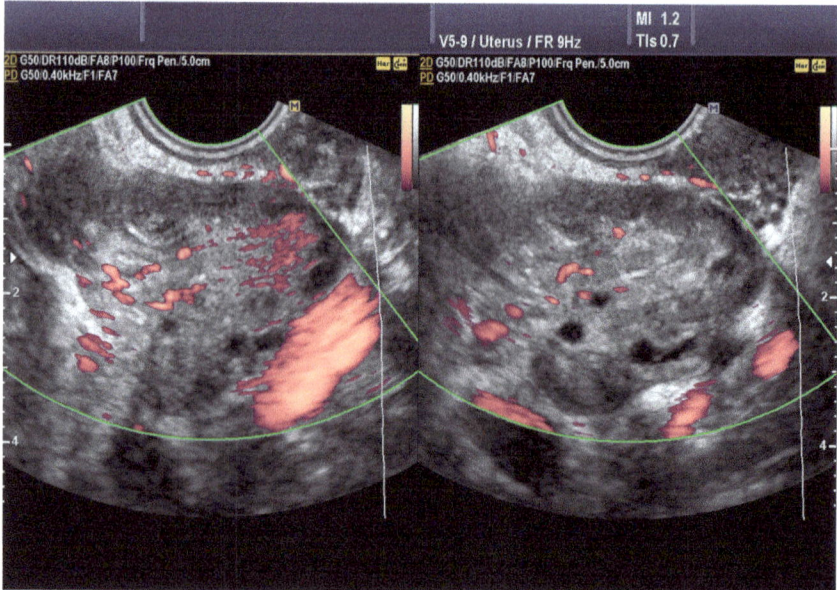

Fig. 7.8.8: Patient with symtoms, enlarged ovary, cysts distribution is characteristic of polycystic ovaries

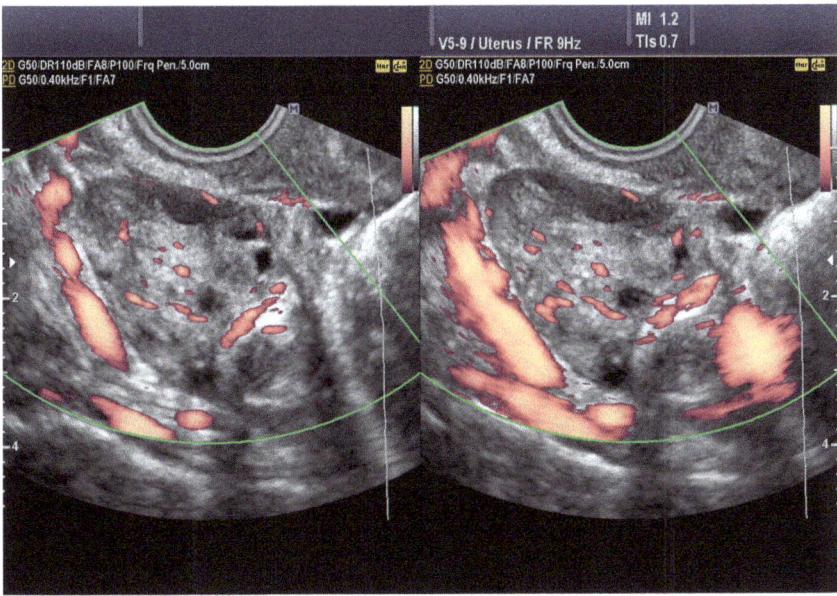

Fig. 7.8.9: Stromal hyperemia as seen on color flow mapping and power angio studies

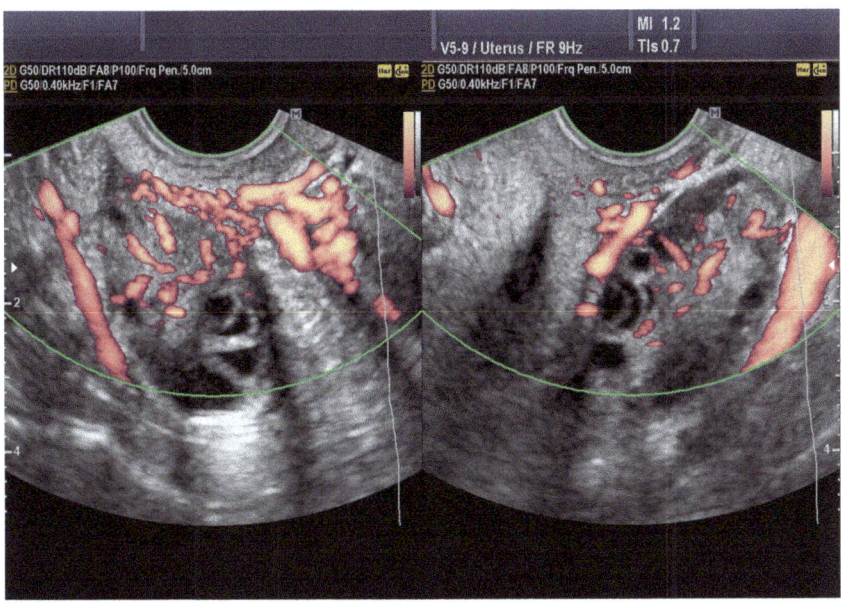

Fig. 7.8.10: Moderate stromal hyperemia

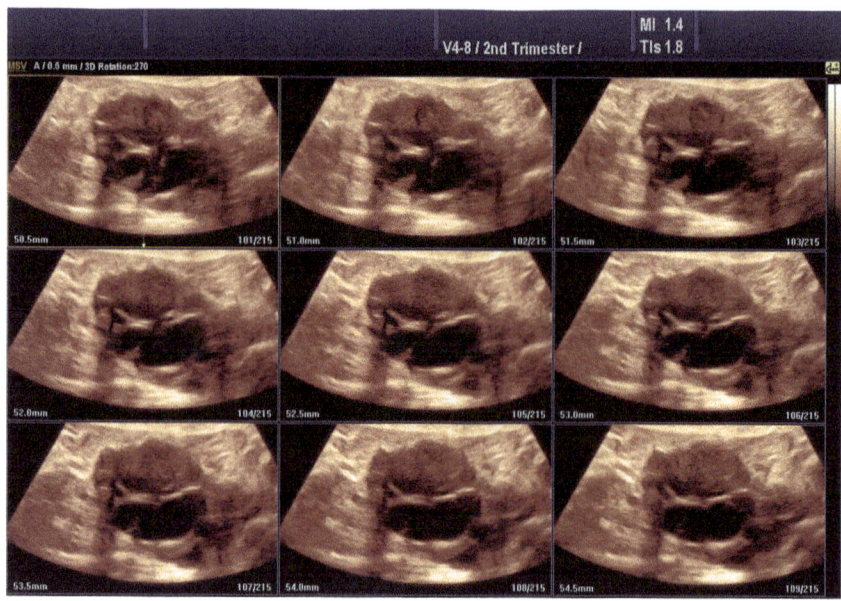

Fig. 7.8.11: As seen on MSV

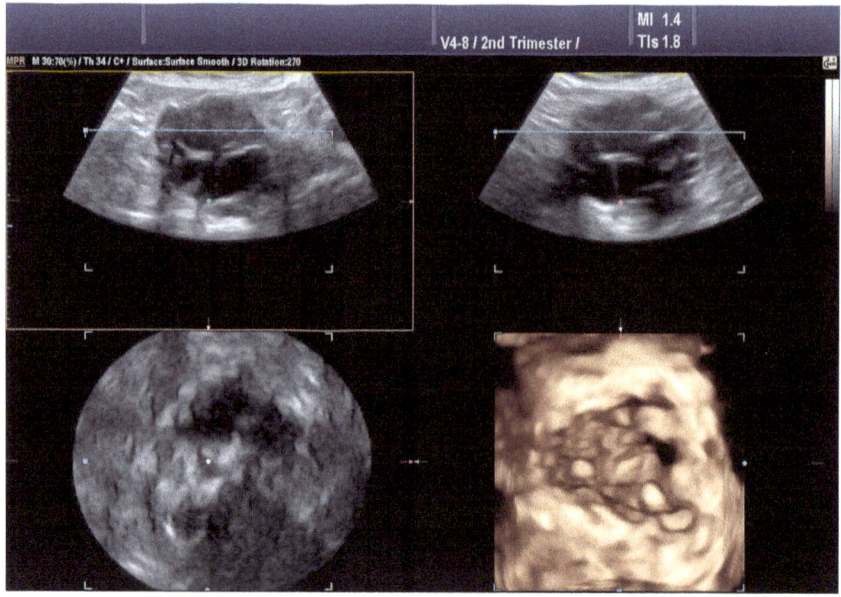

Fig. 7.8.12: Polycystic ovaries as seen on MPR

7.8. Polycystic Ovaries

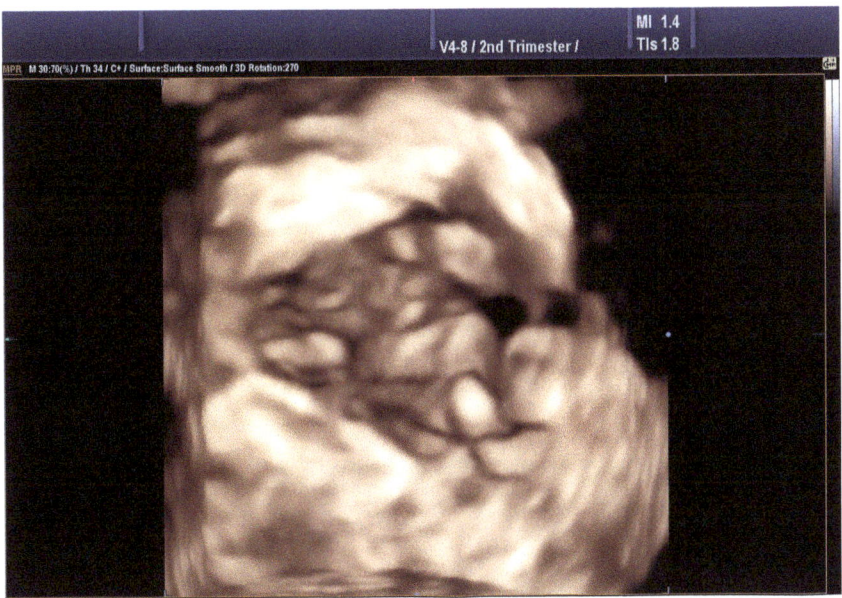

Fig. 7.8.13: As seen on 3D

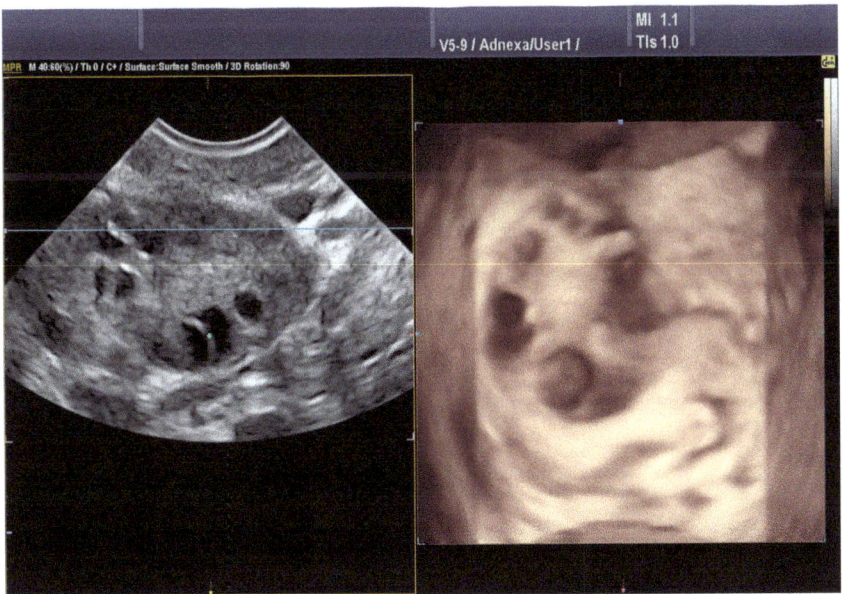

Fig. 7.8.14: Polycystic ovaries as seen on 3D

7.9. ENDOMETRIOSIS

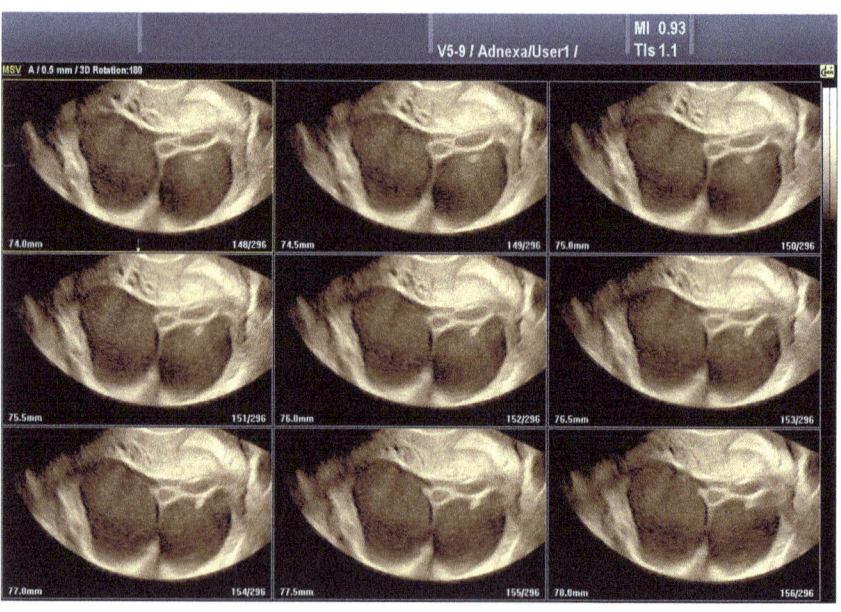

7.9. Endometriosis

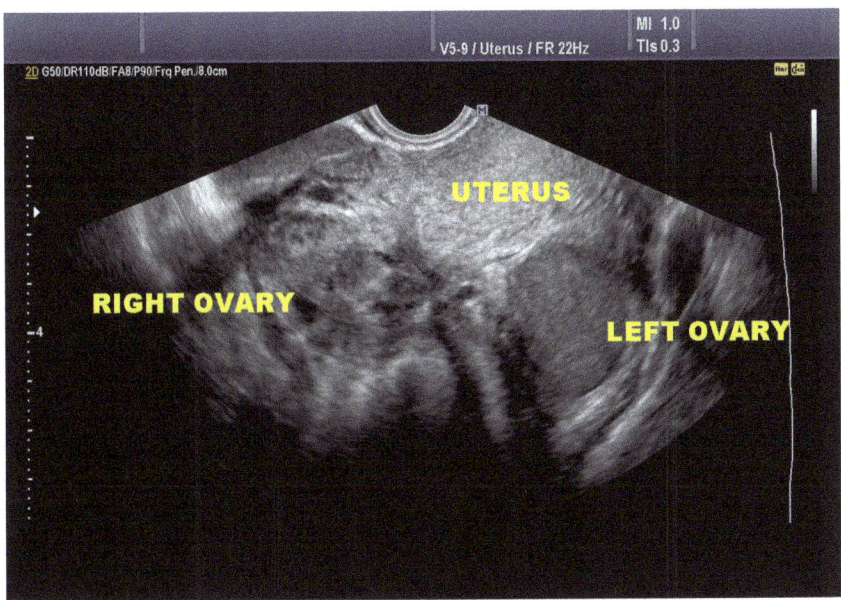

Fig. 7.9.1: TVS Should be the first line imaging technique for endometriosis

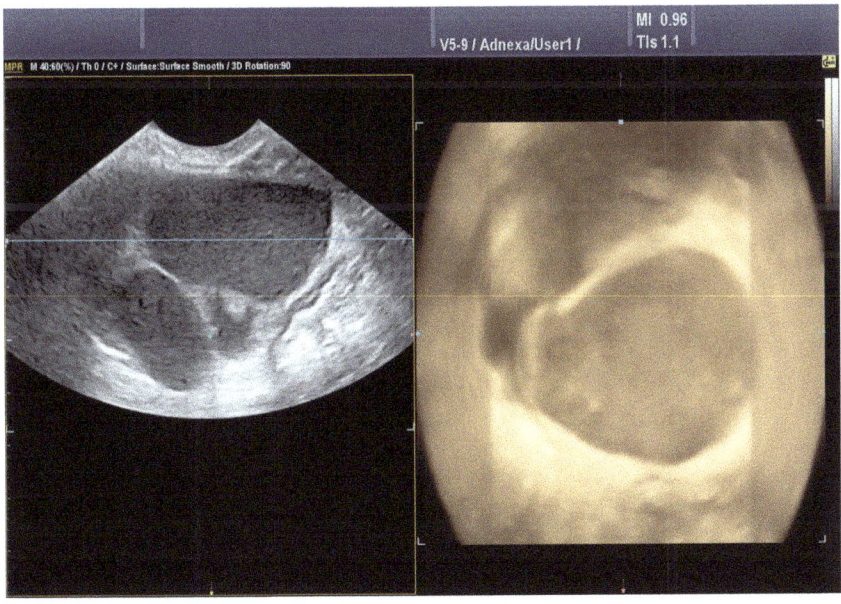

Fig. 7.9.2: Patients with endometriosis can have pelvic pain, dyspareunia, dysmenorrhea or chronic pelvic pain

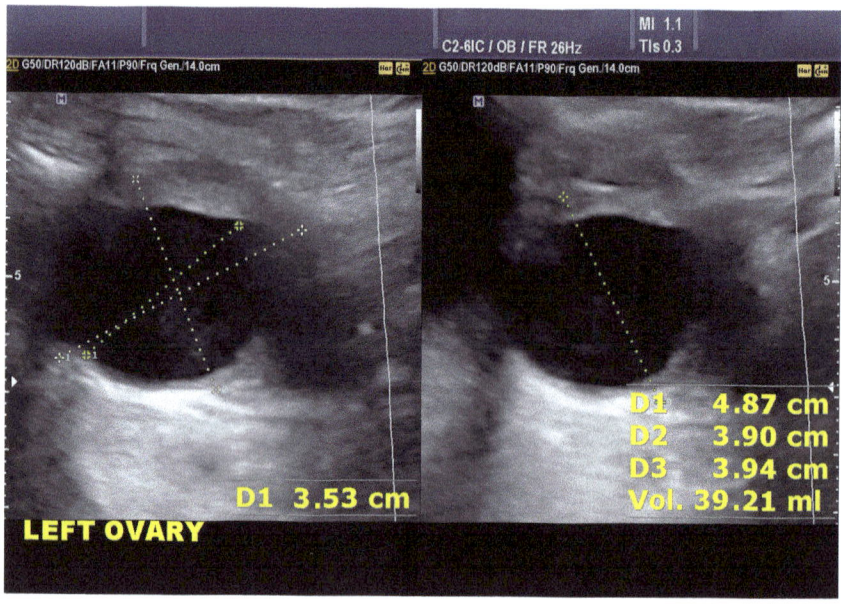

Fig. 7.9.3: Look for ovarian mobility, can be seen sliding (while moving the probe) or whether they are fixed with the uterus or adjacent structures

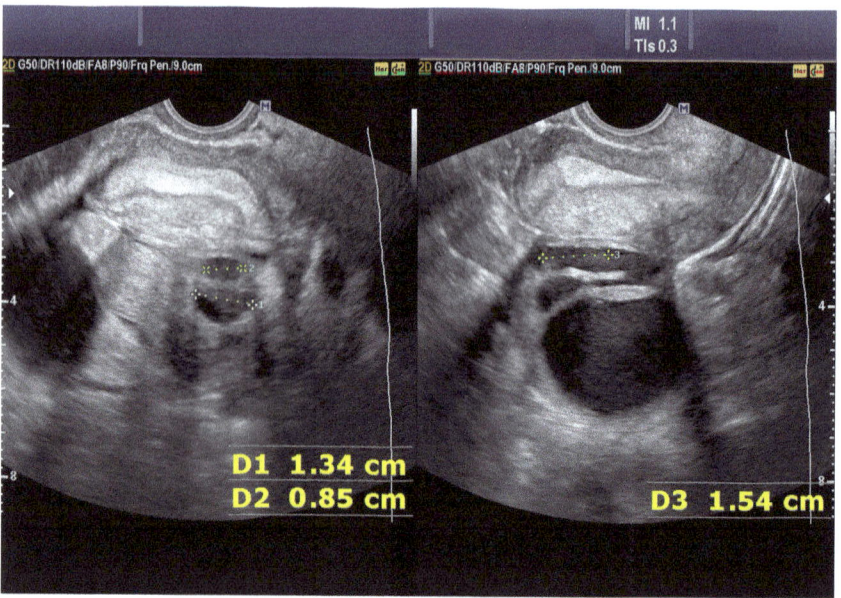

Fig. 7.9.4: With the TVS probe always look for mobility of the ovary

7.9. Endometriosis

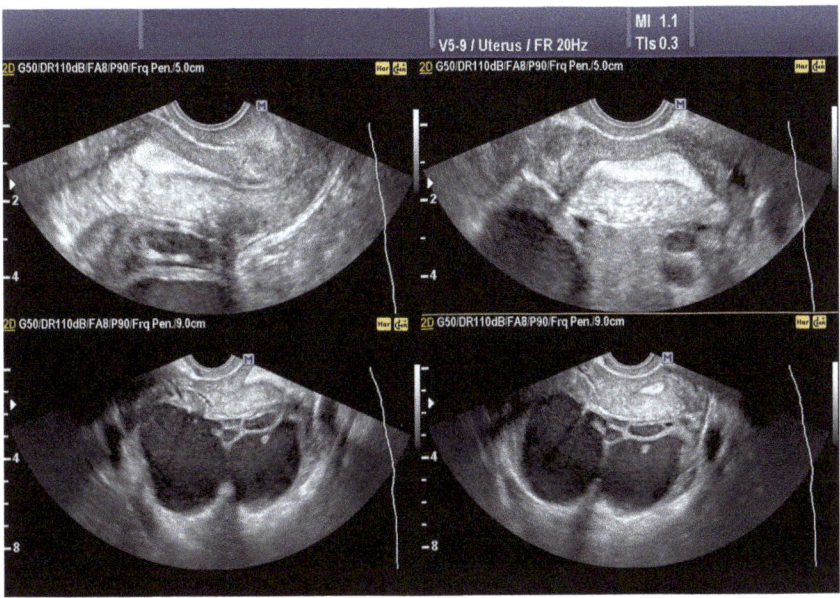

Fig. 7.9.5: Both ovaries are prolapsed posteriorly and are seen as kissing ovaries

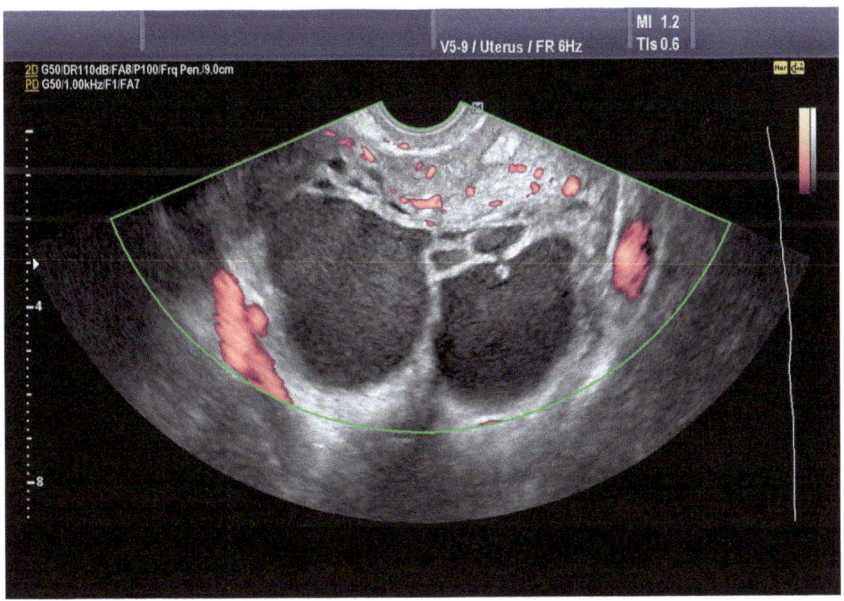

Fig. 7.9.6: On color flow mapping no internal vascularity is delineated

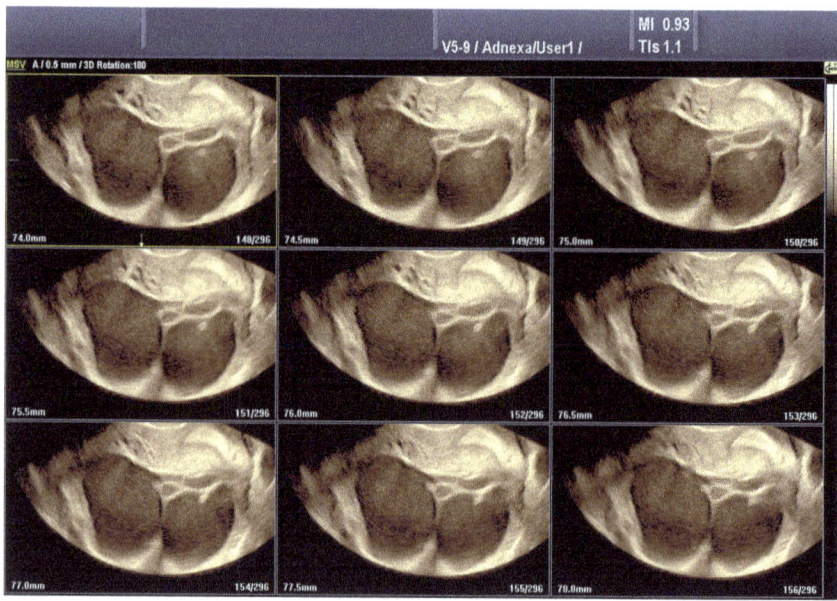

Fig. 7.9.7: As seen on 3D

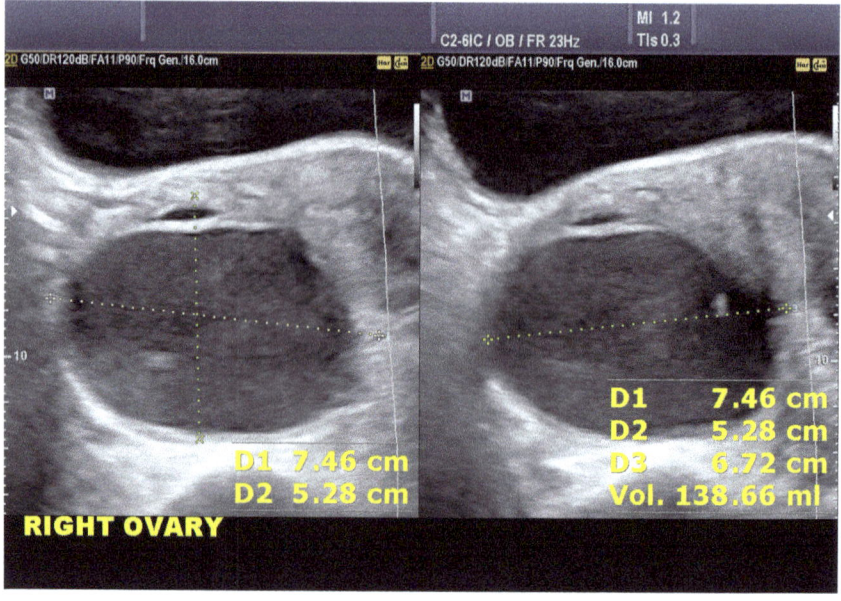

Fig. 7.9.8: Endometriotic cysts are typically unilocular

7.9. Endometriosis

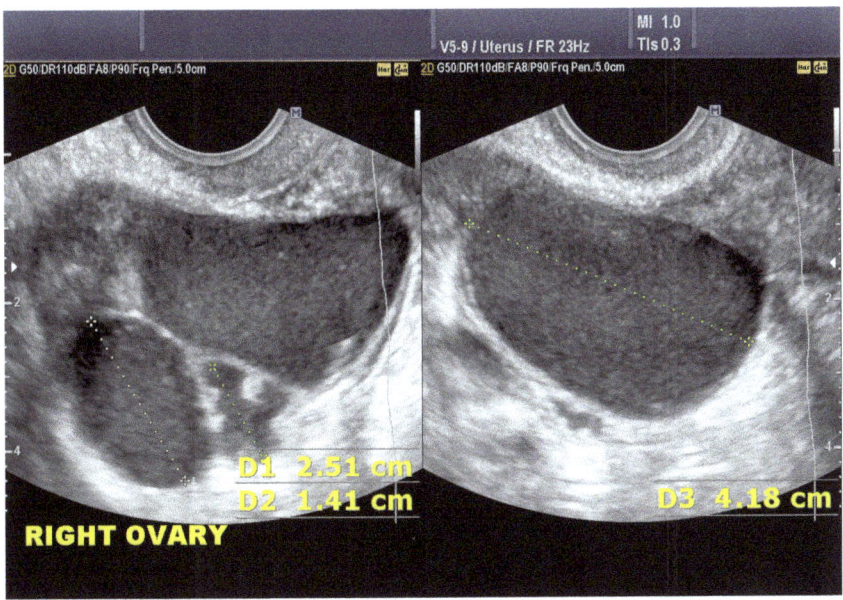

Fig. 7.9.9: The cyst may have thin or thick septation

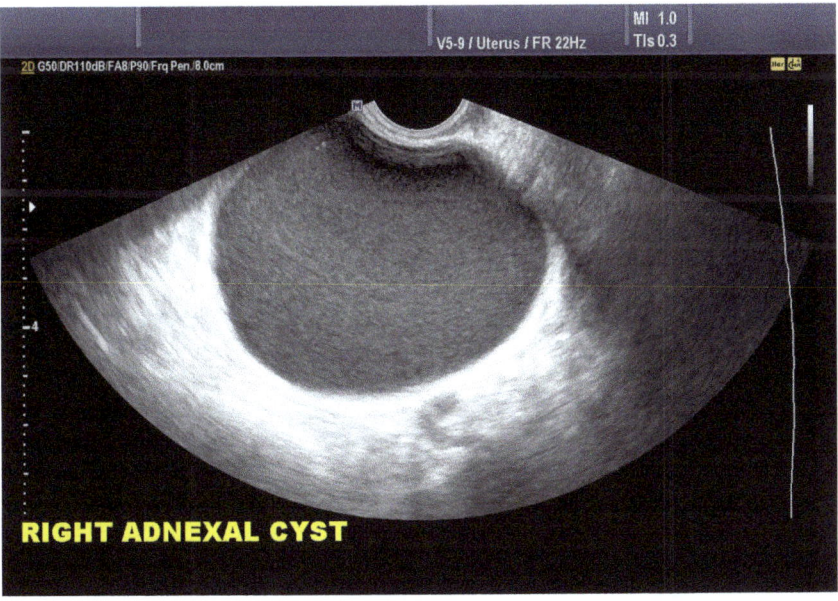

Fig. 7.9.10: Ovarian cyst, thin or thick walled with diffuse fine internal echoes

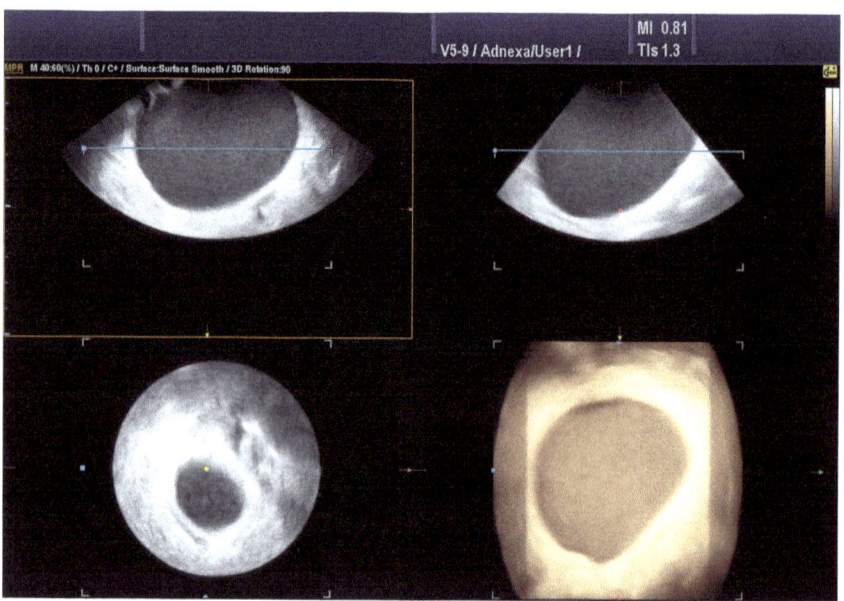

Fig. 7.9.11: Homogeneous low level echoes as seen on 3D

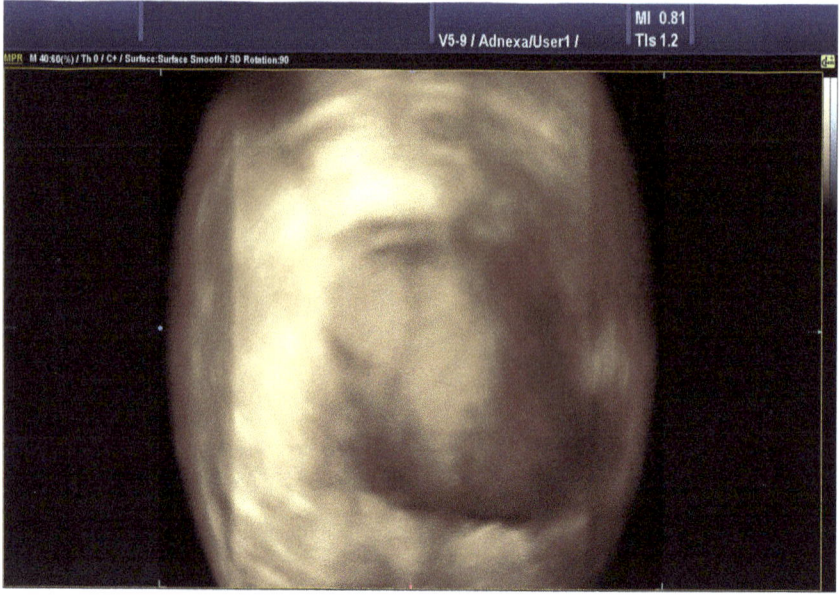

Fig. 7.9.12: Endometrioma as seen on 3D

7.9. Endometriosis

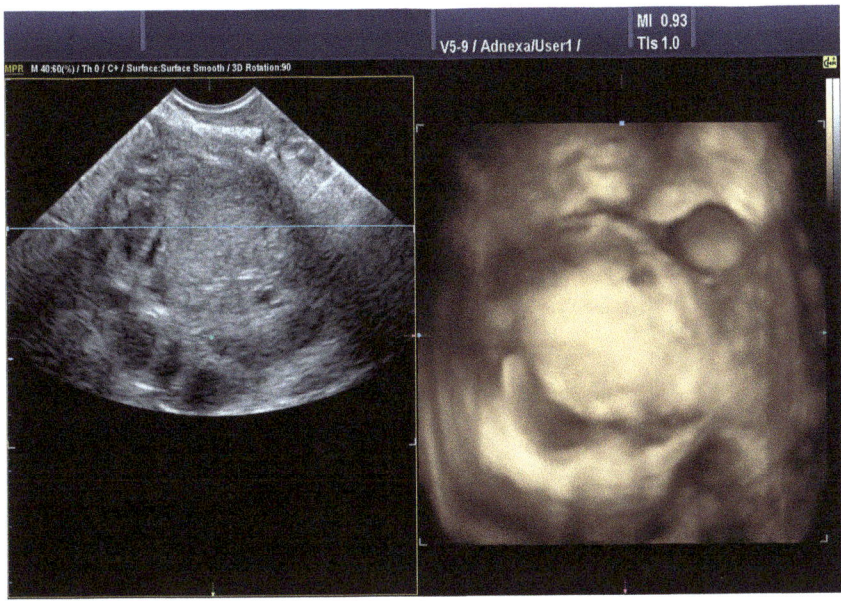

Fig. 7.9.13: Cyst as seen on 3D

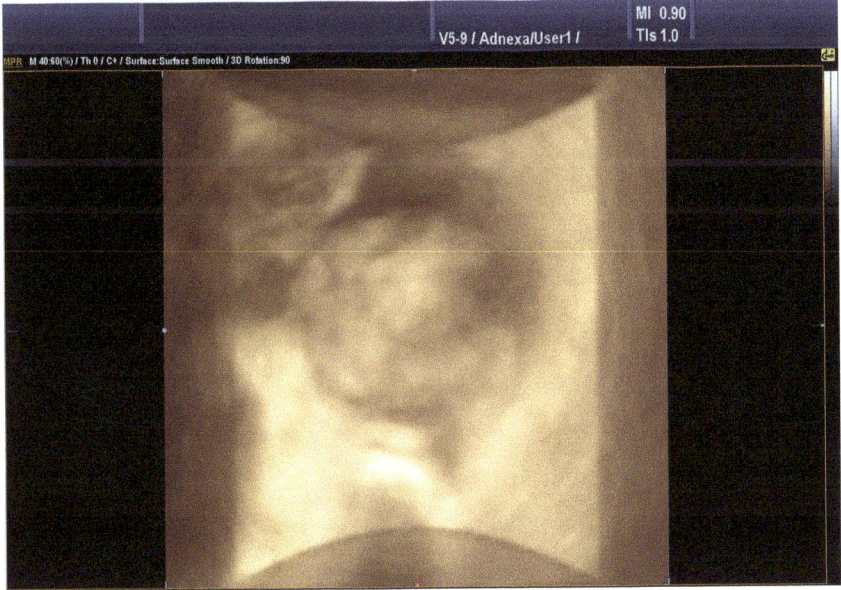

Fig. 7.9.14: Endometrioma as seen on 3D

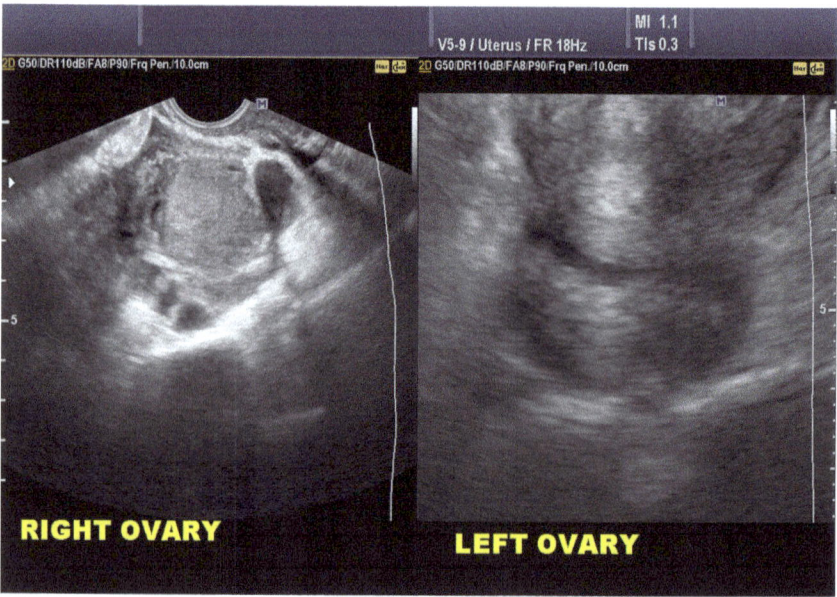

Fig. 7.9.15: Ovarian cyst with multiple fine internal echoes

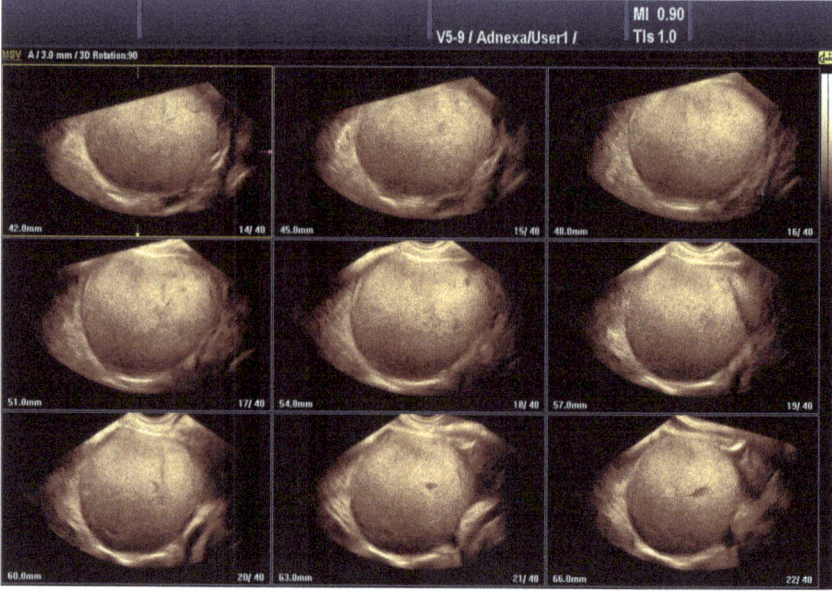

Fig. 7.9.16: Endometriotic cyst as seen on MSV

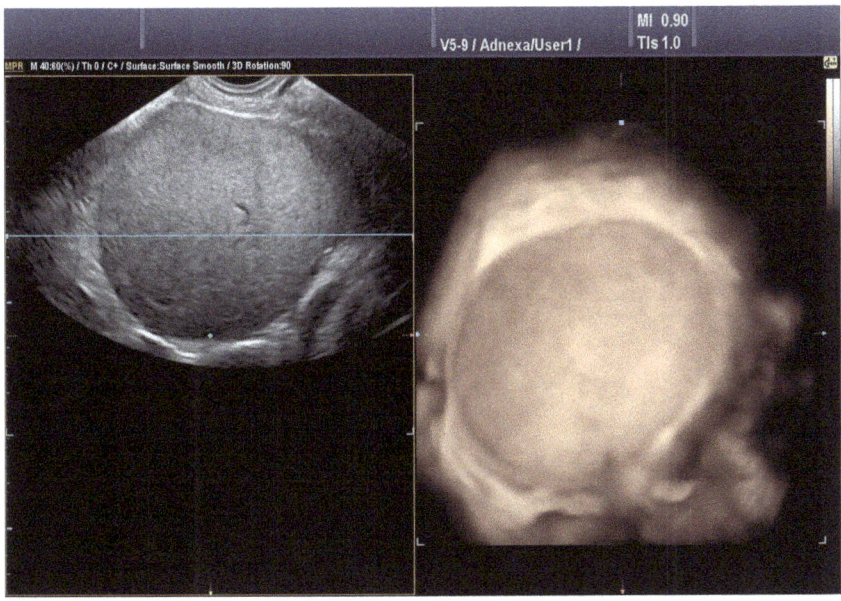

Fig. 7.9.17: As seen on 3D

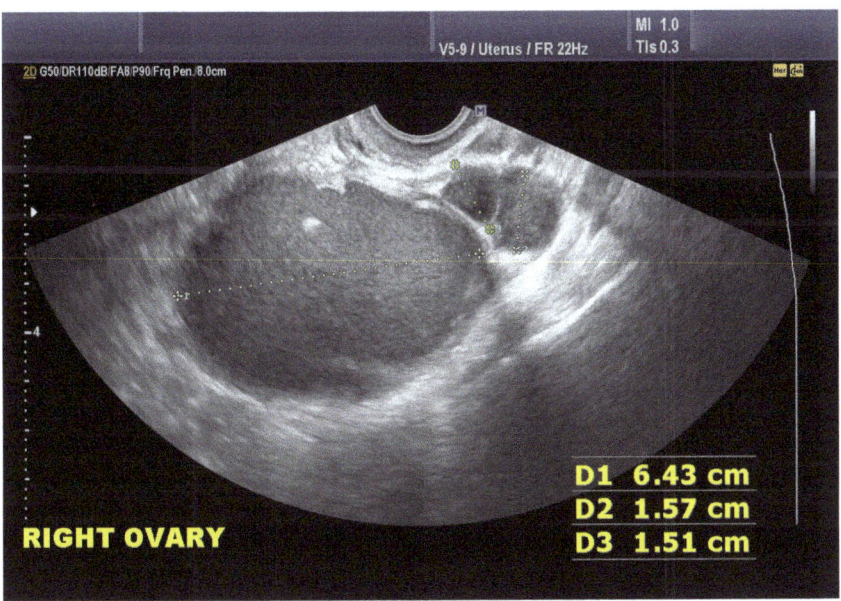

Fig. 7.9.18: Few hyperechoic nodules can be seen within the cyst

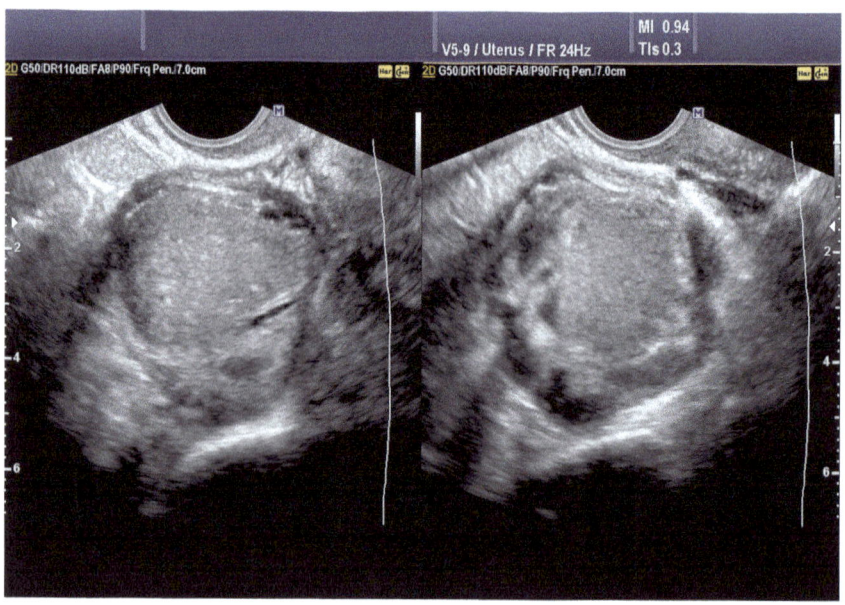

Fig. 7.9.19: Ovarian cyst within the ovary with homogeneous low level echoes

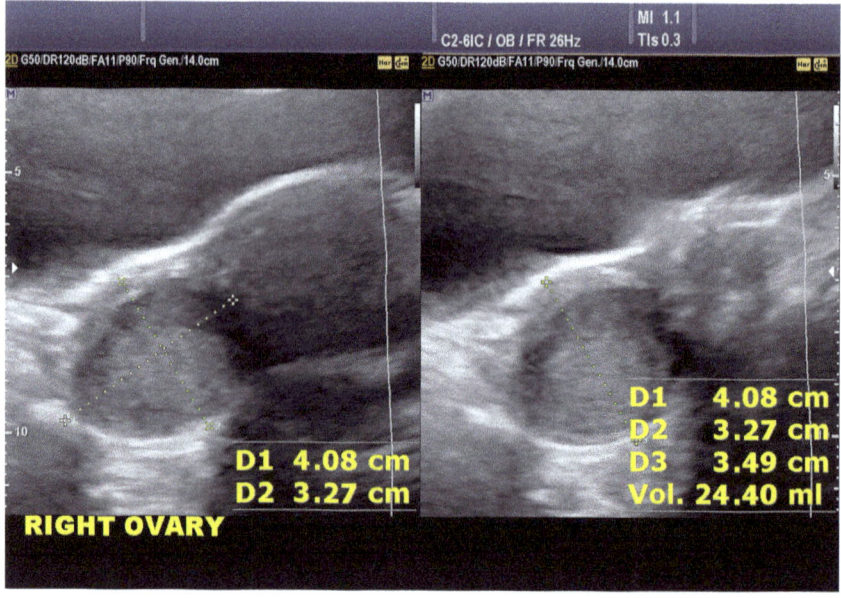

Fig. 7.9.20: Endometriotic cyst can be small or large

7.9. Endometriosis

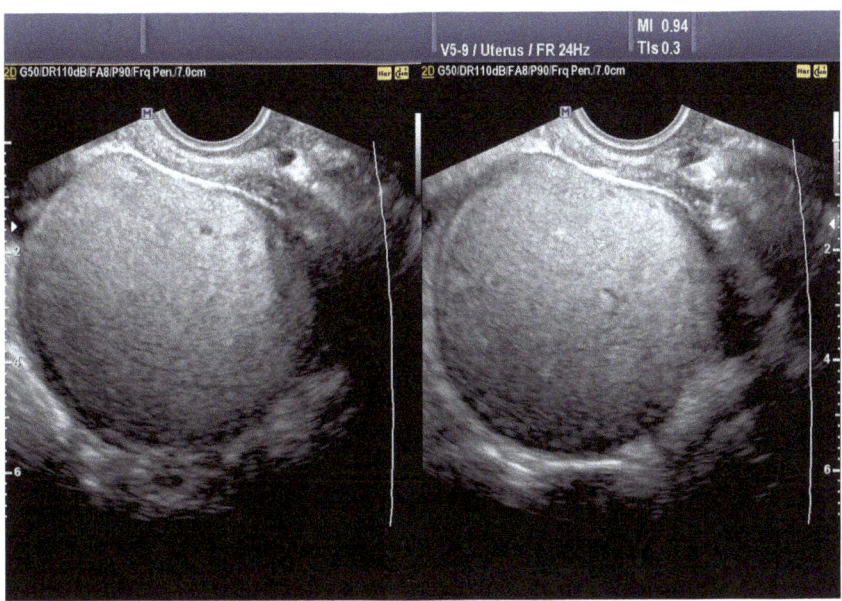

Fig. 7.9.21: Unilocular endometriotic cyst

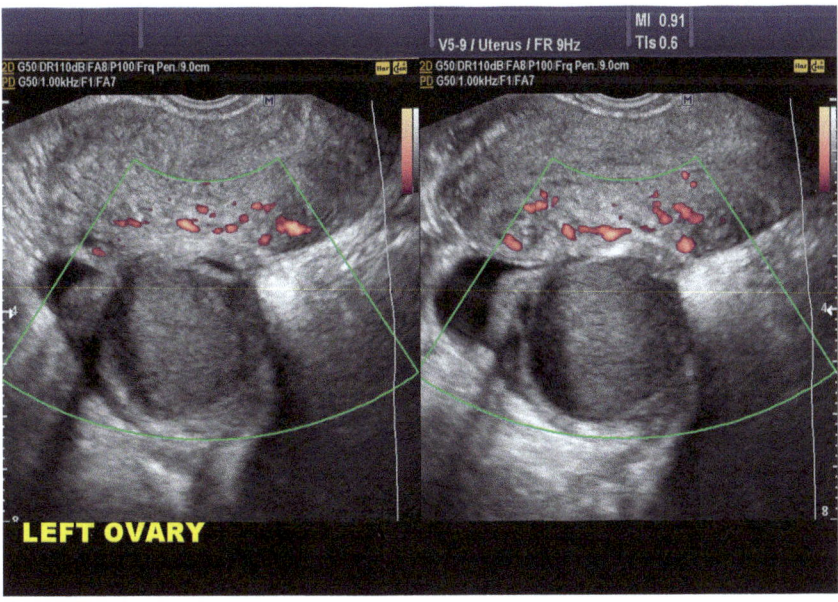

Fig. 7.9.22: Endometriotic cysts seen in the ovary which is prolapsed posteriorly and obliterates the pouch of Douglas

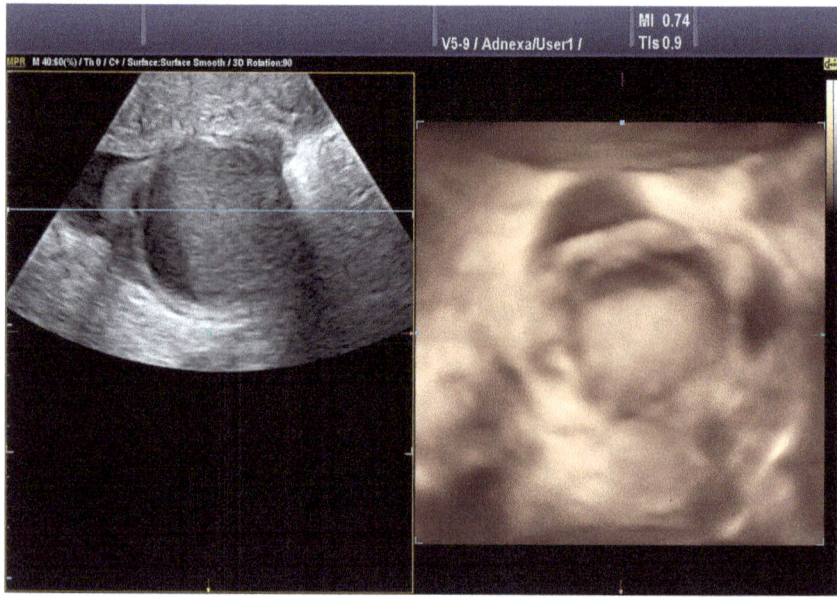

Fig. 7.9.23: One can see nodules in the pouch of Douglas and restricted mobility of the ovary

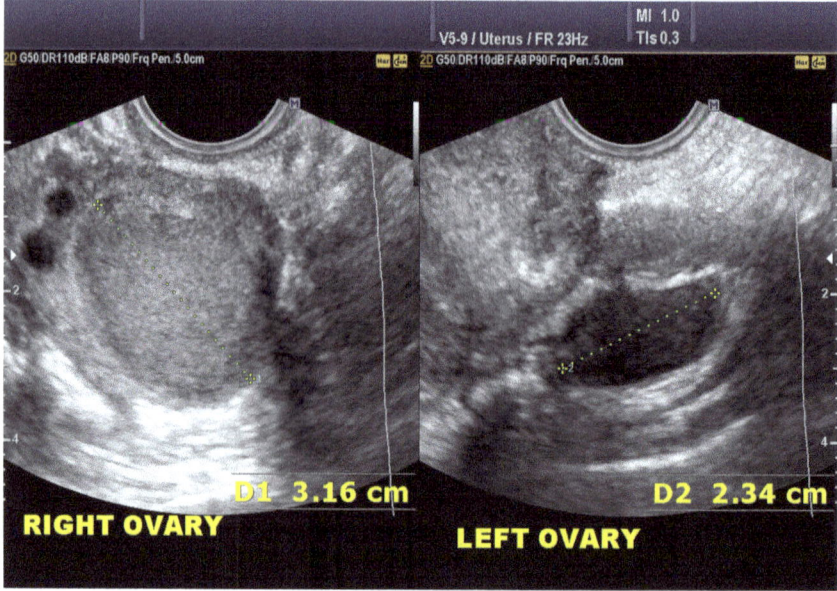

Fig. 7.9.24: Be careful of not labeling every cyst as endometriotic. See for contents within the cyst, day of the cycle. Endometriotic cyst in the right ovary and corpus luteum in the left ovary

7.9. Endometriosis

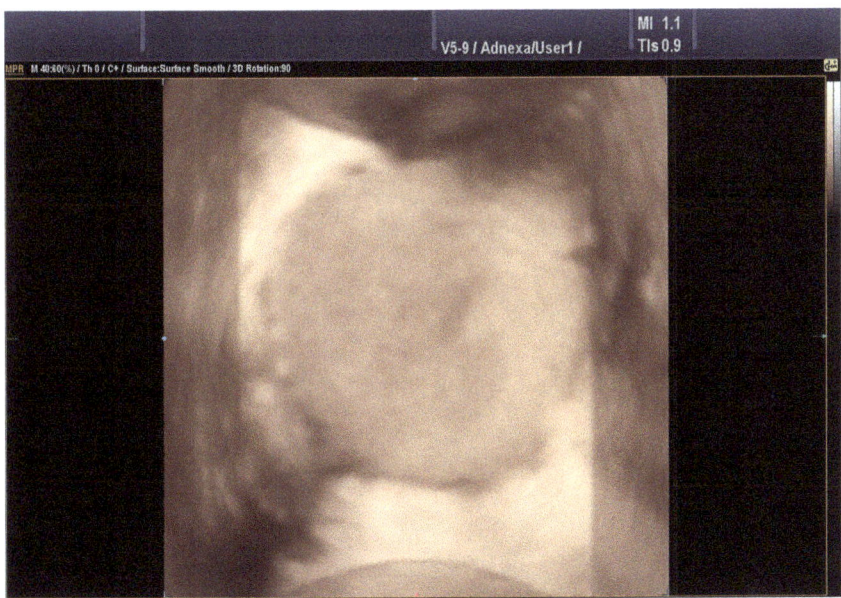

Fig. 7.9.25: As seen on 3D

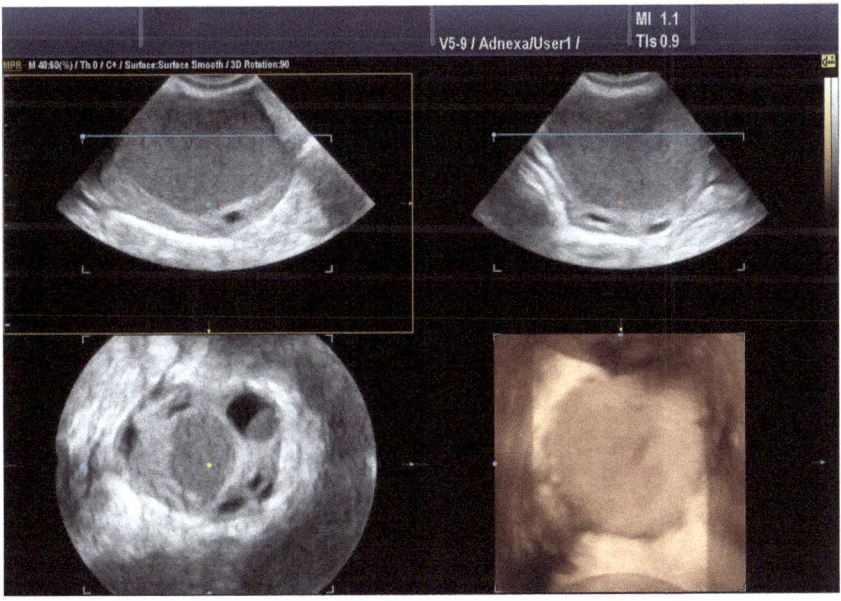

Fig. 7.9.26: Endometriotic cyst as seen on MPR

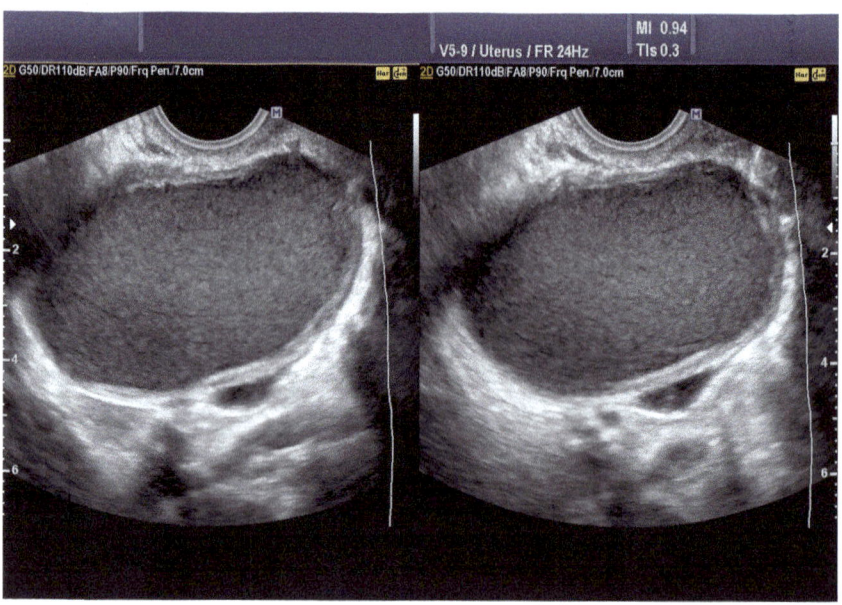

Fig. 7.9.27: Patient with complaints of infertility and dysmenorrhea would require further workup with a cyst as seen on TVS

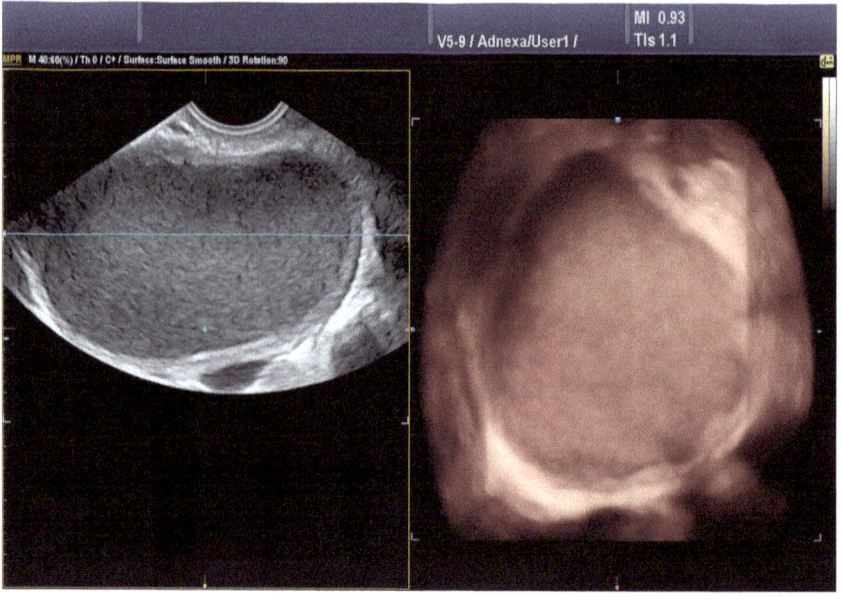

Fig. 7.9.28: Endometriotic cyst as seen on MPR

7.9. Endometriosis

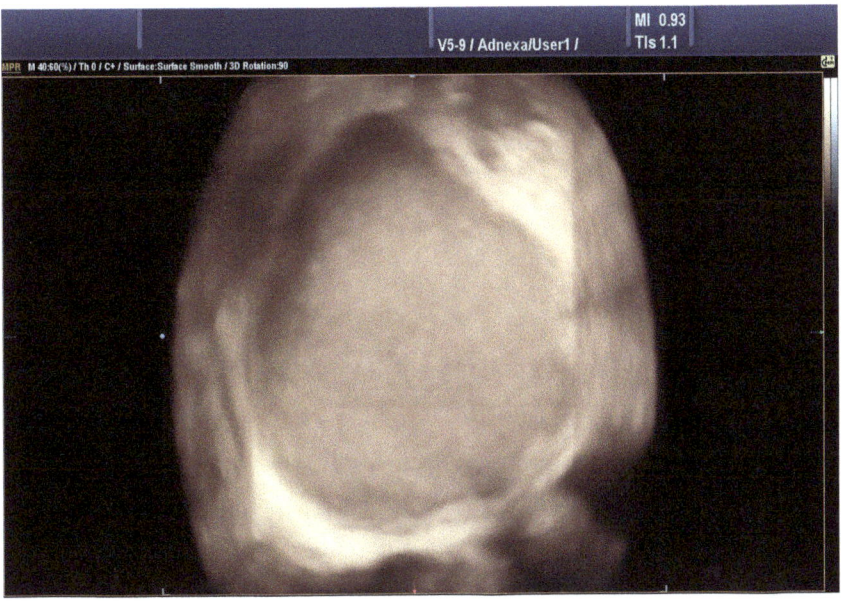

Fig. 7.9.29: As seen on 3D

7.10. ADNEXAL MASS

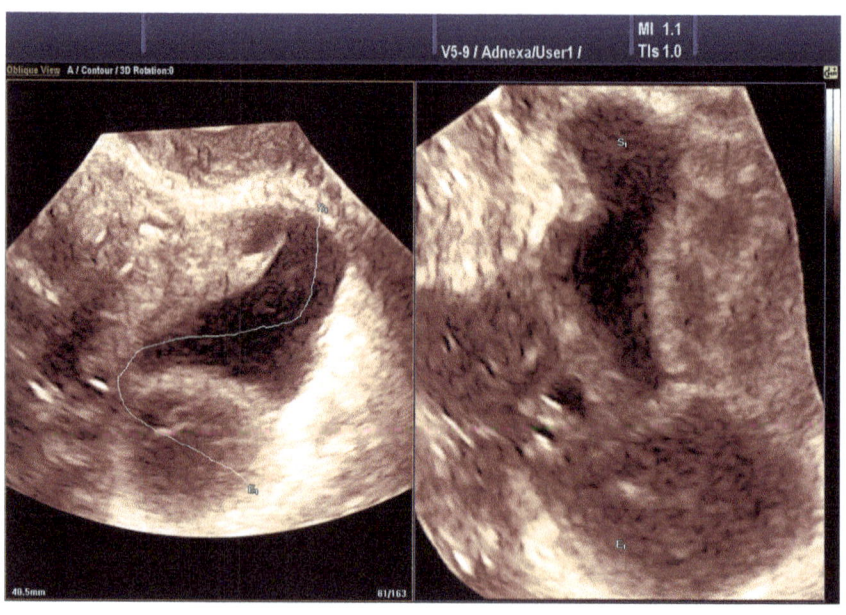

7.10. Adnexal Mass

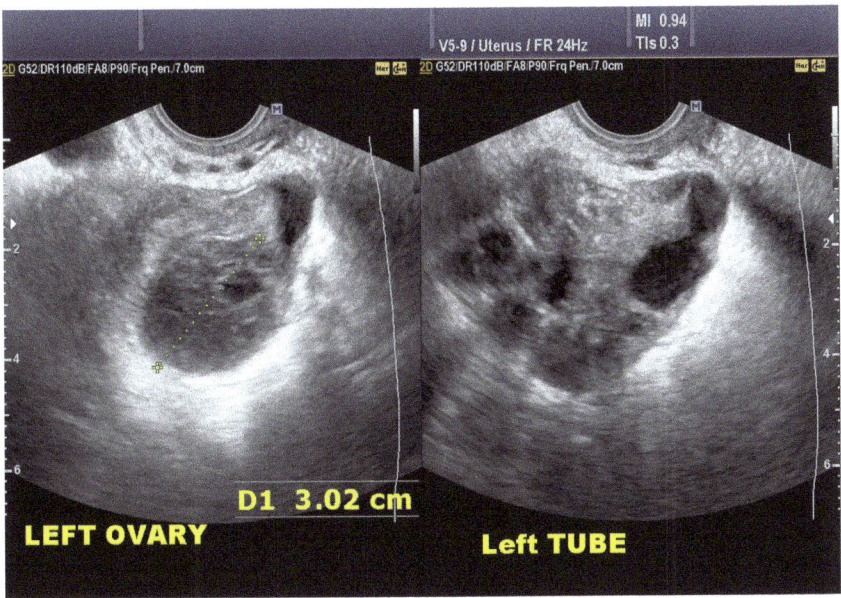

Fig. 7.10.1: Ovary and tube seen in a patient with acute symptoms. This is always not possible

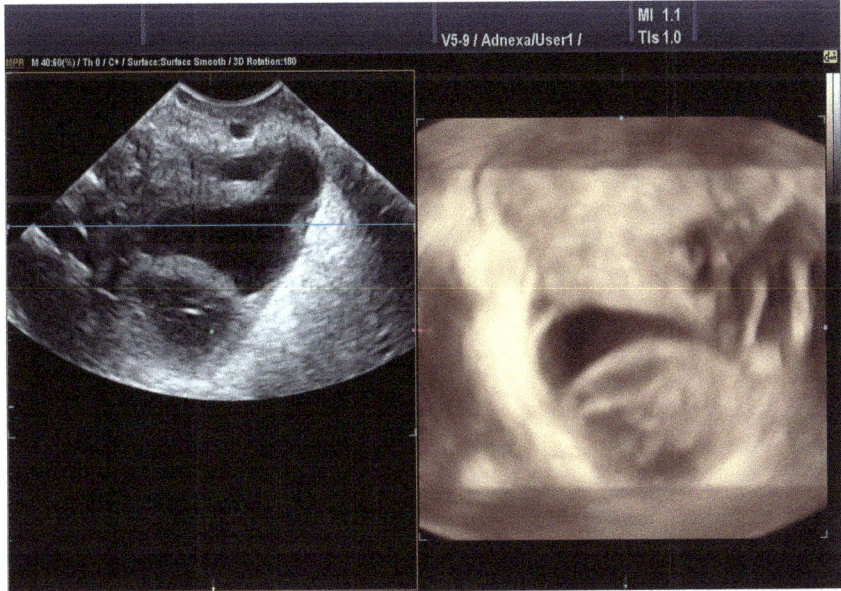

Fig. 7.10.2: One can delineate the dilatation of the tube and the adjacent ovary stuck to it on 3D

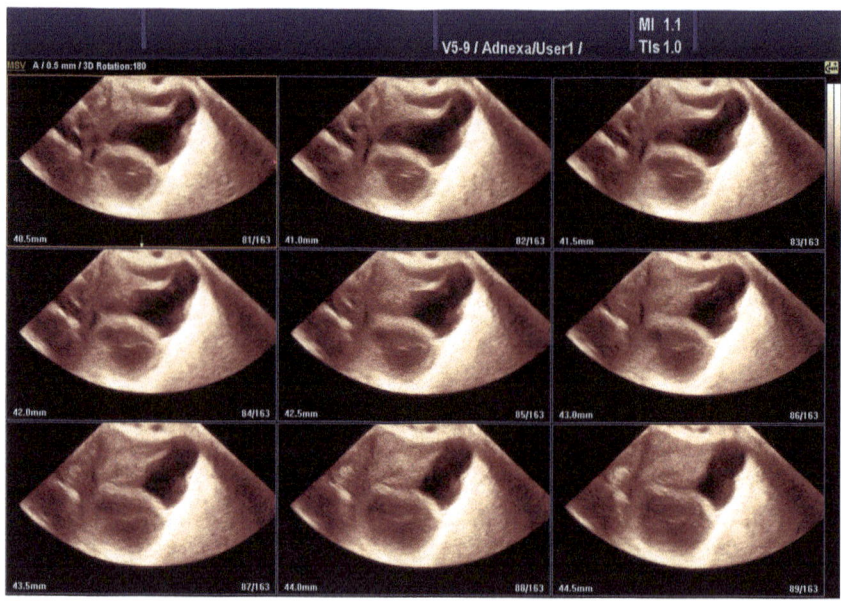

Fig. 7.10.3: Tubo-ovarian mass as seen on MSV

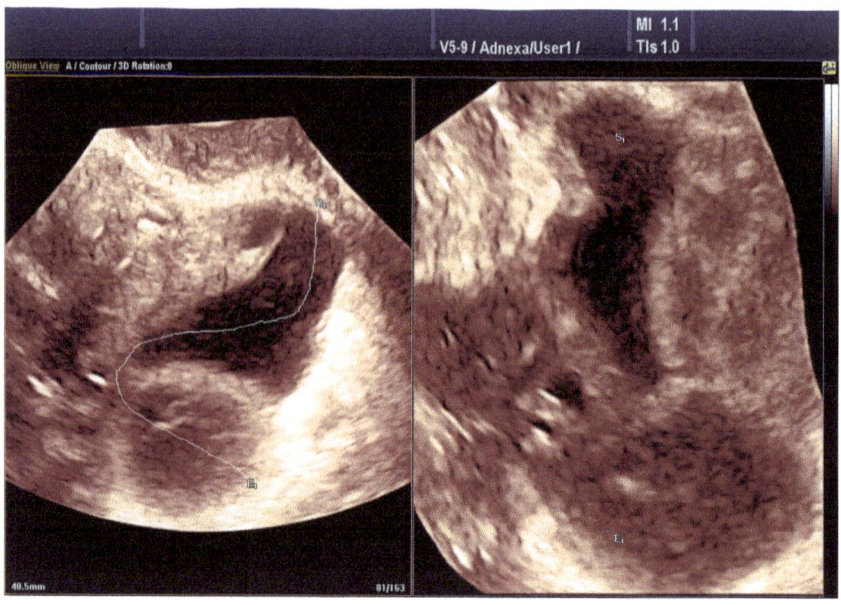

Fig. 7.10.4: Tube and ovary traced on a 3D scan

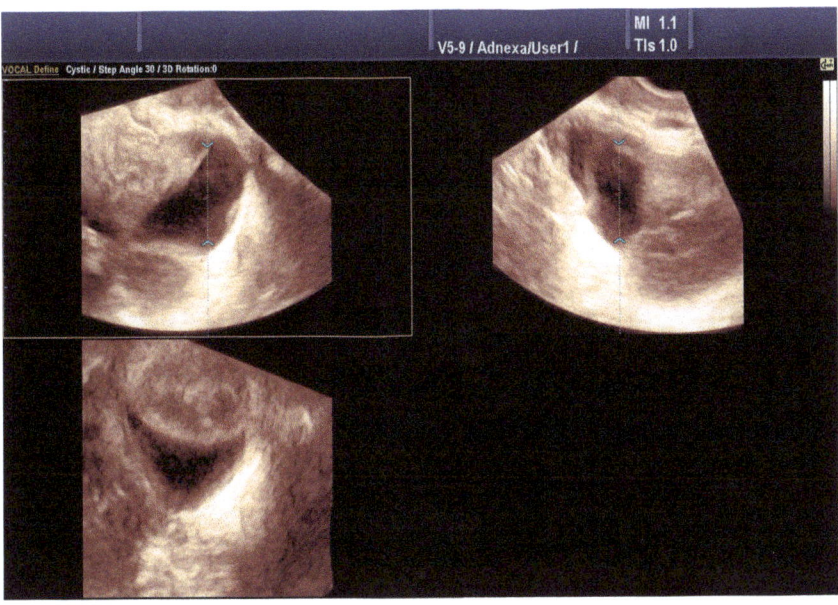

Fig. 7.10.5: Tubo-ovarian mass as seen on MPR

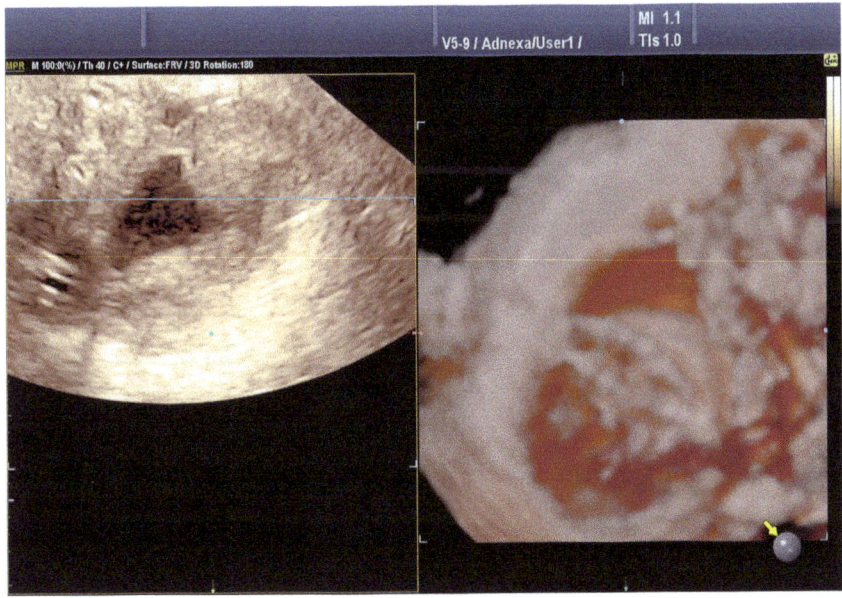

Fig. 7.10.6: As seen on 3D

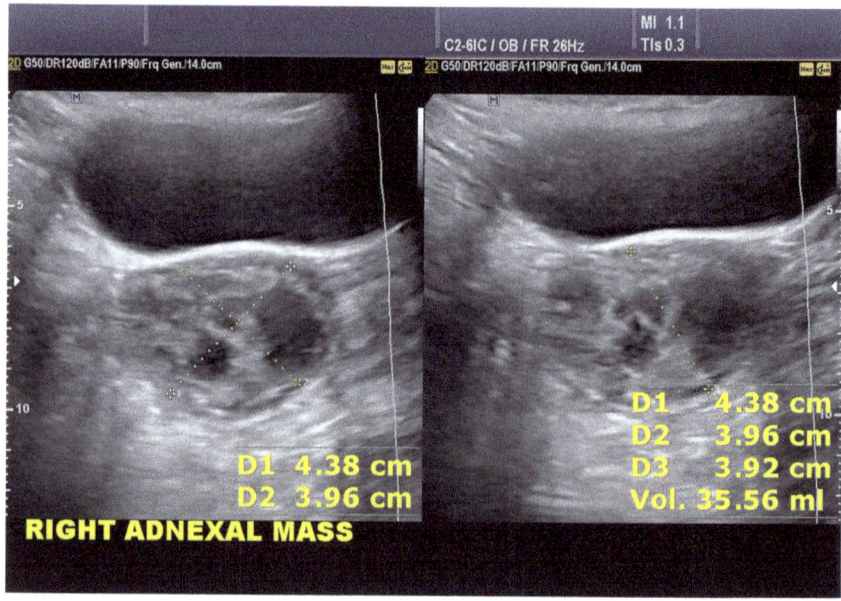

Fig. 7.10.7: On a TAS one can suspect an adnexal mass

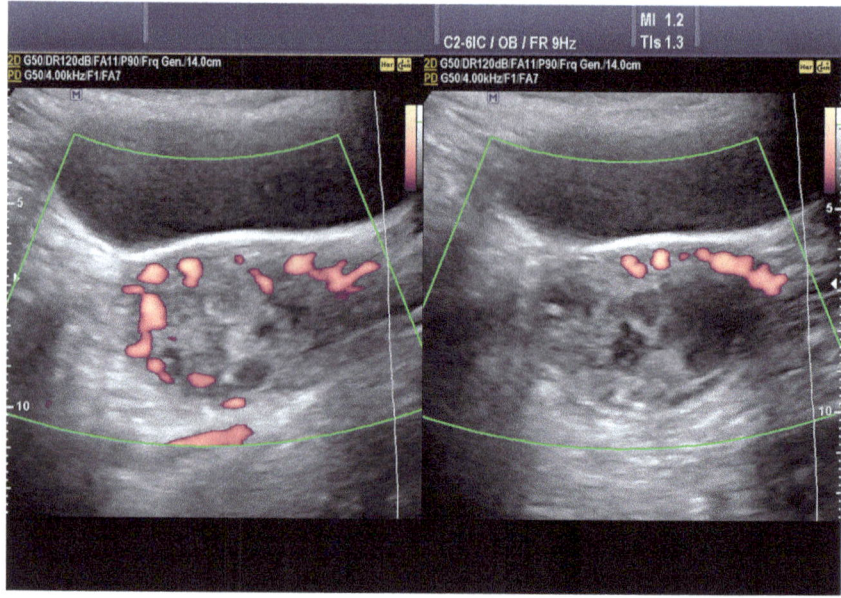

Fig. 7.10.8: Vascularity of the mass as seen on color flow mapping

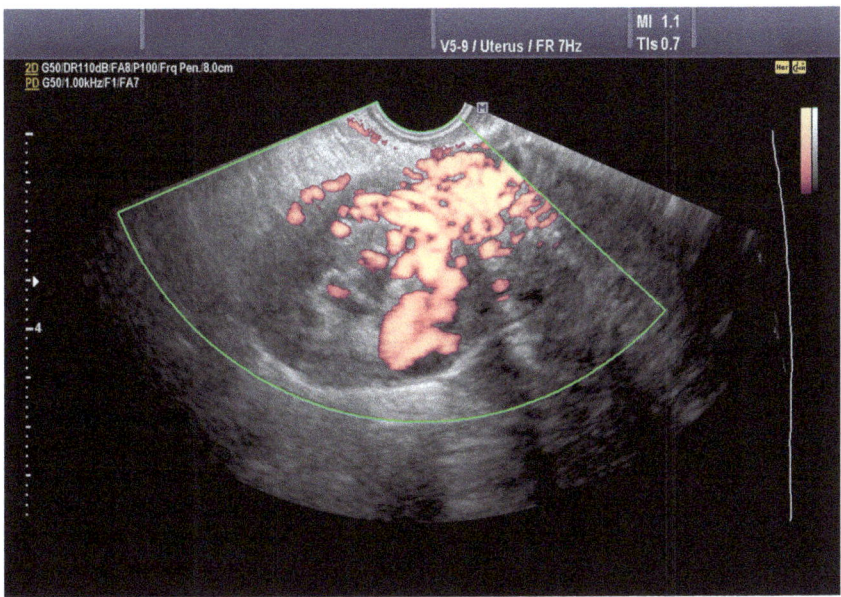

Fig. 7.10.9: Moderate vascularity as seen on power angio studies

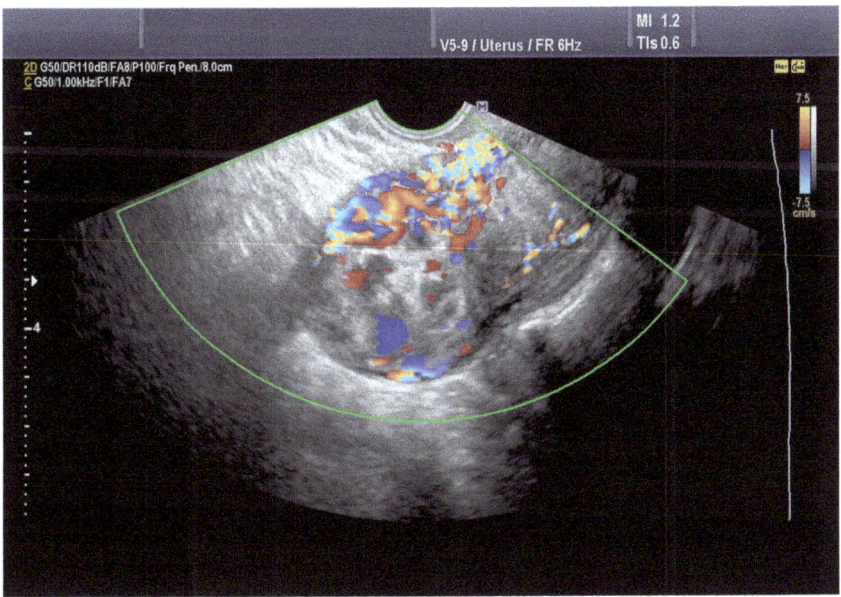

Fig. 7.10.10: Look for probe tenderness and check with the patient

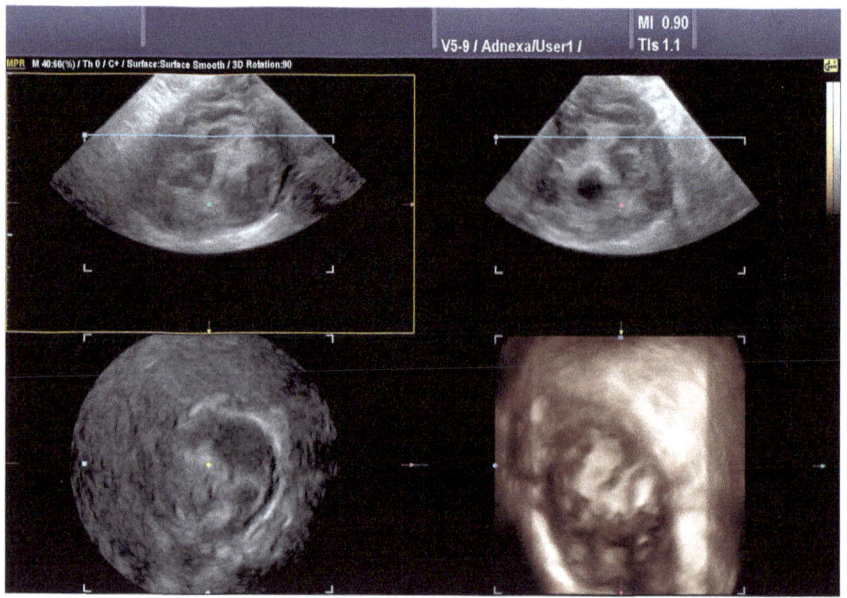

Fig. 7.10.11: Mass as seen on MPR

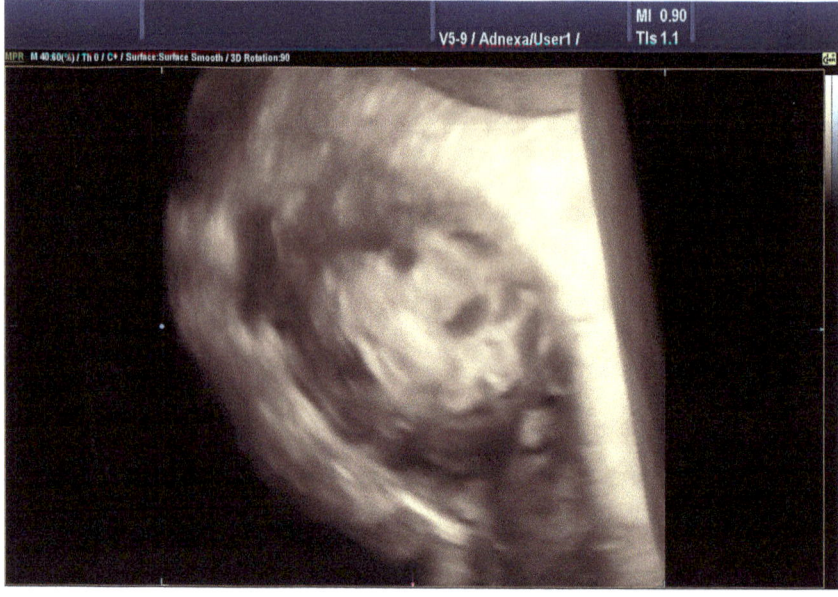

Fig. 7.10.12: As seen on 3D

7.10. Adnexal Mass

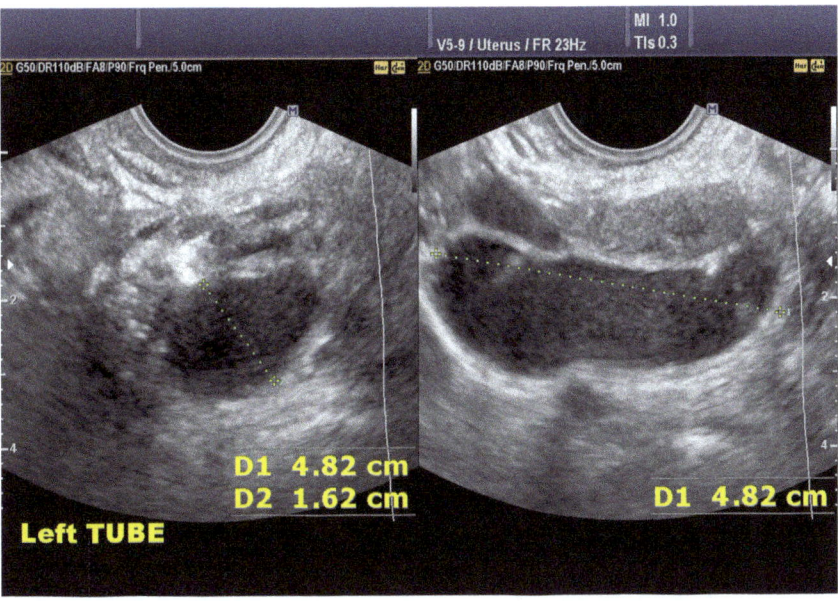

Fig. 7.10.13: Pyosalpinx seen as a tubular mass which is thick walled with internal echoes seen separate from the ovary

7.11. HYDROSALPINX

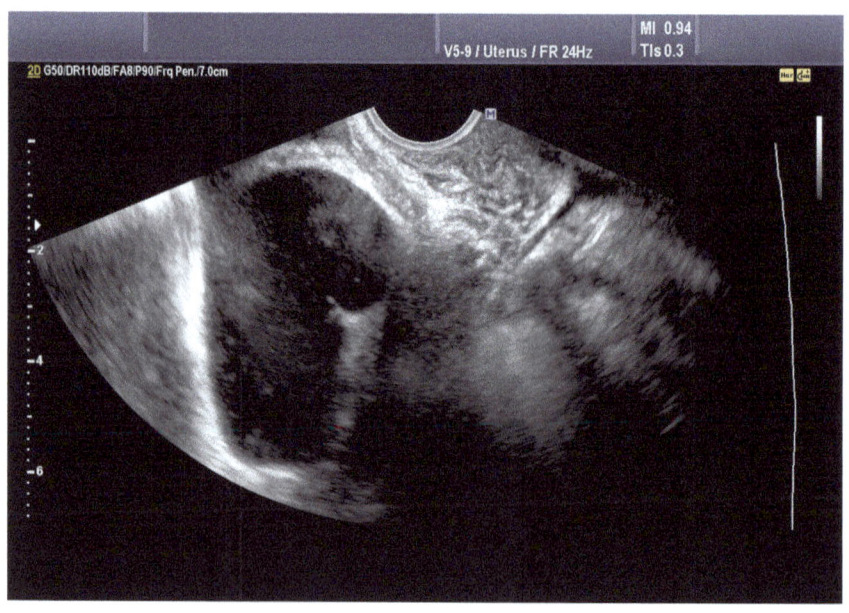

7.11. Hydrosalpinx

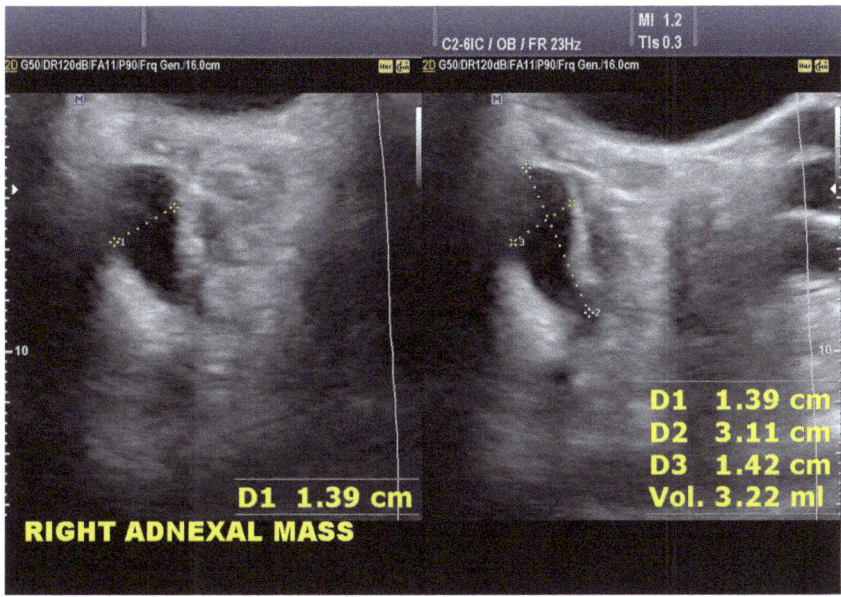

Fig. 7.11.1: An extraovarian cystic adnexal mass should always raise the suspicion of a tubal mass

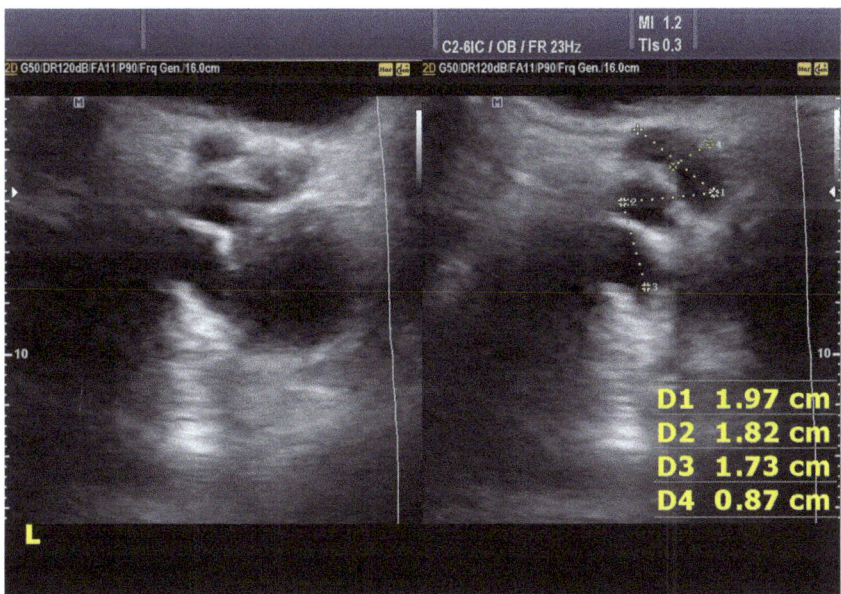

Fig. 7.11.2: Folded tubular elongated cystic structure, hydrosalpinx should be suspected

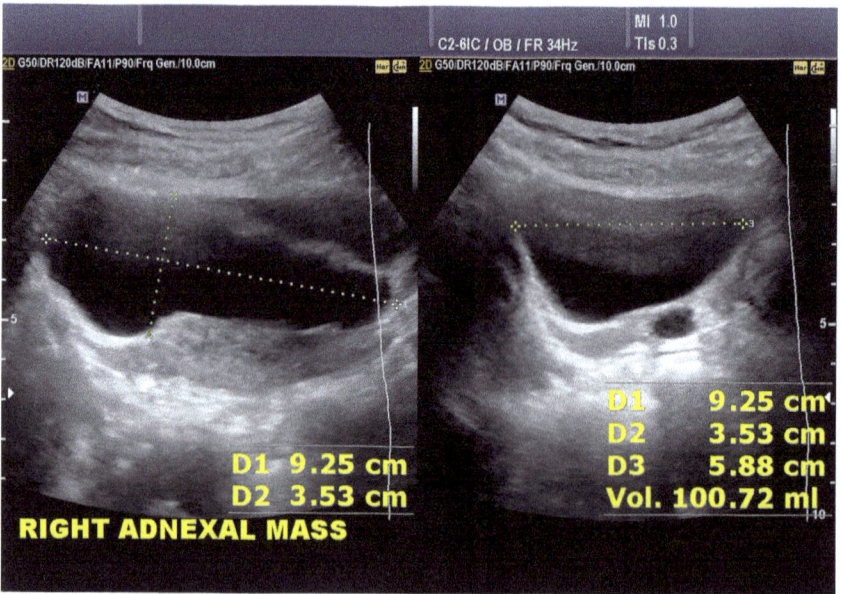

Fig. 7.11.3: Tubular structure is identified with the ovary seen separately

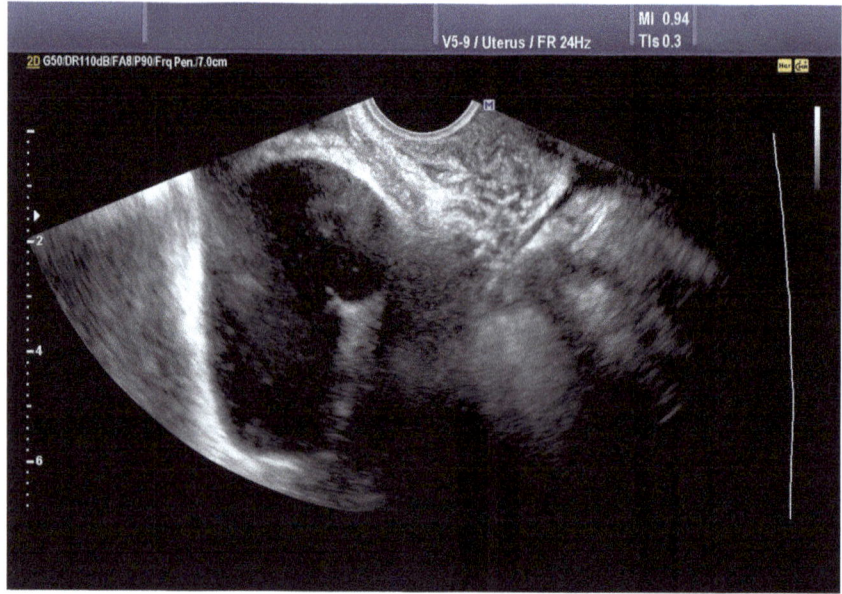

Fig. 7.11.4: Usually anechoic but echoes, floating or attached can also be seen

7.11. Hydrosalpinx

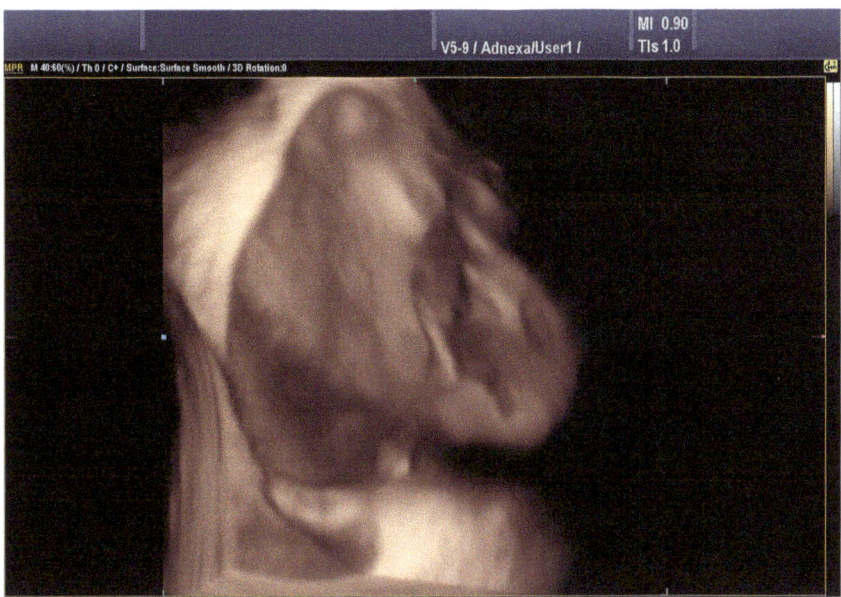

Fig. 7.11.5: Hydrosalpinx as seen on 3D

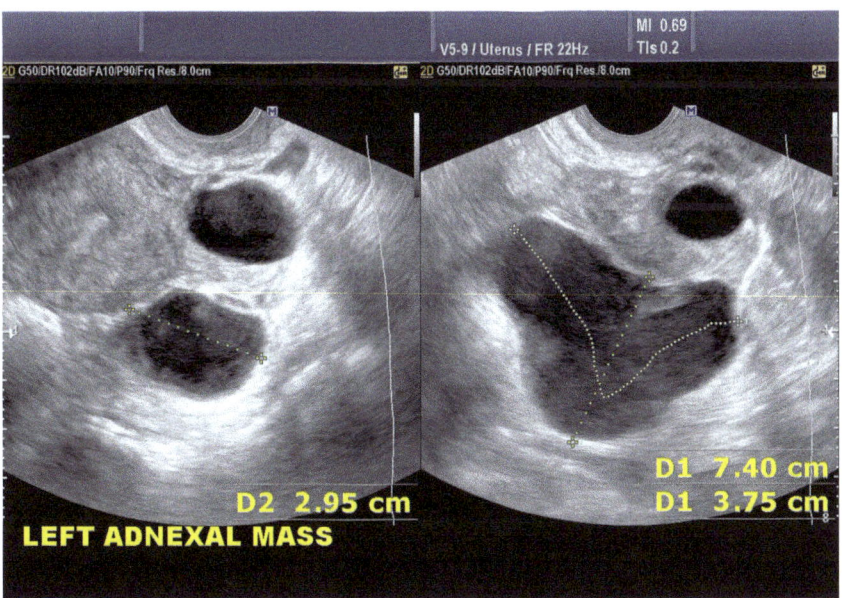

Fig. 7.11.6: Ovary and dilated tube seen separately

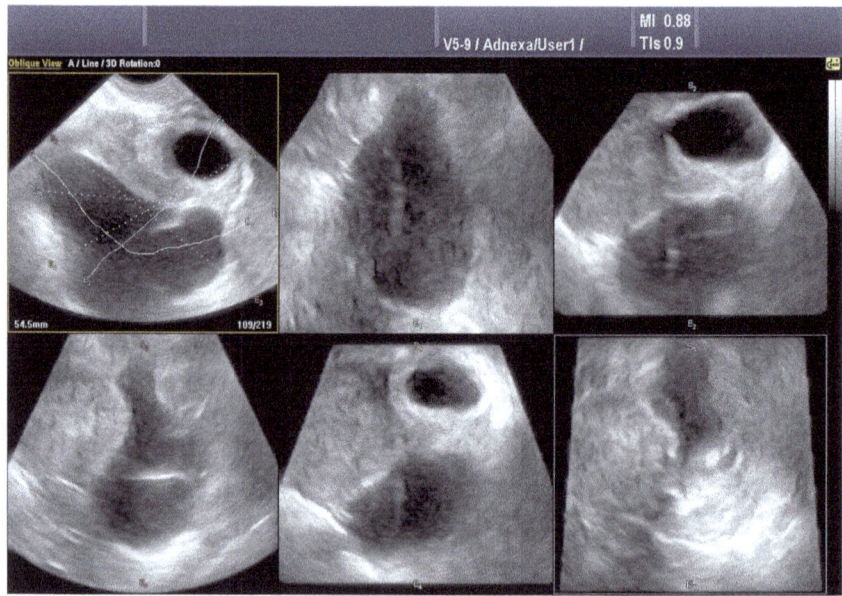

Fig. 7.11.7: As seen on oblique views

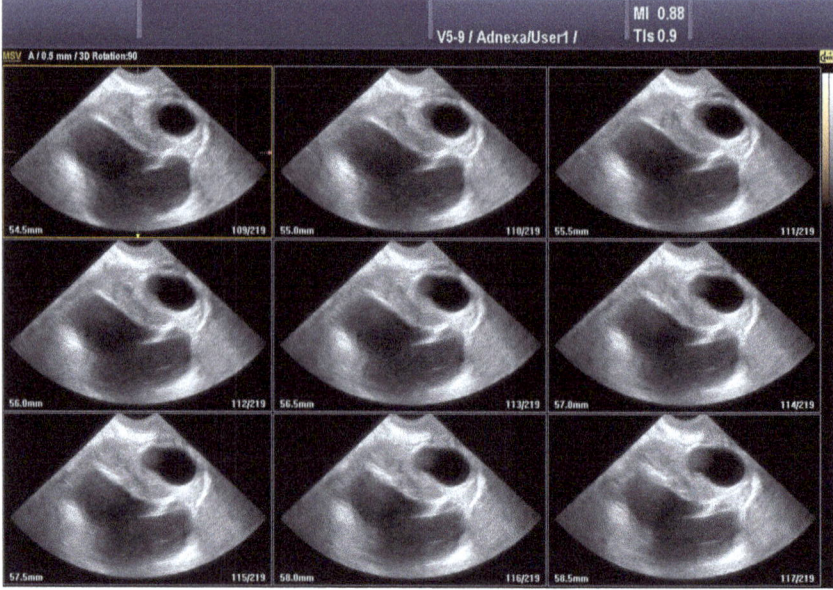

Fig. 7.11.8: As seen on MSV

7.11. Hydrosalpinx

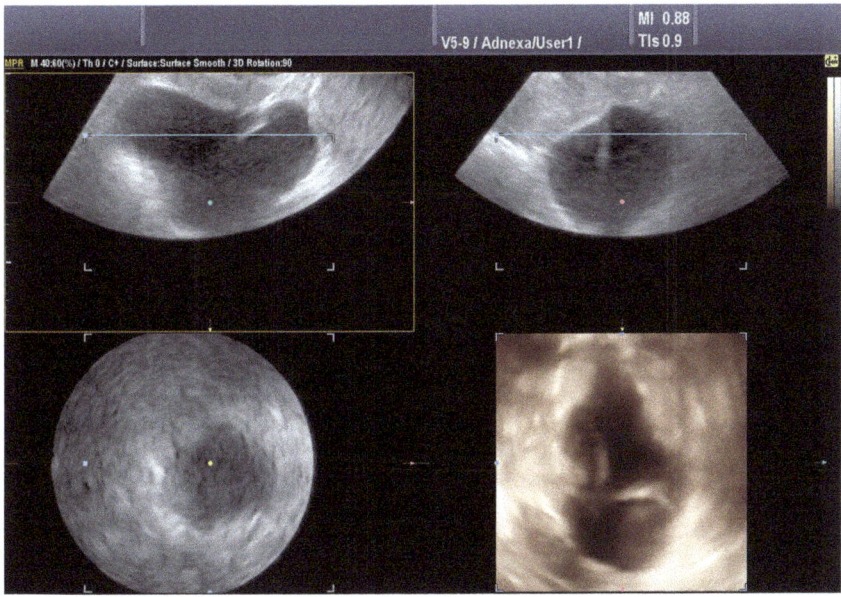

Fig. 7.11.9: As seen on MPR

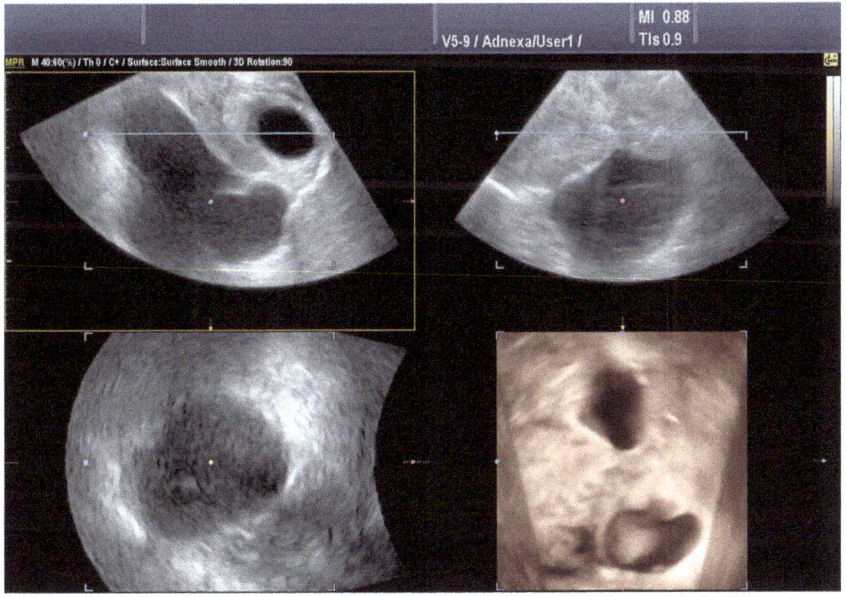

Fig. 7.11.10: As seen on MPR

7.12. POUCH OF DOUGLAS

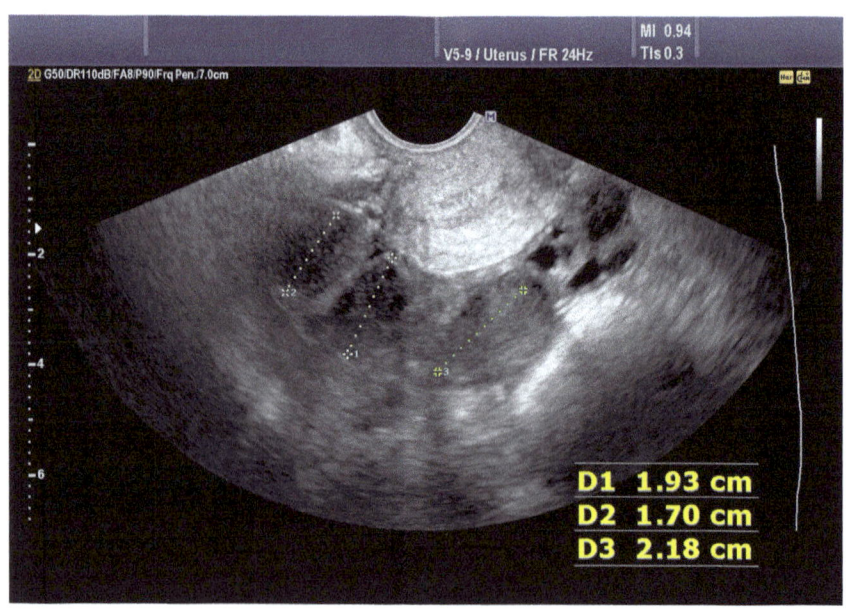

7.12. Pouch of Douglas

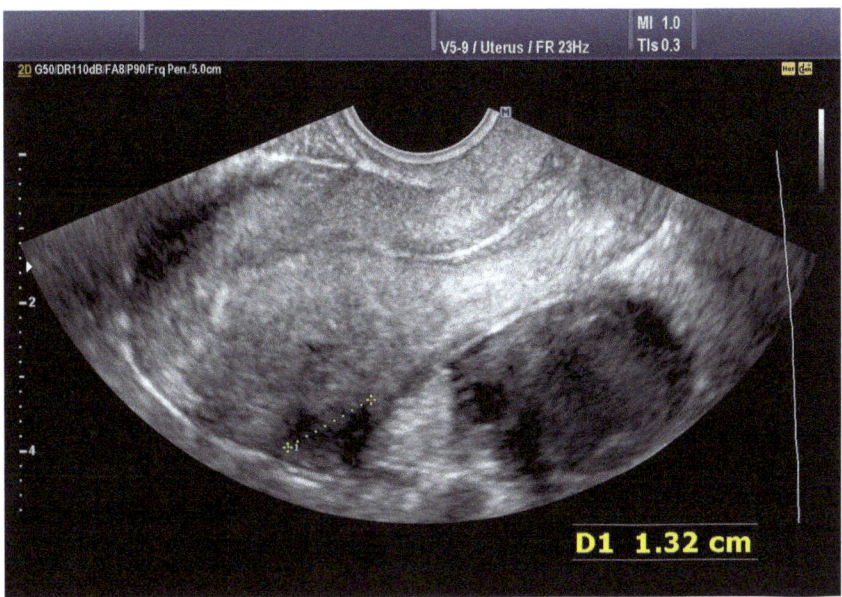

Fig. 7.12.1: Fluid loculi seen in the pouch of Douglas

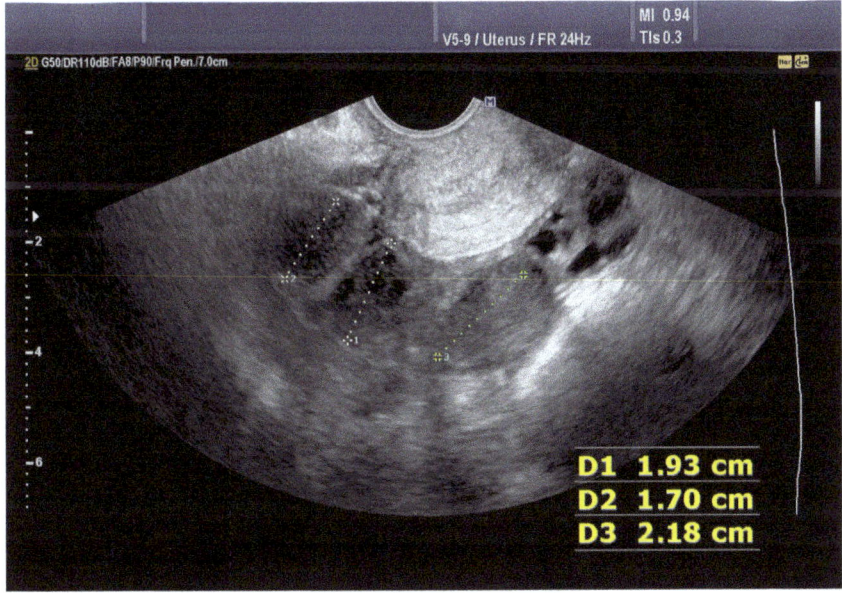

Fig. 7.12.2: Evaluate for ovarian and uterine mobility with slide and glide

7.13. ECTOPIC

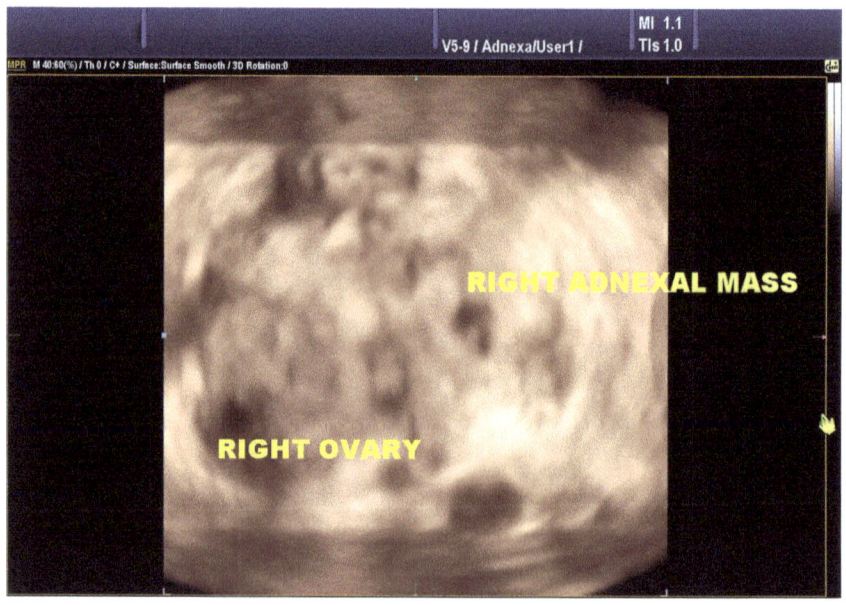

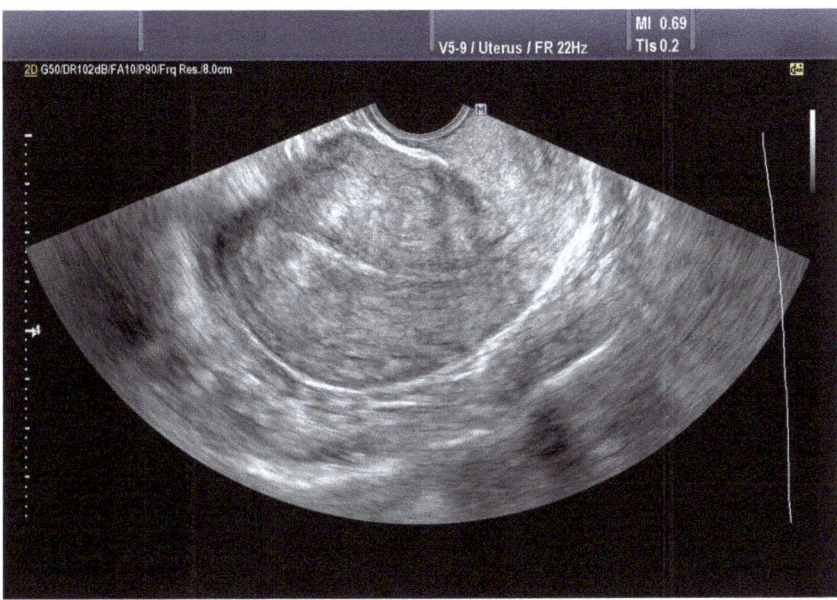

Fig. 7.13.1: Empty uterus (no intrauterine) gestational sac seen in a patient with beta hCG values above the discriminatory zone should have a suspicion of ectopic pregnancy

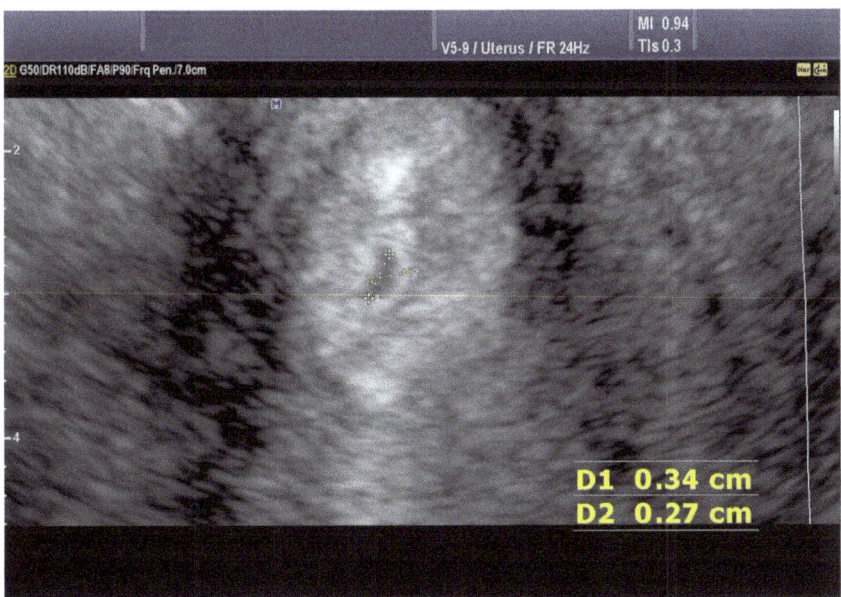

Fig. 7.13.2: Pseudogestational sac is a central anechoic area in the uterus mimicking a gestational sac

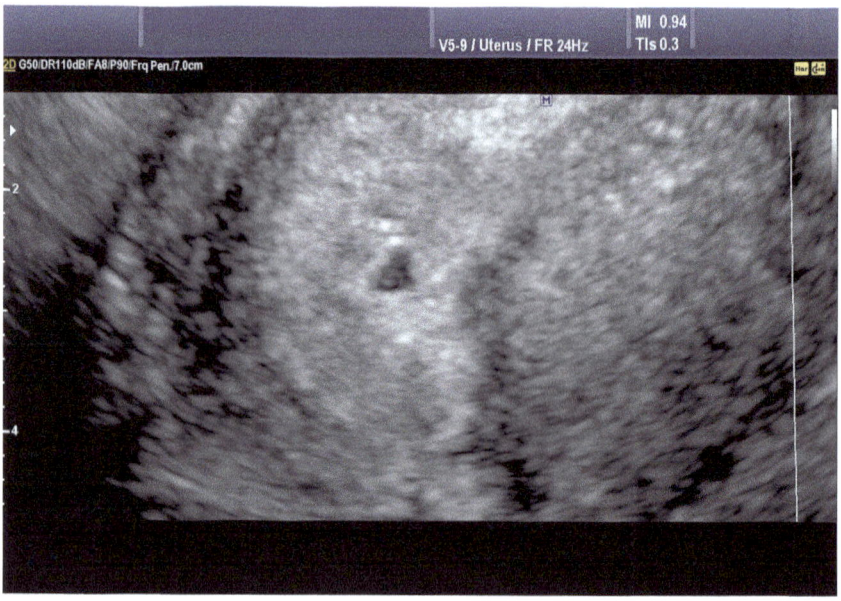

Fig. 7.13.3: Strong suspicion of a pseudogestational sac

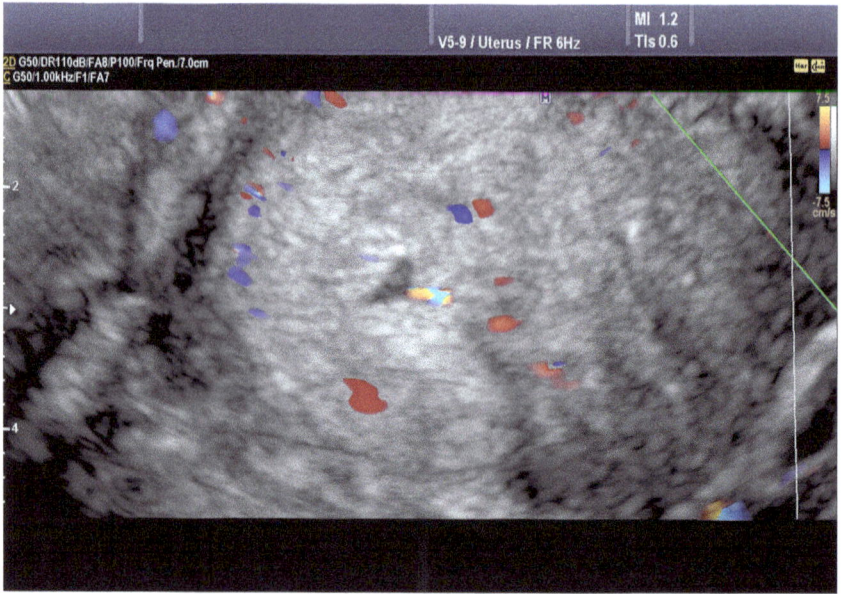

Fig. 7.13.4: Switch on color and see a vessel going towards the gestational sac and you know it is not a pseudogestational sac

7.13. Ectopic

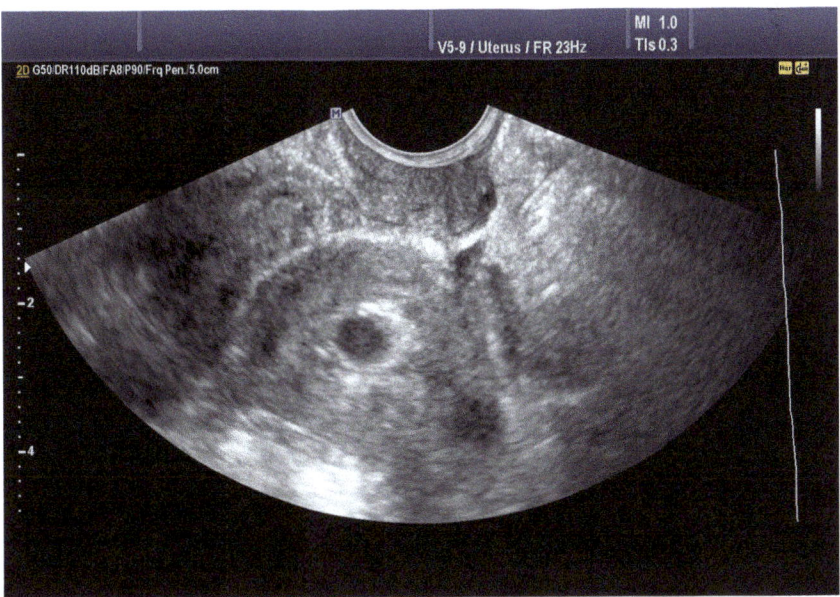

Fig. 7.13.5: Gestational sac seen in the adnexa is the perfect marker for ectopic pregnancy

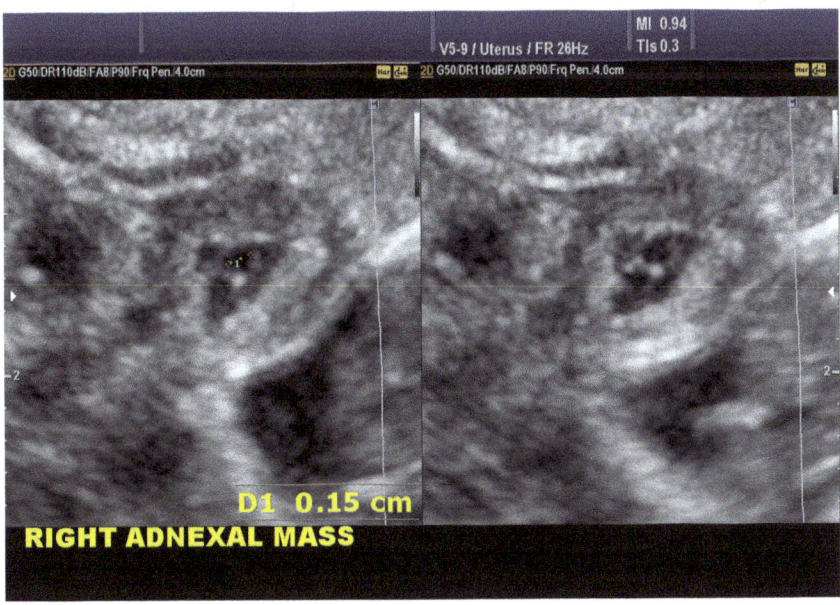

Fig. 7.13.6: Gestational sac showing yolk sac and embryonic cardiac activity can be seen

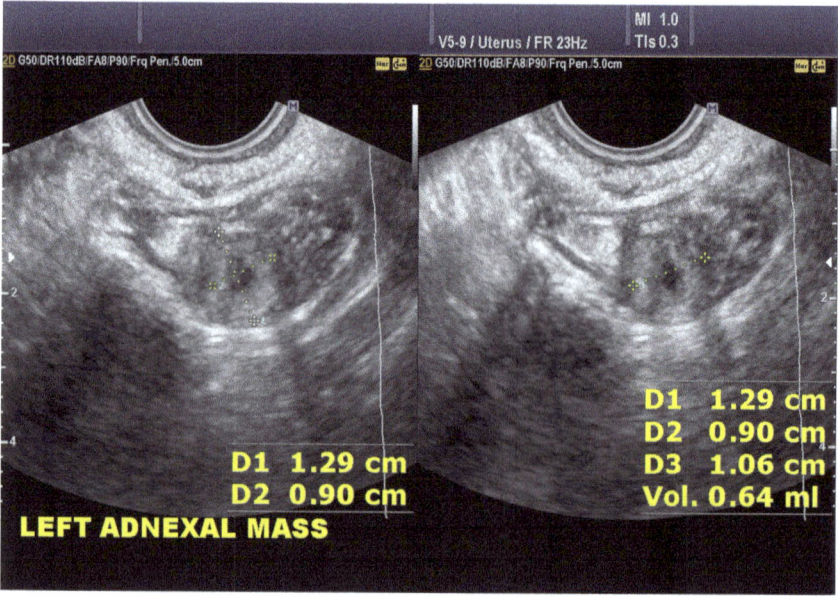

Fig. 7.13.7: Left adnexal mass, extraovarian showing a gestational sac with beta hCG value much above the discriminatory zone

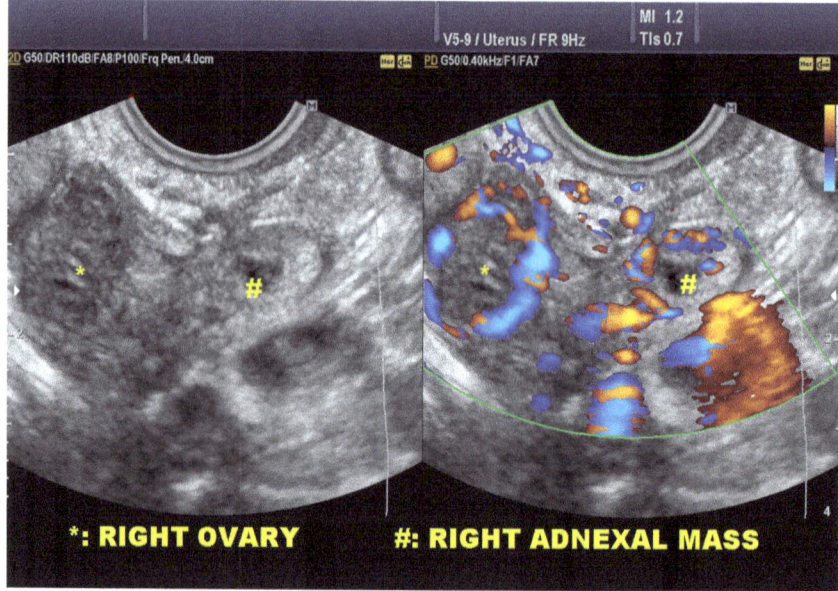

Fig. 7.13.8: Ectopic pregnancies can be seen mostly on the side of the corpus luteum

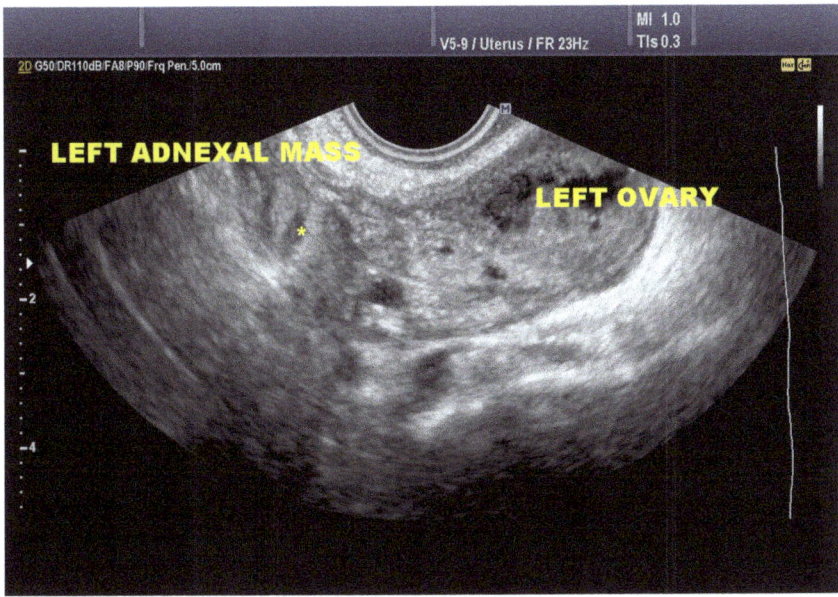

Fig. 7.13.9: Corpus luteum in the left ovary with a left adnexal mass

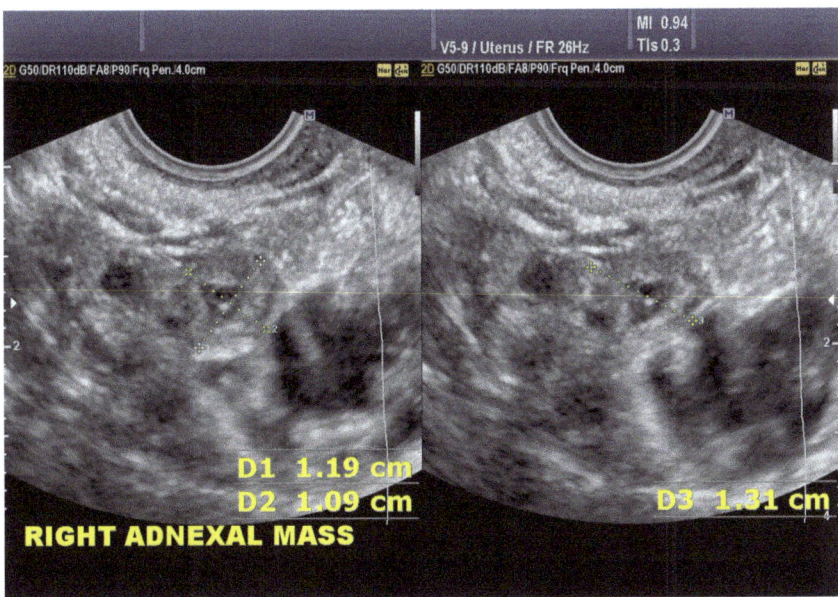

Fig. 7.13.10: TVS to diagnose an ectopic pregnancy

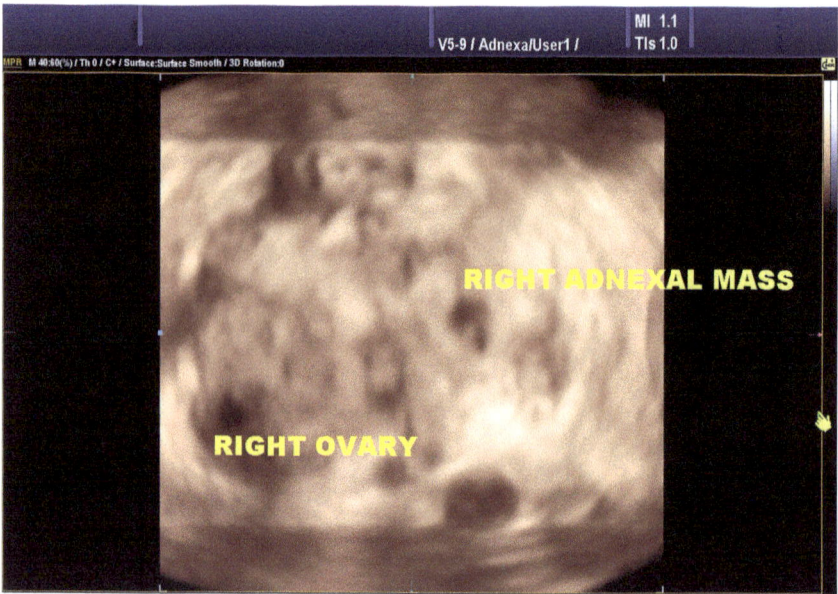

Fig. 7.13.11: Ectopic gestation (adnexal) mass as seen on 3D

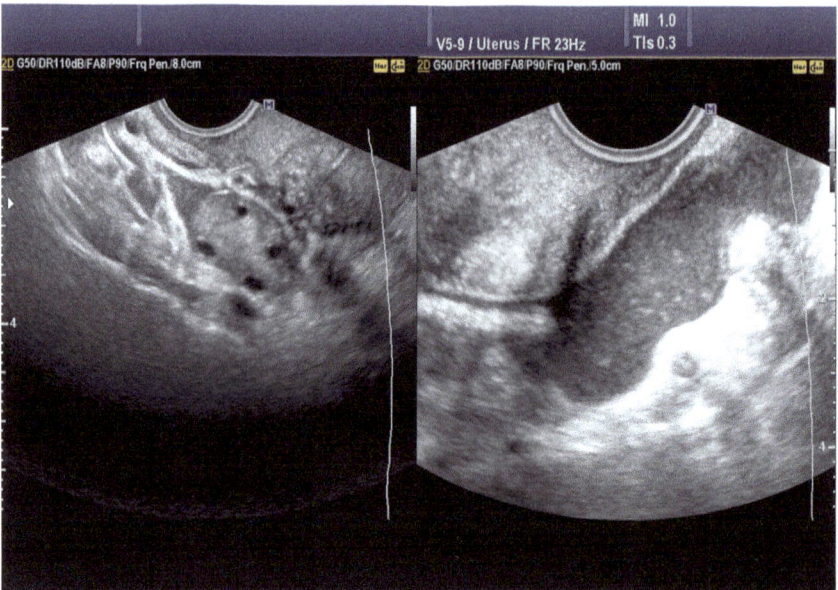

Fig. 7.13.12: Free fluid in the pouch of Douglas with concurrent symptoms, history and beta hCG findings can make you suspect an ectopic

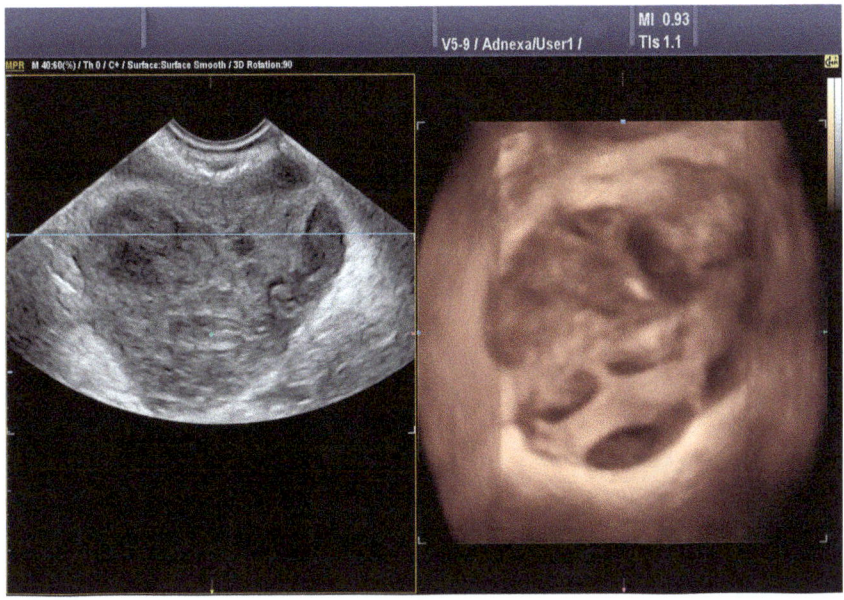

Fig. 7.13.13: Be careful of not labeling the corpus luteum as an ectopic pregnancy

7.14. FREE FLUID

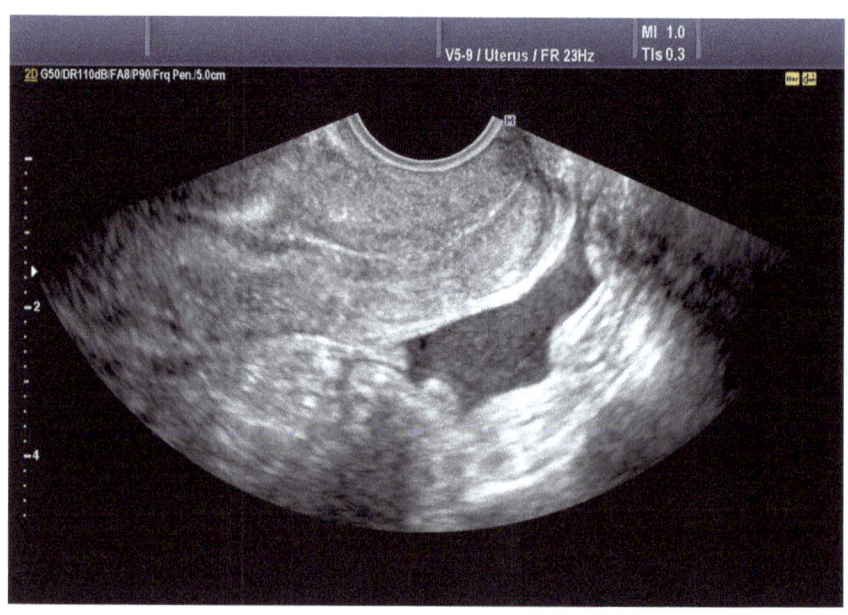

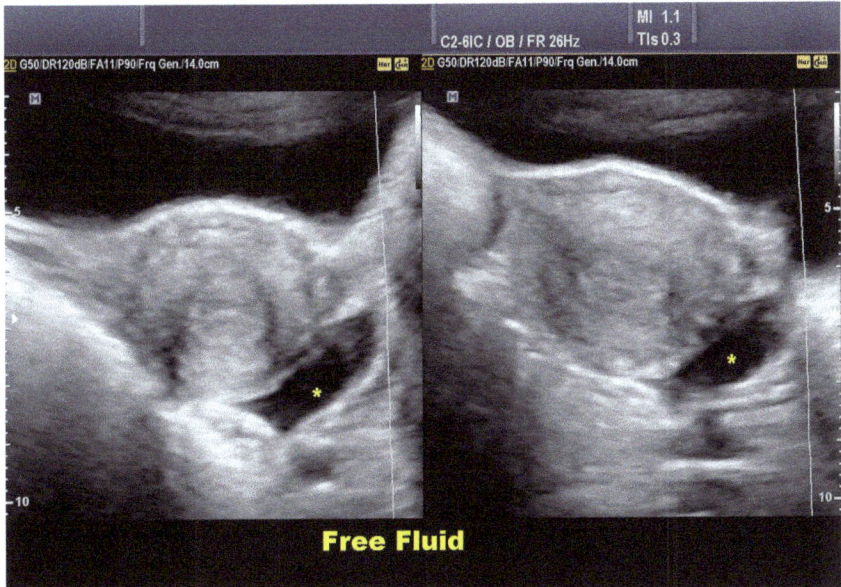

Fig. 7.14.1: Minimal free fluid is normally seen at any stage of the cycle

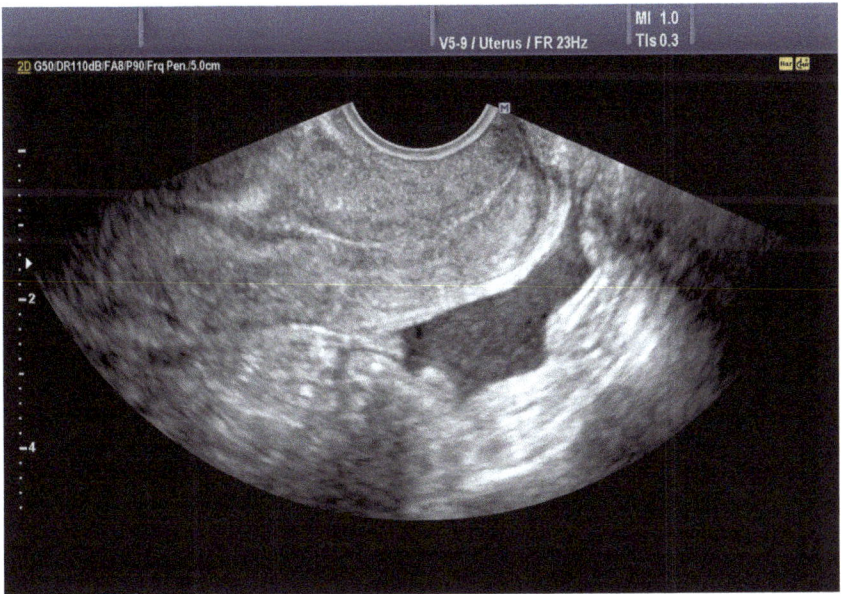

Fig. 7.14.2: Free fluid in the pouch of Douglas

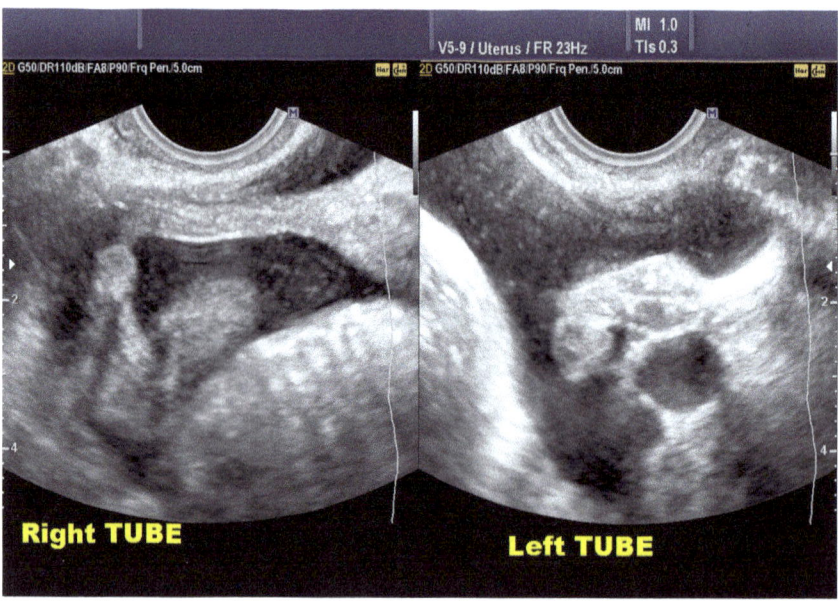

Fig. 7.14.3: With free fluid evaluate the upper abdomen go through all the investigations, should not be a part of ascites, pleural and pericardial effusion

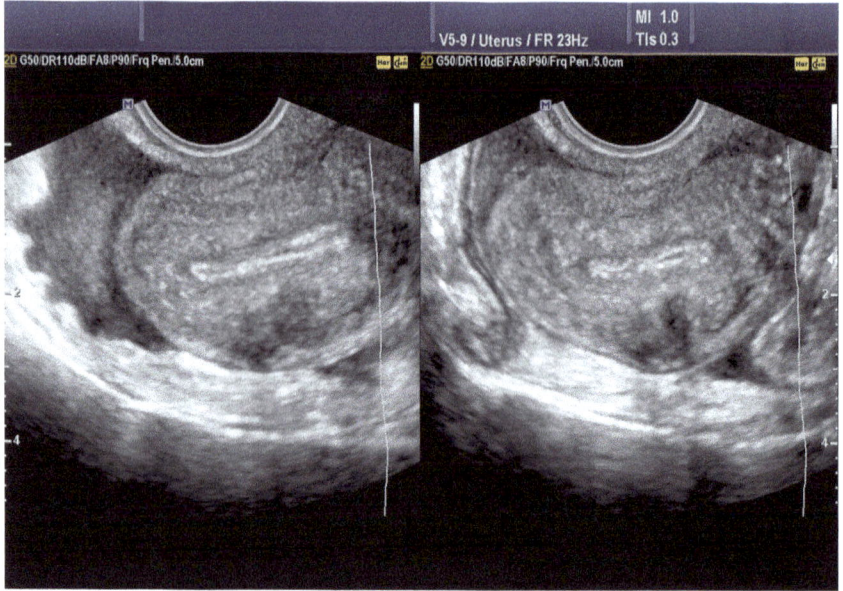

Fig. 7.14.4: Patient with severe pain, amenorrhea, echogenic free fluid evaluate carefully for an ectopic

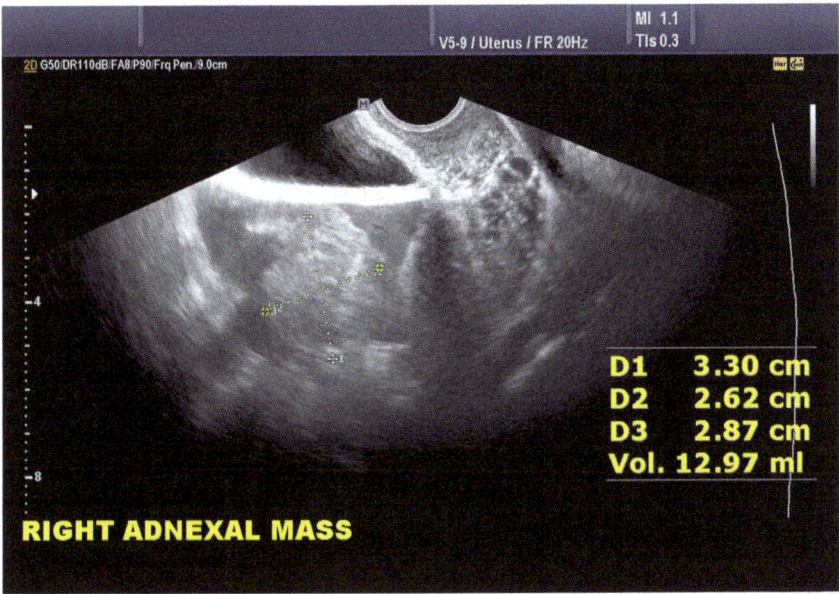

Fig. 7.14.5: With pregnancy test positive, no gestational sac in the uterus evaluate the tubal area very carefully for an ectopic gestation

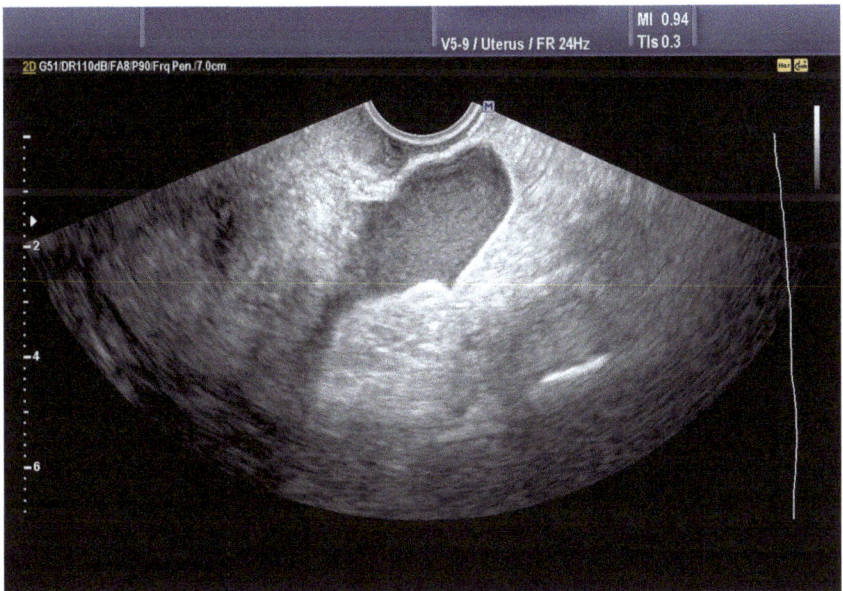

Fig. 7.14.6: Free fluid, evaluate for other adnexal pathology especially infective

EU GSPR Authorised Reprsentative
Logos Europe, 9 rue Nicolas Poussin
1700, La Rochelle, France
Phone: +33 (0) 6 67 93 73 78
E-mail: contact@logoseurope.eu

www.ingramcontent.com/pod-product-compliance
Ingram Content Group UK Ltd.
Pitfield, Milton Keynes, MK11 3LW, UK
UKHW050427150426
5217IPUK00019B/1272